The Clinical Anaesthesia Viva Book
Second edition

D1388696

WITHDRAWN
FROM LIBRARY
BRITISH MEDICAL ASSOCIATION

0944303

The Clinical Anaesthesia Viva Book

Second edition

Julian M. Barker
Simon L. Maguire
Simon J. Mills

and

Abdul-Ghaaliq Lalkhen
Brendan McGrath
Hamish Thomson

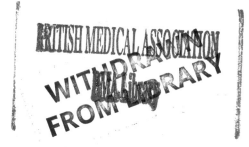
BRITISH MEDICAL ASSOCIATION
WITHDRAWN FROM LIBRARY

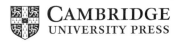

CAMBRIDGE
UNIVERSITY PRESS

CAMBRIDGE UNIVERSITY PRESS
Cambridge, New York, Melbourne, Madrid, Cape Town, Singapore, São Paulo, Delhi

Cambridge University Press
The Edinburgh Building, Cambridge CB2 8RU, UK

Published in the United States of America by Cambridge University Press, New York

www.cambridge.org
Information on this title: www.cambridge.org/9780521720182

© J. Barker, S. Maguire, S. Mills *et al.*, 2009

This publication is in copyright. Subject to statutory exception
and to the provisions of relevant collective licensing agreements,
no reproduction of any part may take place without
the written permission of Cambridge University Press.

First edition published 2002
© Greenwich Medical Media
This edition published 2009

Printed in the United Kingdom at the University Press, Cambridge

A catalogue record for this publication is available from the British Library

ISBN 978-0-521-72018-2 Paperback

Cambridge University Press has no responsibility for the persistence or
accuracy of URLs for external or third-party Internet websites referred to
in this publication, and does not guarantee that any content on such
websites is, or will remain, accurate or appropriate.

Every effort has been made in preparing this publication to provide accurate and
up-to-date information which is in accord with accepted standards and practice at
the time of publication. Although case histories are drawn from actual cases, every
effort has been made to disguise the identities of the individuals involved.
Nevertheless, the authors, editors and publishers can make no warranties that the
information contained herein is totally free from error, not least because clinical
standards are constantly changing through research and regulation. The authors,
editors and publishers therefore disclaim all liability for direct or consequential
damages resulting from the use of material contained in this publication. Readers
are strongly advised to pay careful attention to information provided by the
manufacturer of any drugs or equipment that they plan to use.

Contents

List of contributors

Julian M. Barker is a Consultant in Cardiothoracic Anaesthesia and Intensive Care at Wythenshawe Hospital, Manchester, UK.

Simon L. Maguire is a Consultant Anaesthesist and Royal College Tutor, University Hospital of South Manchester, Manchester, UK.

Simon J. Mills is a Consultant Anaesthetist at Blackpool Victoria Hospital, Blackpool, UK.

Abdul Ghaaliq Lalkhen is a Consultant in Anaesthesia and Pain Medicine at Hope Hospital, Salford, UK.

Brendan A. McGrath is a Consultant in Anaesthetics and Intensive Care at Wythenshawe Hospital, Manchester, UK.

Hamish Thomson is a locum Consultant in Cardiothoracic Anaesthesia and Intensive Care at Wythenshawe Hospital, Manchester, UK.

Foreword

In the 7 years since this popular book was first published, there have been a number of changes in the Final FRCA Examination. In accordance with the standards laid down by the Regulator, the Postgraduate Medical Education and Training Board (PMETB), these changes have been intended to increase the reliability of the examination, particularly the vivas, which are now known as 'structured oral examinations' reflecting the changes introduced.

However, to the aspiring candidate entering the examination hall, these changes are of little concern; the knowledge and presentation skills needed when answering a question are the same as they have always been. And, that is where this book will be of immense assistance.

There are excellent tips on revising for the examination, how to present a case or answer a direct question, and useful hints on interpreting the chest X-ray and other data. With an excellent index to help, there is a huge amount of clinical material to work through for the Long Cases and Short Cases. Because no two vivas are ever the same, even with identical opening questions, the authors have provided much more information than would be expected during the actual vivas. This allows for revision in areas where the Examiners may, or may not, lead you depending on how well you are doing.

The authors rightly stress the need to structure your answers and that there may be no right or wrong answer to some of the clinical questions. What the Examiners want to know is what would you do, and why.

Successful candidates at the vivas are those who are knowledgeable, have seen a lot of clinical cases in a variety of specialties and who can distil and communicate the essence of a clinical case to their supervisors. Although reading this book will not prepare you completely for the Clinical Structured Oral Examination, it will go a long way towards making sure you know what is expected and can present yourself well on the day.

Dr Peter Nightingale
Consultant in Anaesthesia & Intensive Care
University Hospital of South Manchester

Preface

Welcome to the second edition of *The Clinical Anaesthesia Viva Book*. We are extremely grateful for all the positive feedback that we received for the first edition, both from candidates for the FRCA and from examiners and consultant colleagues. We actually set about writing a 'Book 2' several months ago and two things became apparent. Firstly, was the fact that the first book needed some updating, especially with regard to some aspects of peri-operative care; examples of this are investigation of high-risk patients for non-cardiac surgery and the recommendations for peri-operative beta-blockade. Secondly, after questioning the current batch of trainees about what they had been asked in their clinical vivas, it became clear that while there were some new questions, they weren't in abundance. This is good news if you are about to take the exam and reaffirms a point we made in the first edition – there aren't many 'new' diseases, just patients still suffering from bad hearts, bad chests and difficult airways that need anaesthesia! The clinical problems remain very much the same, and this explains why it can't be an easy job to write new questions for the exam! For these reasons we decided to add to, and update, the first book.

Having been consultants for 5 years or so now, the three of us felt a bit more distanced from the exam than we did when we wrote the first edition. For that reason we enlisted the help of three excellent senior trainees who have enabled us to keep the book fresh. This has, however, led to a small rugby team of authors; still, someone has to compete with the numbers on a professorial general surgical ward-round and it may as well be the anaesthetists!

We have endeavoured to write the book in the same style as the first edition. The questions were constructed after asking candidates from recent viva examinations what they had been asked. Some of the long cases in particular may cover a few topics in any given scenario (e.g. obesity and a difficult airway) and to keep the flow of the line of questioning we have answered these questions as they occurred. We have cross-referenced some of the questions but there is a slight element of repetition. We decided to leave this in for the sake of completeness and so the whole question represented what the candidate experienced.

We hope that you find the book useful and we wish you success in the Final FRCA.

Julian Barker
Simon Maguire
Simon Mills

Acknowledgements

Rowan Pollock
Samantha Pool
Keith Pearce

- Technicians in the Cardiology Department at University Hospital of South Manchester, Wythenshawe
- For help with the ECGs

Dr Elaine Smith, Consultant Radiologist, University Hospital of South Manchester, Wythenshawe

Dr Claire Barker, Consultant Radiologist, Christie NHS Foundation Trust, Manchester

– for their help with the X-rays

Chapter 1

Preparation for the Clinical Viva

Examination format

You need to be aware of the format of the vivas.
The day consists of two viva sessions:

1. **The clinical viva**
   This lasts 50 minutes and consists of a long case and three short cases or scenarios. During the first 10 minutes, you will have the opportunity to view clinical information related to the long case consisting of history, examination findings and investigations, e.g. ECG, chest X-ray, pulmonary function tests and blood results. This is followed by 20 minutes of questioning related to this case. During the final 20 minutes, the examiners will question you on three further unrelated topics.
2. **The clinical science viva**
   This is a 30-minute viva consisting of 4 questions on applied pharmacology, anatomy, physiology and physics. This viva is not within the scope of this book.

An approach to revision for the clinical vivas

The period between the written paper and viva examination is a stressful time. For the first 2 weeks you do not even know if you have a viva. This makes it difficult to find the motivation to carry on working until the results are posted. The last thing you want to do is continue the cold, factual learning that has made your life such a misery over the last few weeks. You want to go to the pub instead! However, if you are 'invited' to attend for the vivas, you will find yourself wishing you had worked solidly for the 2 weeks since the written paper! What is needed is a change of tack in order to sustain the flagging momentum. We found sitting around in armchairs (cups of tea in hand) discussing anaesthetic topics far preferable to the 'textbook and solitary desk-lamp at midnight' scenario.

It is important to realise that the viva requires a different approach to revision. This book aims to give you a strategy for viva revision that will hopefully make it less tedious.

We initially found our viva technique left much to be desired, despite adequate knowledge. There is a particular 'knack' to passing this type of

The Clinical Anaesthesia Viva Book, Second edition, ed. Julian M. Barker, Simon L. Maguire and Simon J. Mills. © J. M. Barker, S. L. Maguire, S. J. Mills 2009.

examination, and possessing a well-honed technique can enable you to appear confident and knowledgeable (even if you don't feel it!). With the experience you have gained as a trainee, your knowledge base is very likely to be good enough to tackle most questions. However, it is the way in which you *communicate* your knowledge that will need to impress the examiners. As in all branches of anaesthesia, there are many ways to skin a cat, and revising for the clinical viva is no exception. We found the following techniques extremely valuable in the run-up to the vivas:

- **Group revision**
- **Frequent practice**
- **Practise categorising**
- **Card system**

Group revision

It is extremely useful to team up with some friends or colleagues regularly in the weeks before the viva and practise talking about anaesthetic topics. Practising with friends has several advantages:

- The whole exam period is very stressful and seeing your friends on a regular basis will help keep you sane. This is better than locking yourself in a small room with a pile of books and trying to learn the coagulation cascade for the fifth time since qualification!
- Your morale will remain in better shape than if you were revising on your own because you will be able to encourage each other. You will also be more aware of the progress you are making.
- As a group, you can pool your resources in terms of reference books and previous questions. During the working day, one of you may have had a practice viva with a consultant who asked an awkward question or a common question asked in a different way. You can then discuss with your friends how they would have answered it.
- Different people revise in different ways and, consequently, will have their own way of talking about a subject. This means that others in the group will benefit from listening to the practice viva. They may have a particular piece of knowledge that really helps an answer gel together or they may use a particular turn-of-phrase that succinctly deals with a potential minefield.
- You can practise phrasing your answers in a particular way in the knowledge that, if it all falls apart halfway through, it won't matter and you can have another go. This is less easy to do in front of consultants who might write your reference!
- By being 'the examiner', you will gain insight into the pitfalls of the viva process. You can usually see someone digging a hole for themselves a mile off!

Frequent practice

Repetition of clinical scenarios

During your revision, you will find the same clinical situations coming up time and time again (as in the exam). Over the years, anaesthetic techniques may change but new techniques are all aimed at trying to solve particular *clinical problems*, for example, the fibre-optic scope to help with the difficult airway or new drugs that provide more cardiovascular stability. However, the *problems* remain the same! Patients will still present with difficult airways, ischaemic heart disease, COAD, obesity, hypertension, etc. The more you practise, the more often you will find yourself repeating the problems each of these scenarios presents and thus the more confident and slick you will become at delivering the salient points.

There are obviously a few exceptions, e.g. MRI scanners and laser surgery, where the advancement of technology has presented new challenges to the anaesthetist. These situations are in the minority and as long as you are aware of them and the associated anaesthetic problems, you should be well-equipped to deal with questions on them in the exam.

The clinical scenarios break down into a few categories:

- **Medical** conditions that have anaesthetic implications, e.g.
  Aortic stenosis
  Diabetes
  Hyperthyroidism.
- **Surgical** procedures that have anaesthetic implications, e.g.
  Oesophagectomy
  CABG
  Pneumonectomy.
- **Anaesthetic** emergencies/difficult situations, e.g.
  Anaphylaxis
  Malignant hyperthermia
  Failed intubation.
- **Paediatric** cases. These represent a limited range of cases the examiners are likely to ask you about, e.g.
  Upper airway obstruction
  Pyloric stenosis
  Bleeding tonsil.

Having repeatedly practised these clinical scenarios, you will soon realise that the problems of anaesthetising an obese patient with diabetes, ischaemic heart disease, porphyria and myasthenia for an abdominal aortic aneurysm repair (!) can be broken down into the problems that the respective conditions present to the anaesthetist, plus the problems of the specific operation. You may then approach what seems to be a nightmare question with a degree of confidence and structure.

Phrasing

It cannot be over-emphasized that frequent practice will improve your viva technique. As already mentioned, some topics crop up again and again in different situations, such as part of a long case or even a complete short case (e.g. obesity, anaesthesia for the elderly or the difficult airway). With regular practice, you will soon develop your own 'patter' to help you deal with these common clinical scenarios. These can then be adopted at opportune moments to buy yourself easy marks whilst actually giving you time to gather your thoughts.

Practise categorising

Putting order to your answers demonstrates to the examiners that you conduct your clinical practice in a systematic and safe way. If you do not mention the most important points first (e.g. airway problems in a patient presenting with a goitre), then this may suggest to the examiners that you are disorganized. An 'ABC' (order of priority) approach to many of the questions may be helpful. For example, in obese patients, managing the airway has a higher priority than difficulty with cannulation.

It is often a good idea to use your opening sentence to tell the examiners how you are going to categorize your answer.

Example 1:

'Tell me about the anaesthetic implications of rheumatoid arthritis'.

'Patients with rheumatoid arthritis may have a difficult airway and secondary respiratory and cardiovascular pathology. They are frequently anaemic, taking immunosuppressant drugs and the severe joint pathology leads to problems with positioning'.

Example 2:

'What are the important considerations when anaesthetising a patient for a pneumonectomy'?

'These may be divided into three broad areas: the *pre-operative* assessment of fitness for pneumonectomy and optimisation, the *conduct of anaesthesia* with particular reference to one-lung anaesthesia, positioning, intra-operative monitoring and fluid balance and finally *post-operative care*'.

Card system

We formatted postcards to summarise the main problems associated with different anaesthetic situations. These proved to be a good starting point for viva practice and a quick source of reference. They also encouraged us to deliver the first few points in a punchy manner.

For example:

'What problems do you anticipate with anaesthetising a patient with Down's syndrome'?

'These patients present the following problems for the anaesthetist. They may have a difficult airway, an unstable neck, cardiac abnormalities, mental retardation, epilepsy and a high incidence of hepatitis B infection'.

Viva technique

■ **Think first**
■ **The opening sentence**

■ **Categorise or die!**
■ **The long case**

Think first

Don't panic. If you are unlucky enough to be asked a question about an obscure subject such as lithium therapy (as two of us were in our science viva), remember the examiners have only just seen the questions as well. It may also be of some comfort to know that there will be at least ten other candidates being asked the same question at the same time. Keep things simple at first and think about how you are going to structure your answer. Categorising your answer may allow you to deliver more information about the topic than you thought you knew. Conversely, do not dwell on what you do not know, e.g. the pH and dose!

Example: *'Tell me about lithium'*

Think...	'What is it used for'?
Say...	'Lithium is a drug used in the treatment of mania and the prophylaxis of manic depression'.
Think...	'What is the presentation and dose?...I don't know the dose'.
Say...	'It is presented in tablet form'.
Think...	'What is its mode of action?...I have no idea but I know it is an antipsychotic'!
Say...	'Its main action is as an antipsychotic'.
Think...	'Why are they asking me this question? What is the relevance to anaesthetic practice'?
Say...	'It has a narrow therapeutic range and therefore toxicity must be looked for. Side effects may include nausea, vomiting, convulsions, arrhythmias and diabetes insipidus with hypernatraemia'.

A similar approach can be used for the clinical viva.

The opening sentence

This will set the tone of the viva. If the first words to come from your mouth are poorly structured, ill thought-out or just plain rubbish, then you are likely to annoy the examiners and will face an uphill struggle. If, on the other hand, your first sentence is coherent, succinct and structured, then you will be half-way there. With a bit of luck, the examiners will sit back, breathe a sigh of relief (because it has been a very long day for them) and allow you to demonstrate your obvious knowledge of the subject in hand!

For example:

'*What are the problems associated with anaesthesia for thyroid disease*'?

'Anaesthesia for patients with thyroid disease has implications in the pre-, intra- and post-operative periods'.

You are then able to expand in a logical way from here.

'Pre-operatively, assessment of the airway and control of the functional activity of the gland is essential . . . '

Categorise or die!
Remember this lends structure to your answer and gives the examiners the impression you are about to talk about the subject with authority. If you categorise your answer well enough, they may actually stop you and move onto something else.

The long case
The above points relate to the short and long cases but there are aspects of the long case that can be anticipated. Some answers can therefore be prepared in advance.

Opening question
You will be asked to summarise the case so prepare your opening sentence beforehand.

For example:

You may be asked to summarise the scenario of a 75-year-old man with chronic obstructive pulmonary disease who is scheduled to undergo an elective cardio-oesophagectomy the following day.

'Would you like to summarise the case'?

One possible answer may begin:

'This is an elderly gentleman with complex medical problems who is scheduled for a cardio-oesophagectomy. He has evidence of chronic obstructive pulmonary disease, ischaemic heart disease and diabetes. There will be substantial strain on his cardio-respiratory system. This operation is a major procedure that involves considerable fluid shifts, a potential for large blood loss and requires careful attention to analgesia. These are the main issues that I would concentrate on in my pre-operative assessment'.

Even though a cardio-oesophagectomy involves other considerations (e.g. double-lumen tube / one-lung ventilation) it can be seen that this opening sentence could be adapted to suit other clinical scenarios such as:

Pneumonectomy

Laparotomy

CABG / valve replacement

Cystectomy

Open prostatectomy

Analyse *all* the investigations

You will be asked for your opinion on the ECG, chest X-ray, blood results, etc., so make sure you have decided on the abnormalities and the most likely causes for them in the 10 minutes you have to view the data. Try to make your answers punchy and authoritative.

For example, 'The ECG shows sinus rhythm with a rate of 80 and an old inferior infarct' is better than going through the ECG in a painstaking 'The rate is ... the rhythm is ... the axis is ... '

Don't waste valuable time waffling on about the normal-looking bones on a chest X-ray if there is a barn-door left lower lobe collapse. This does not necessarily imply you are not thorough, providing you demonstrate that you have looked for and excluded other abnormalities.

Anaesthetic technique

You will usually be asked how you would anaesthetise the patient in the long case. There will often not be a right or wrong answer, but you should try to decide on *your* technique and be able to justify it. The examiners may only be looking for the principles of anaesthesia for a particular condition such as aortic stenosis, although this is probably more likely in the short cases.

For example:

> *'You are asked to provide an anaesthetic for a 77-year-old lady who needs a hemi-arthroplasty for a fractured neck of femur. She had a myocardial infarction 3 months ago and has evidence of heart failure'.*

You should be able to summarise the principles involved and choose an anaesthetic technique appropriate to the problems presented. You could, for example, give this patient a general anaesthetic with invasive monitoring (PAFC, A-line, etc.), you could use TIVA with remifentanil or a neuroaxial block. All of these techniques could be justified, but to simply say that you would use propofol, fentanyl and a laryngeal mask without saying why, may be asking for trouble!

In some circumstances it may be the options for management rather than a *specific* technique that is required. You may find it appropriate to list the options for analgesia in a patient having a pneumonectomy, for example, and then say why you would use one technique over the others.

You should try to address the anaesthetic technique for the long case BEFORE you face the examiners. You will not look very credible if you have had 10 minutes to decide on this and have not reached some kind of conclusion.

Overall, most candidates felt that the examiners were pleasant and generally helpful. If you are getting sidetracked they will probably give you a hint so you do not waste time talking about something for which there are no allocated marks. If they do give you a hint, take it!

Good luck.

Chapter 2

The Short Cases

Abdominal aortic aneurysm rupture

You are called to the ward to see a 74-year-old man with a ruptured aortic aneurysm. His blood pressure is 70/40.

What are the major problems in managing a ruptured AAA?

Pre-operatively
- Severe hypovolaemia
- Initial fluid resuscitation must be cautious
- Assessment of concomitant medical problems
- Patients are usually 'arteriopaths' with significant coronary disease
- No time for lengthy investigations
- Access to vascular surgery – may need to transfer out

Intra-operatively
- Cardiovascular instability   Induction
  Before aortic cross-clamping
  When the clamp is removed
- Large blood losses   Blood, FFP and platelets required
- Effects of massive transfusion
- Temperature control
- Metabolic acidosis

Post-operatively
- **Respiratory support** may be required for poor gas exchange and metabolic acidosis.
- **Cardiovascular complications** include haemorrhage, myocardial and lower limb ischaemia.
- **Renal failure** is common due to peri-operative hypotension, aortic cross-clamping (infra-renal clamp still significantly reduces renal blood flow by about 40%), atheromatous emboli, surgical insult, intra-abdominal hypertension (>12 mmHg) or compartment syndrome (>20 mmHg).

The Clinical Anaesthesia Viva Book, Second edition, ed. Julian M. Barker, Simon L. Maguire and Simon J. Mills. © J. M. Barker, S. L. Maguire, S. J. Mills 2009.

■ **Neurological sequelae** such as paraplegia or stroke may occur secondary to damaged spinal arteries or embolic/ischaemic events.

What is your immediate management on the ward?

■ ABC approach – highest FiO_2 obtainable should be commenced.
■ Two large-bore intravenous cannulae should be inserted and fluids given.

How much fluid would you use?

This would depend on the blood pressure and the clinical state of the patient. A patient who has an unrecordable blood pressure and is about to arrest should be given fluids quickly, but in this man **fluids should be given cautiously**. Repeated 250 ml fluid boluses titrated to physiological endpoints (consciousness, base deficit, lactate) should be used. One should not necessarily aim to restore blood pressure to 'normal' as this may reverse vasoconstriction and disrupt fibrin clots that were contributing to haemostasis.

What else would you do?

■ Take blood for full blood count, urea and electrolytes, clotting screen, blood gas.
■ Cross-match for 10 units, consider type O-negative or group-specific blood.
■ Second anaesthetist (preferably consultant) is required.
■ Haematology should be alerted to the need for large volumes of blood, FFP and platelets.
■ An assessment of co-existing medical problems and the likelihood of difficult intubation should be made.
■ **Do not delay surgery** whilst awaiting lengthy investigations.
■ Transfer the patient to the operating theatre as soon as possible.
■ **Only haemodynamically stable** patients can be taken for CT scanning to diagnose rupture and assess suitability for open or endovascular repair.

What monitoring would you use?

■ ECG, non-invasive BP, SpO_2 and capnography initially.
■ **Surgery should not be delayed by prolonged attempts to insert arterial and central lines at this stage.**

How would you proceed with anaesthesia?

■ **Big drips**
■ All vaso-active drugs should be drawn up prior to induction.
■ Blood should be immediately available.

- A method of delivering warmed fluids rapidly and continuously is beneficial such as a 'Level-1™ infusor'.
- **Anaesthetise in theatre on the table**
- A rapid sequence induction is performed with the **surgeon scrubbed** and the **patient already cleaned and draped** (muscle relaxation may release the tamponade on the aorta worsening bleeding and the combined effects of induction agents and IPPV can cause profound hypotension).
- Anaesthesia is maintained with an appropriate agent in oxygen/air.
- Avoid nitrous oxide because bowel distension may increase intra-abdominal pressure post-operatively.
- When the cross-clamp is on and there is 'relative' stability, invasive lines may be inserted if not already in place.
- Temperature probe
- Nasogastric tube
- Urinary catheter
- Active warming such as with a warm air blower over the chest helps to maintain temperature, but should be avoided on the legs during clamping.
- Loop diuretics (e.g. furosemide), dopamine, mannitol, fenoldapam and N-acetylcysteine have been proposed as renoprotective agents. There is no Level 1 evidence to support their use. The mainstay of renal preservation is maintenance of renal oxygen delivery and the avoidance of nephrotoxins (e.g. non-steroidal anti-inflammatory drugs, angiotensin-converting enzyme inhibitors, contrast and aminoglycosides).

How would you control the hypertension associated with cross-clamping?

SVR may rise by up to 40% resulting in myocardial ischaemia. If increasing the inspired **volatile** concentration and giving **opioid** and/or **propofol** are not effective, then **GTN** can be used, especially if myocardial ischaemia is present.

How would you manage the patient at the end of the operation?

- **Intensive care** is usually required.
- Sedation and ventilation may need to be continued until the temperature is corrected, cardiovascular stability is established and acid/base status and gas exchange are acceptable.
- Predictors of survival to discharge include patient age, total blood loss and post-operative hypotension.

Bibliography

Cowlishaw P, Telford R. (2007). Anaesthesia for abdominal vascular surgery. *Anaesthesia and Intensive Care Medicine*, **8**(6), 248–52.

Leonard A, Thompson J. (2008). Anaesthesia for ruptured abdominal aortic aneurysm. *Continuing Education in Anaesthesia, Critical Care and Pain*, **8**(1), 11–15.

Sakalihasan N, Limet, R, Defawe O. (2005). Abdominal aortic aneurysm. *Lancet*, **365**, 1577–89.

Acromegaly

An acromegalic patient presents for surgery to a pituitary tumour.

What are the common surgical approaches?

There are two main approaches to surgery:

(1) Over 90% of pituitary adenomas will be treated by the **trans-sphenoidal approach**. This approach, in which an incision is made in the nasal septum, is well tolerated and gives good cosmetic results. Complications are uncommon but include:

- Haemorrhage
- Visual loss
- Persistent CSF leak
- Panhypopituitarism
- Stroke

(2) The other surgical option is a **frontal craniotomy**.

How can pituitary tumours present?

Most pituitary tumours are benign and arise from the anterior pituitary. They can be secreting (around 70%) or non-secreting and may present in a number of ways:

- Mass effect of the tumour: Headache
  Nausea and vomiting
  Visual field defects
  Cranial nerve palsies
  Papilloedema
  Raised ICP (rare, but more common with non-functioning macroadenomas)
- Effects from the secretion of one or more hormones
- Non-specific – headache, infertility, epilepsy
- Incidental, e.g. during imaging ('incidentalomas')

Classification of pituitary tumours:

1. **Non-functioning (25%)**	Commonly null-cell adenomas, craniopharyngiomas and meningiomas	
2. **Functioning (75%)**	Prolactin	30%
	Prolactin + GH	10–12%
	GH	20%
	ACTH	12–15%
	FSH/LH	1–2%
	TSH	1%

What are the features of acromegaly?

There is hypersecretion of growth hormone with resultant soft tissue overgrowth.

Clinical features include:

■ **Face**	Increased skull size
	Prominent supraorbital ridge
	Prognathism
	Headaches
■ **Mouth**	Macroglossia
	Soft tissue overgrowth in larynx/pharynx
	Obstructive sleep apnoea
■ **Skeleton**	Large hands and feet
	Thick skin
	Osteoporosis
	Kyphosis
■ **Neuromuscular**	RLN palsy
	Peripheral neuropathy
	Proximal myopathy
■ **Cardiovascular**	Hypertension
	Heart failure
■ **Endocrine**	**Diabetes**

Diagnostic tests for acromegaly:

■ Random serum growth hormone > 10 mU/l – can give false-positives due to its short half-life and pulsatile pattern of release.
■ Failure of growth hormone suppression following a glucose load.
■ Elevated IGF-1 – growth hormone exerts many of its effects through insulin-like growth factor-1 (IGF-1) which also has a longer half-life than growth hormone.

Which features are of concern to the anaesthetist?

■ **Upper airway obstruction**	This may result from a large mandible, tongue and epiglottis together with generalised mucosal hypertrophy. Laryngeal narrowing may cause difficulty with tracheal intubation and post-operative respiratory obstruction can occur. A history of stridor, hoarseness, dyspnoea or obstructive sleep apnoea should be specifically asked for.
■ **Cardiac**	Hypertension and congestive cardiac failure requiring pre-operative investigation and treatment.
■ **Endocrine**	Commonly glucose intolerance and diabetes mellitus. Other associations include thyroid and adrenal abnormalities that may necessitate thyroxine and steroid replacement.

What post-operative management problems may you encounter?

■ **Surgical** complications
  such as: Haemorrhage
                              Stroke
                              Visual loss
                              Cerebral oedema leading to impaired consciousness

■ **Hormonal**
  supplementation
  Steroids   Surgery may reduce the function of the pituitary
                              gland and hydrocortisone is often prescribed in the
                              immediate peri-operative phase.
  Thyroxine   Prescribed with caution due to the risk of cardiac
                              ischaemia.
  Insulin   Titrated to the required serum glucose
                              concentration.

■ **Diabetes insipidus**   This occurs in 40% of patients and is transient,
                              typically occurring in the first 12–24 hours due to
                              oedema around the surgical site. It presents as
                              polyuria with a low urine osmolality despite
                              normal/high serum osmolality. Treatment is by
                              estimating and replacing the fluid deficit (which is
                              hypo-osmolar) and the administration of
                              desmopressin (DDAVP), a synthetic ADH analogue.

■ **CSF rhinorrhoea**   Generally, no treatment is required, although the
                              risk of infection is probably increased. CSF drainage
                              (e.g. lumbar drain) may reduce the pressure
                              sufficiently to allow the leak to seal.

■ **Post-operative pain**
■ **Hypertension on**   May contribute to post-operative bleeding but is
  emergence   often short-lived. Ensure adequate analgesia. May
                              require short-acting agents to control such as
                              labetalol.

Bibliography

Nemergut E, Dumont A, Barry U, Laws E. (2005). Perioperative management of patients undergoing
    trans-sphenoidal pituitary surgery. *Anesthesia and Analgesia*, **101**, 1170–81.
Smith M, Hirsch NP. (2000). Pituitary disease and anaesthesia. *British Journal of Anaesthesia*, **85**(1),
    3–14.

Acute asthma

*You are called to the accident and emergency department to see a
31-year-old lady, known to have asthma, who has been admitted with
acute shortness of breath.*

How would you make a clinical assessment of the severity of this attack?

> This is a common clinical scenario and therefore requires a punchy answer because you will have seen it frequently. Don't forget that, before examining for specific physical signs, a brief history should be obtained if possible.

- History   From patient/relative/paramedic
            Speed of onset
            Previous and current treatment (steroids, home nebulisers)
            Previous attacks requiring artificial ventilation

Clinical features of **acute severe** asthma include:

- **Inability to complete sentences in one breath**
- Tachycardia > 110 beats/min
- Respiratory rate > 25/min
- PEFR < 50% of predicted or best

Clinical features of **life-threatening** asthma include any one of:

- Silent chest
- Cyanosis (SpO_2 <92% or PaO_2 <8 kPa)
- Bradycardia or arrhythmias
- Exhaustion, confusion, coma
- A normal $PaCO_2$ (4.6–6.0 kPa)
- PEFR < 33% of predicted or best

What investigations might be helpful?

Asthma is primarily a clinical diagnosis, but further information may be gained from a few investigations.

- **Peak expiratory flow rate** – as outlined above
- **CXR** – performed to exclude a pneumothorax and may show pulmonary hyperinflation
- **Arterial blood gases** – initially these may show hypocarbia with some degree of hypoxia. As the acute attack progresses, worrying results include a normal/high $PaCO_2$ as ventilation worsens and PaO_2 < 8 kPa. Some degree of metabolic acidosis is inevitable
- **ECG** – this invariably shows a tachycardia, but may also reveal P pulmonale, right axis deviation, arrhythmias and ST elevation.

Apart from an acute exacerbation of asthma, what would you include in your differential diagnosis?

The two most common differential diagnoses in adults would probably be **left ventricular failure** and **chronic obstructive airways disease**.

Others include:

- Pulmonary embolism
- Upper airway obstruction
- Inhaled foreign body
- Aspiration
- Churg–Strauss syndrome (allergic granulomatosis)
- Aspergillosis

What would be your immediate management of this lady?

Sit the patient up	
Oxygen	As high a concentration as possible from a facemask (reservoir)
β_2 agonists	Starting with 2.5–5 mg of salbutamol nebulised in oxygen and repeated as required. If there is no response (or a deterioration), this may be given intravenously at a dose of 3–20 μg/min. It should be noted, however, that some investigators have concluded that intravenous β_2 agonists may be less effective than nebulised. Side effects include tachycardia, arrhythmias, tremor, hyperglycaemia, hypokalaemia and lactic acidosis.
Anticholinergics	Ipratropium bromide 0.5 mg nebulised in oxygen if initial response to salbutamol is poor. These agents may be synergistic with the β_2 agonists.
Steroids	The role of steroids in acute severe asthma is now well established and they should be given soon after presentation. Normal practice is to give 200 mg of intravenous hydrocortisone. Peak response is at 6–12 hours.
Magnesium	IV magnesium sulphate (1.2–2 g IV infusion over 20 minutes) single bolus for those with life-threatening asthma or a poor response to inhaled bronchodilators. (Mechanism of action: Ca^{2+} antagonist effect in bronchial smooth muscle, reduces Ach release at the neuromuscular junction, may increase sensitivity of β receptors to catecholamines.)
Aminophylline	In acute asthma, the use of intravenous aminophylline does not result in any additional bronchodilatation compared with standard care with beta-agonists. No subgroups in which aminophylline might be more effective could be identified in a recent Cochrane review and the frequency of adverse effects was higher.
Fluids and electrolytes	These patients will have both reduced intake and increased losses and careful fluid replacement is indicated. Hypokalaemia is relatively common.
Regular reassessment	

What other less well-established treatments do you know about?

- **Adrenaline** — No benefit from nebulised route, may be of benefit in refractory bronchospasm. Beware arrhythmias.
- **Ketamine** — No conclusive evidence. May have a sedative role in the ITU if a trial bolus helps with bronchospasm.
- **Inhalational agents** — These have bronchodilator effects but there is the risk of cardiovascular side effects.
- **Helium** — This reduces the work of breathing by reducing gas density and therefore turbulent flow. Fi O_2 limited.
- **ECMO**

What are the indications for mechanical ventilation?

- Respiratory arrest
- Reducing level of consciousness or coma
- Exhaustion
- Increasing hypoxaemia despite maximal medical treatment
- Increasing acidosis despite maximal medical treatment

Mechanical ventilatory support is required in 1%–3% of acute admissions with asthma.

What are the important points of the ventilator settings in asthmatics?

There are many changes in lung physiology that cause problems for mechanical ventilation:

- Airflow obstruction means lung overinflation is a hazard – risk of barotrauma/pneumothorax
- Lung units will have variably increased time constants, so long inspiratory times may be necessary to provide time for adequate gas exchange. This is not as commonly appreciated as the need for long expiratory times.
- Lung overinflation reduces venous return, compresses the heart and increases pulmonary vascular resistance

> The principles in ventilation are to limit peak and mean airway pressures, allow a prolonged expiratory time and maintain adequate oxygenation in the face of a high $PaCO_2$.

Strategies include:

- Low respiratory rate
- Low tidal volumes may be necessary to avoid barotrauma.
- Prolonged expiratory time (I:E ratio)
- Low inspiratory flow rate (with volume-controlled ventilators)
- The use of extrinsic PEEP remains controversial.
- Permissive hypercapnia. *Very* high $PaCO_2$ levels may have to be tolerated.

If it becomes impossible to ventilate the patient or there is a precipitous drop in cardiac output, the ventilator should be disconnected from the endotracheal tube and the lungs manually deflated by compression on the chest.

Bibliography

British Thoracic Society Scottish Intercollegiate Guidelines Network. (2008). British Guideline on the Management of Asthma. *Thorax*, **63**(Suppl. 4), iv1–iv121.

Burburan, S, Xisto D, Rocco P. (2007). Anaesthetic management in asthma. *Minerva Anestesiologica*, **73**(6), 357–65.

Cowman, S, Butler J. (2008). The use of intravenous aminophylline in addition to beta-agonists and steroids in acute asthma. *Emergency Medicine Journal*, **25**, 289–90.

Acute C2 injury

You are asked to anaesthetise a 68-year-old patient for fixation of an unstable C2 fracture.

Discuss the anaesthetic management.

This patient is going to have a difficult airway. The fracture is either due to trauma, in which case the patient may have other injuries, or it may be due to an underlying medical condition such as rheumatoid arthritis.

There are several important issues that require more information, both from the patient and the surgeon. An ABC approach to the pre-op assessment may be useful:

- Airway – the neck will be immobilised in, for example, a hard collar (mouth opening limited) or a halo (unobstructed mouth opening). A thorough airway assessment is essential.
- Breathing – Has the patient any associated chest injuries? Does the patient look easy to ventilate? Has the patient got a cord injury that has compromised ventilation? Consider post-operative respiratory monitoring or support with high cervical lesions affecting the intercostal or phrenic nerves.
- Circulation – there is a possibility of cardiac arrhythmia and autonomic dysfunction (hypotension with lesions above T6, bradycardia with lesions above T1).
- Neurological assessment and documentation of any deficit is vital.
- Associated injuries – a secondary survey should have been completed (10% of patients will have another vertebral column fracture).
- Other usual pre-op information should be sought in terms of previous GAs, allergies, past medical history, etc.
- Proposed surgical plan
  - Approach – anterior (via neck or mouth) or posterior or both
  - Positioning – supine or prone

> **Some patterns of spinal cord injury:**
>
> - Complete injury   Motor and sensory loss below a certain level
> - Central cord   Arms paralysed > legs
>   Variable sensory disturbance
>   Bladder dysfunction
> - Anterior cord   Paralysis below level of lesion
>   Proprioception, touch and vibration sense preserved
> - Posterior cord   Touch and temperature sensation impaired
> - Hemisection   Brown–Séquard syndrome:
>   Ipsilateral paralysis, loss of proprioception, touch
>   and vibration sensation
>   Contralateral loss of pain and temperature
>   sensation

Would you use an arterial line?

Yes. Invasive monitoring is necessary with cord compromise. Spinal cord perfusion pressure will be affected by both oedema and anatomical displacement and any drop in mean arterial pressure (MAP) could compromise the cord further. In addition, prone positioning can affect MAP and cord perfusion.

> **Spinal cord monitoring**
>
> - Increasingly used.
> - Evoked potentials – motor and sensory can be used.
> - These are affected by volatile agents and NMBs.
> - The spinal cord is most likely to suffer ischaemic events at C2/C3.

How would you manage the patient's airway?

This depends on the immobilisation measures in place, the degree of cord compromise and the risk of aspiration. The proposed technique should be discussed with the surgeon. Skull traction or a Halo frame limits neck movements, while full immobilisation in a hard collar with sandbags limits both neck movement and mouth opening.

    Awake fibre-optic intubation (AFO) is probably the technique of choice for a number of reasons:

- Minimises neck movements.
- Does not necessitate good mouth opening.
- Checking for intact neurological function immediately after intubation helps to exclude this as a cause of any post-operative neurological deterioration.

AFO in these patients is, however, not without potential problems as coughing may be disastrous in this setting. Careful preparation with local anaesthesia and the judicious use of opioids such as a Remifentanil infusion will help to suppress coughing. An experienced operator is essential.

If the stomach is empty and the airway accessible, the following may be considered:

- Asleep fibre-optic intubation (+/− LMA or ILMA)
- Standard laryngoscopy with cervical spine immobilisation

Is there any problem using certain muscle relaxants?

Suxamethonium can potentially cause hyperkalaemia by an exaggerated release of potassium ions from denervated muscles, especially if surgery occurs >72 hours after the injury. NMBs will interfere with spinal cord monitoring – see box below.

If the surgeon wants to position this patient prone, what are the considerations?

- The deleterious effects of prone positioning are:
  - V/Q mismatching
  - Reduced venous return
  - Reduction in cardiac output
- General precautions:
  - Meticulous care of pressure points
  - Ensure that the abdomen is free for respiration
  - Avoid pressure on the eyes
- Specifically for this procedure:
  - More personnel will be required for a log roll to ensure that the axial skeleton remains neutral.
  - A plan for fixing the head in position (usually involving a Mayfield frame) must be made.

Eye injury under anaesthesia

- Corneal abrasion – drying/eyes not taped – may take months to heal.
- Ischaemic optic neuropathy (ION) – more common with prone position as increased intra-ocular pressure. Not due to external pressure.
- Central retinal artery occlusion (CRAT) – caused by external pressure (often due to horseshoe headrest) or emboli from the carotid artery.

What would you use for post-operative analgesia?

The surgeons use local anaesthetic with adrenaline to vasoconstrict the operative field and longer-acting local anaesthetic could be instilled at the end of surgery. Regular paracetamol in addition to PCA morphine will provide adequate analgesia. NSAIDs should be carefully considered after discussion with the surgeon, as a haematoma could be catastrophic for the patient.

Bibliography

Meek, S. (1998). Fractures of the thoracolumbar spine in major trauma patients – clinical review. *British Medical Journal*, **317**(21), 1442–3.

Sidhy VS, Whitehead EM, Ainsworth, P, Smith M, Calder I. (1993). A technique of awake fibre-optic intubation. Experience in patients with cervical spine disease. *Anaesthesia*, **48**, 910–13.

Yentis SM, Hirsch NP, Smith GB. (2004). *Anaesthesia and Intensive Care A–Z – An Encyclopaedia of Principles and Practice*, 3rd edition. London: Butterworth Heinemann, Elsevier.

Acute myocardial infarct

You are asked to assess a 55-year-old male patient for an open reduction and internal fixation of a wrist fracture. He gives a history of acute myocardial infarction (AMI) 4 years ago, but does not remember which tablets he is on. He gives no recent history of chest pain, his previous AMI was painless. A routine pre-operative ECG has been done.

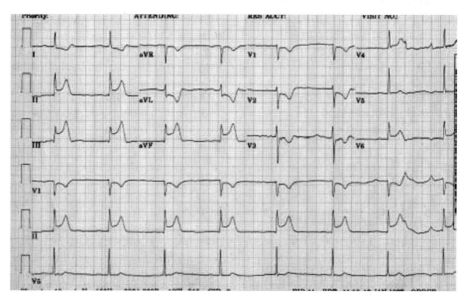

What does it show?

The findings on this ECG are:

- Rate: 50 bpm (300/6)
- Rhythm: Normal sinus rhythm with borderline first-degree heart block. The PR interval is just over five small squares.
- Axis: + 45 degrees (see atrial flutter question for method).
- P waves: Normal.
- QRS: Normal.
- ST: **ST elevation in leads II, III and aVF in keeping with acute inferior myocardial infarction. There is ST elevation in V6 suggesting lateral involvement. There are reciprocal ST changes in V1–V3.**
- T waves: There is T wave inversion in V1–V3.

In summary, the ECG shows an acute inferior (infero-lateral) myocardial infarction.

What medication would you expect the patient to be on?

The NICE guidelines 2001 for the management of patients post myocardial infarction indicate:

- Anti-platelet therapy (aspirin), ACE inhibitor, and beta-blockade should be started early as an inpatient post-AMI and continued indefinitely unless there is a clear indication to discontinue them.
- In patients with heart failure, beta-blockade should be started after ACE inhibitors and started at a low dose, which is gradually increased.
- Patients with NYHA grade III or IV heart failure should be started on spironolactone.
- Symptomatic treatment of heart failure may require the use of loop diuretics.
- Statin therapy should be continued if already in place. If not, assessment for statins should be performed 12 weeks post-infarct.
- Nitrates and calcium channel blockers may be used for symptomatic control.
- Clopidogrel (ADP mediated platelet aggregation inhibitor) improves outcome in NSTEMI/ACS when given with aspirin. NICE guidance 2004 suggests that it should be continued for 12 months. It is also often given post-ST elevation AMI and is shown to improve outcome. In this situation it is usually given for 28 days.

What are the anaesthetic implications of these drugs?

Aspirin	Potential to increase bleeding. Usually stopped 7 days before surgery with high risk of bleeding
Clopidogrel	Increases bleeding risk and is best stopped at least 7 days before surgery and peripheral or central nerve blockade
ACEI	Increase the incidence of hypotension during induction of general anaesthesia. Some authors suggest omitting the day before surgery

Beta-blockers	While they may increase the risk of bradycardia, beta-blockers have been shown to reduce cardiac mortality post-non-cardiac surgery in patients with, and at risk of ischaemic heart disease (Mangano *et al.*, 1996). This is thought to be via their favourable effects on cardiac oxygen demand and by attenuation of the stress response.
Diuretics	May result in hypovolaemia and electrolyte disturbance
Statins	May have cardio-protective properties, but further research is needed to assess efficacy.

How would you assess this patient?

Perform an ABC assessment of the patient and take a history.

Airway:	Administer oxygen via reservoir bag at 15 litres per minute
Breathing:	Look, listen and feel. Looking for signs of left ventricular failure
Circulation:	Look, listen and feel. Check HR, BP, JVP, capillary refill, heart sounds and urine output assessing for signs of cardiac insufficiency.
History:	Symptoms that may suggest time of recent AMI – chest pain, jaw pain, arm pain, SOB, nausea, sweating.
	Symptoms of cardiac failure and functional limitation – SOB, orthopnoea, PND, swelling.
	Previous cardiac history.
	Risk factors for AMI – smoking, hypertension, diabetes, hypercholesterolaemia, obesity, and family history.
	Previous medical history.
	Drug history and allergies.
	Anaesthetic history.

What are the symptoms and signs of heart failure?

Right heart failure symptoms:

- Fatigue
- SOB
- Nausea
- Swelling

Right heart failure signs:

- Raised JVP
- Hepatic engorgement
- Pitting oedema
- Ascites and pleural effusions
- Third heart sound
- Tricuspid regurgitation (dilation of ventricle).

Left heart failure symptoms:

- Fatigue
- Exertional dyspnoea
- Orthopnoea
- Paroxysmal nocturnal dyspnoea
- Respiratory distress if pulmonary oedema.

Left heart failure signs:

- Cardiomegaly with displaced apex
- Third or fourth heart sounds
- Mitral regurgitation
- Basal crackles
- Frank pulmonary oedema.

Congestive heart failure occurs when right ventricular failure occurs, secondary to left ventricular failure. It will present as a combination of the above.

NYHA classification of cardiovascular disease	
Class	**Patient symptoms**
Class I (Mild)	No limitation of physical activity. Ordinary physical activity does not cause undue fatigue, palpitation, or dyspnoea (shortness of breath).
Class II (Mild)	Slight limitation of physical activity. Comfortable at rest, but ordinary physical activity results in fatigue, palpitation, or dyspnoea.
Class III (Moderate)	Marked limitation of physical activity. Comfortable at rest, but less than ordinary activity causes fatigue, palpitation, or dyspnoea.
Class IV (Severe)	Unable to carry out any physical activity without discomfort. Symptoms of cardiac insufficiency at rest. If any physical activity is undertaken, discomfort is increased.

Reprinted with permission © 2007, American Heart Association, Inc.

Bibliography

American Heart Association. (1994). *Revisions to Classification of Functional Capacity and Objective Assessment of Patients with Diseases of the Heart.* http://www.americanheart.org/presenter. jhtml?identifier=1712.

Comfere T. (2005). Angiotensin system inhibitors in a general surgical population. *Anaesthesia and Analgesia*, **100**(3), 636–44.

Coriart P. (1994). Influence of chronic ACEI on anaesthetic induction. *Anaesthesiology*, **81**(2), 299–307.

Feringa HH, Bax JJ, Poldermanns D. (2007). Perioperative management of ischemic heart disease in patients undergoing noncardiac surgery. *Current Opinions in Anaesthesiology*, **20**(3), 254–60.

Mangano DT, Layug EL, Wallace A *et al.* (1996). Effects of Atenolol on mortality and cardiovascular morbidity after noncardiac surgery. *New England Journal of Medicine*, **335**(23), 1713–21.

NICE. (2001). Prophylaxis for patients who have experienced a myocardial infarction.

Poldermans D, Boersma E, Bax JJ *et al.* (1999). The effect of bisoprolol on perioperative mortality and myocardial infarction in high-risk patients undergoing vascular surgery. *New England Journal of Medicine*, **341**(24), 1789–94.

Airway assessment

How do you assess a patient's airway prior to anaesthesia?

Remember:
- History
- Examination
- Investigations

This is easy to forget in examination conditions.

■ **History**	Any history of previous problems with airway management must be elicited and the anaesthetic charts reviewed.
■ **Examination**	
Anatomical problems	Obesity
	Large breasts
	Prominent teeth
	Short, thick neck
	Syndromes associated with difficult intubation
	Trauma, local infection, radiotherapy
Mallampati score	This assesses the visibility of the pharyngeal structures and assumes the view is related to the size of the tongue base. The further assumption is that a large tongue base may hinder exposure of the larynx.
	Initially there were three proposed classes, but Samsoon and Young added a fourth in 1987 and this has gained common acceptance.

Mallampati score
Technique – patient sitting, head neutral, mouth fully open and tongue fully extended, no phonation. Some suggest conducting the test twice.

- Class I   Exposure of soft palate, uvula and tonsillar pillars
- Class II   Exposure of soft palate and base of uvula
- Class III   Exposure of soft palate only
- Class IV   No visualisation of pharyngeal structures except hard palate

Forward mandibular movement

Cervical spine movement	Assesses atlanto-occipital and atlanto-axial joint mobility. The patient is asked to extend the head with the neck in full flexion.
Thyromental distance	Described in 1983 by Patil *et al.* and defined as the distance from the chin to the notch of the thyroid cartilage with the head fully extended. If this is less than 6 cm, it may be associated with difficult intubation.
Sternomental distance	Described in 1994 by Savva and defined as the distance from the tip of the chin to the sternal notch. If this is less than 12 cm, it may be associated with difficult intubation
Prayer sign	Difficult intubation has been associated with the inability to place both palms flat together and seems to be more common in diabetics

Wilson risk score

Wilson risk score:

This gives a score from 0–2 for each of the following risk factors:

- Weight
- Head and neck movement
- Jaw movement
- Receding mandible
- Buck teeth

A score of 3 or more predicts 75% of difficult intubations (with 12% incidence of false-positives).

Individually, these tests have only moderate sensitivity and specificity. More recently, investigators have looked at combined predictors to try and increase the usefulness of these tests.

The combination of Mallampati class III/IV with a thyromental distance of less than 7 cm is predictive of a grade IV laryngoscopy with high sensitivity and specificity.

- **Investigations**
  Plain X-rays of head and neck
  CT scan
  Fibre-optic laryngoscopy

Some useful terms

Difficult intubation	When placement of an endotracheal tube requires more than 3 attempts and/or more than 10 min (ASA)
Difficult laryngoscopy	As described by Cormack and Lehane

Difficult mask ventilation	Less clearly defined but certainly a different entity to the concepts above. One study showed a 15% incidence of difficult mask ventilation in patients who had difficult or failed intubation.
Failed oxygenation	$SpO_2 < 90\%$ with FiO_2 1.0 (DAS)

How would you manage a difficult airway?

A difficult airway may be recognised pre-operatively as described above or may be unrecognised, presenting itself when the patient is anaesthetised +/− paralysed. These two situations warrant different management. The basic principles common to both include:

- Maintain oxygenation
- Call for experienced (in difficult airway) senior anaesthetic help
- Call for experienced surgical help
- Ensure difficult airway adjuncts are available
- Have working knowledge of a difficult airway algorithm.

Recognised difficult airway

With anticipated difficult airway management, the airway should be secured with the patient awake. Preparation in this case is essential. Consideration should be given to the following:

- Psychological preparation of the patient
- Monitoring
- Drying agents
- Aspiration prophylaxis
- Sedation
- Oxygen supplementation
- Topical local anaesthesia +/− nerve blocks
- Topical vasoconstrictors
- Appropriate equipment

If intubation fails in these circumstances, options include:

1. Cancellation of surgery
2. Regional anaesthesia   It must be recognised that this could result in the need for general anaesthesia and airway control in suboptimal conditions should the regional block fail.
3. Surgical airway

Unrecognised difficult airway

This scenario occurs when 'Plan A' for conventional intubation has failed and presents a very different scenario. Management depends on whether mask ventilation is possible or not and whether the intubation was part of a rapid-sequence induction.

If mask ventilation is possible, 'Plan B' intubation techniques can be attempted. Options include alternative rigid or fibre-optic laryngoscope blades, blind oral or nasal techniques, flexible fibre-optic laryngoscope, retrograde intubation, illuminating stylet, rigid bronchoscope or percutaneous dilatational tracheostomy. 'Plan B' is omitted during a rapid sequence induction.

'Plan C' involves maintenance of the airway and oxygenation and waking the patient. One or two person bag-valve-mask systems may be required as may the use of oral or nasal airway adjuncts. Failing oxygenation is an indication to attempt LMA insertion.

'Plan D' is for 'can't intubate, can't ventilate' scenarios and involves cannula or surgical cricothyroidotomy for emergency rescue oxygenation.

It must be noted that the LMA is a supraglottic device and may fail if an obstruction lies at or below the glottic opening.

Bibliography

Difficult Airway Society Website. www.das.uk.com.

Henderson JJ, Popat MT, Latto IP, Pearce AC; Difficult Airway Society. (2004). Difficult Airway Society guidelines for management of the unanticipated difficult intubation. *Anaesthesia*, **59**(7), 675–94.

Lee A, Fan LT, Gin T, Karmakar M, Ngan Kee D. (2006). A systematic review (meta-analysis) of the accuracy of the Mallampati tests to predict the difficult airway. *Anesthesia and Analgesia*, **102**(6), 1867–78.

Mallampati SR, Gatt SP, Gugino LD *et al.* (1985). A clinical sign to predict difficult tracheal intubation: a prospective study. *Canadian Anaesthesia Society Journal*, **32**, 429–34.

Airway blocks in the context of awake fibre-optic intubation

What are the indications for performing an awake fibre-optic intubation?

- Suspected or known difficult intubation
- Patient with a full stomach and an anticipated difficult intubation
- Suspected or known cervical spine injury
- Anticipated difficult mask ventilation (e.g. morbid obesity)

What are the contraindications to performing an awake fibre-optic intubation?

- Patient refusal
- Patient unable to co-operate
- Bleeding upper airway
- Allergy to local anaesthetics
- Upper airway tumours with stridor (scope may completely obstruct the tracheal lumen or cause severe bleeding)

What antisialogogue would you use?

- Glycopyrronium 4–8 mcg/kg im (or iv) an hour before the procedure
- Hyoscine 0,.2 mg im or
- Atropine 0.3–0.6 mg im

What is the nerve supply to the nose?

Mainly from two sources:

- The second division of the trigeminal nerve via the sphenopalatine ganglion. (Also supplies the superior part of the palate, uvula and tonsils.)
- The anterior ethmoidal nerve

How would you anaesthetise the nose?

Options include:

- 4% cocaine pledgets
- Lidocaine spray
- Nebulised lidocaine

How is the oropharynx innervated?

- Plexus derived from the vagus, facial and glossopharyngeal nerves
- The **glossopharyngeal nerve**:
  - Exits the skull via the jugular foramen and enters the pharynx between the superior and middle constrictor muscles of the pharynx.
  - **Sensation** to the posterior third of the tongue (lingual branch), anterior surface of epiglottis, posterior and lateral walls of the pharynx and tonsillar pillars.
  - **Motor** to stylopharyngeus

How could you anaesthetise the pharynx?

- Topical anaesthesia with 10% lidocaine spray or gargled/nebulised 4% lidocaine
- Benzocaine lozenges
- If there is still a marked gag reflex following one of the above procedures, then a glossopharyngeal nerve block can be performed.

Techniques for glossopharyngeal nerve block
Internal: Anterior or posterior approach

Anterior approach
- Mainly blocks the lingual branch.
- Apply topical anaesthesia to the tongue.

- Displace the tongue away from the side to be blocked.
- A gutter forms between the tongue and teeth.
- Use a spinal needle to gain an unobstructed view.
- Insert the needle at the posterior 'cul-de-sac' of the gutter at a depth of 0.25 – 0.5 cm and aspirate.
- If air is aspirated, retract a short distance.
- Inject 2 ml LA.

Posterior approach
- A more proximal block, it blocks sensory (pharyngeal, lingual and tonsillar branches) and motor to stylopharyngeus.
- Apply topical anaesthesia to the tongue.
- Depress the tongue.
- Insert an angled needle behind the middle of the posterior tonsillar pillar to a depth of 1 cm.
- After aspiration, inject 3 ml LA.
- More likely to get intravascular injection with this approach.

External
- Injection deep to and behind styloid process (2–4 cm deep).
- Found midway between the tip of the mastoid process and the angle of the jaw.
- Tiger country with internal carotid and jugular vessels close by.

What is the sensory and motor supply to the larynx

- Innervation of the laryngeal inlet is primarily from the **superior laryngeal nerve**, a branch of the vagus.
- The superior laryngeal nerve leaves the vagal trunk in the carotid sheath and travels anteriorly to the cornu of the hyoid bone.
- Here, it divides to form the internal branch (sensory) and the external branch (motor to cricothyroid muscle).
- The internal branch pierces the thyrohyoid membrane and enters the piriform fossa mucosa. It provides sensory supply to the larynx down to the vocal cords, the base of the tongue, vallecula, aryepiglottic folds and arytenoids.
- The **recurrent laryngeal nerves** (from the vagus) supply sensation below the vocal cords and all the muscles of the larynx except cricothyroid.

How could you anaesthetise the larynx?

The sensory supply above and below the cords needs to be addressed.
 Sensation above the cords:

Superior laryngeal nerve block
May be performed externally by injection or internally by topical anaesthesia.

External
- Seated or semi-recumbent patient
- A wheal is raised 1 cm inferior and 2 cm anterior to the extremity of the prominent cornua of the hyoid bone.
- The needle is walked off the lower border of the hyoid bone to pierce the thyrohyoid membrane.
- 2–3 ml of 2% lidocaine is injected.
- The injection is repeated on the other side.

Internal
- Using Krause's forceps, hold a lignocaine-soaked pledget in the piriform fossa for 2–3 minutes on each side.
- Very simple (if you can find Krause's forceps!)

Sensation below the cords:
Cricothyroid puncture

- Also known as a translaryngeal block.
- Will anaesthetise most of the laryngeal surface.
- The cricothyroid membrane is identified and the skin overlying it fixed with the index and thumb of the operator's non-dominant hand.
- Following disinfection and local anaesthetic infiltration to the skin, a syringe with saline is attached to a 20-gauge cannulae and inserted through the cricothyroid membrane.
- Air is aspirated confirming laryngeal placement of the cannulae.
- The needle is withdrawn and 2–3 ml of 2% lidocaine is injected.
- The induced coughing aids dispersion of the local anaesthetic.

Alternatives are to use nebulised 4% lignocaine as the sole anaesthetic technique or to 'spray as you go' via the bronchoscope (probably the commonest technique for awake fibre-optic intubation). See also Long Case 1 'The one about the woman with a goitre for an emergency laparotomy'.

Bibliography

Allman KG, Wilson IH. (2001). *Oxford Handbook of Anaesthesia*. Oxford, UK: Oxford University Press.

Hagberg CA. (2000). *Handbook of Difficult Airway Management*. University of Texas, Houston, USA: Churchill Livingstone.

Yentis SM, Hirsch NP, Smith GB. (2004). *Anaesthesia and Intensive Care, A–Z – An Encyclopaedia of Principles and Practice*, 3rd edition, London: Butterworth-Heinemann, Elsevier 2004.

Amniotic fluid embolism

You are the anaesthetist on-call for delivery suite. You are called urgently to a delivery room where a woman in the second stage of labour has collapsed. Just prior to this she became extremely breathless and went blue, according to the midwife. She is now not breathing. What is your immediate management?

> **RESUSCITATION – this should be easy marks because it is 'bread and butter'.**
> **ALWAYS follow the ABC approach. You can be talking about this whilst thinking about the differential diagnosis.**

- **Call for immediate help** from a senior obstetrician and anaesthetist.
- If not breathing and no pulse – commence **CPR** and get defibrillator.
- Establish an **airway** – the trachea should be intubated if appropriate.
- Establish **breathing** with 100% oxygen.
- **Circulation** – Large-bore intravenous cannulae should be sited with blood sent for cross-match, coagulation screen, full blood count, urea, electrolytes and blood glucose.
- Commence fluid resuscitation.
- **Left lateral tilt**/Manual uterine displacement.
- After 5 minutes, consideration should be given to **caesarian section** to aid resuscitation attempts.

There is no evidence of blood loss. What is the differential diagnosis?

The causes of sudden cardiovascular collapse in pregnancy are:

- **Amniotic fluid embolism**
- **Pulmonary thrombo-embolism**
- **Venous air embolism**
- **Occult haemorrhage** such as **placental abruption** or **hepatic rupture** in a patient with fulminating pre-eclampsia/HELLP
- **Intra-cerebral bleed**
- **Drug toxicity** (including local anaesthetics)
- **Sepsis**
- **Myocardial infarction**

What do you know about amniotic fluid embolism?

- Rare (1:20 000 deliveries) but devastating complication of labour or early puerperium.

- Presents with **severe dyspnoea, cyanosis and sudden cardiovascular collapse** (with or without bleeding). **Seizures** may also occur.
- **Cardiac arrest** occurs in up to 87%.
- Up to 50% die in the first hour and the overall mortality is 60–80%.
- Most survivors have a neurological injury.
- Amniotic fluid contains fetal debris, prostaglandins and leukotrienes which block pulmonary vessels, cause pulmonary vasoconstriction, pulmonary hypertension and acute right ventricular failure. Hypoxia causes global myocardial ischaemia and acute lung injury. There is widespread complement activation.
- Women who survive these events may enter a second haemorrhagic phase characterized by massive haemorrhage with uterine atony and DIC.
- The US national registry concluded that the **pathophysiology was more in-keeping with an anaphylactoid reaction** rather than purely an embolic process as fetal squames have been found in the lungs of women without AFE syndrome.
- Three major factors contribute to the problems encountered in this condition:

  1. **Acute pulmonary embolism**
  2. **Disseminated intravascular coagulation (DIC)**
  3. **Uterine atony**

- **Extreme hypoxia** is caused by pulmonary and cardiac shunts.
  Pulmonary shunt   The transient increase in PVR may cause a redistribution of blood flow from blocked pulmonary vessels to patent ones, resulting in incomplete oxygenation as the blood-flow through them overwhelms their maximum rate of oxygenation. The fall in cardiac output results in a fall in mixed venous O_2 saturation returning to the heart, compounding oxygenation problems. There may be direct myocardial depression with pulmonary oedema.
  Cardiac shunt   A (potentially) patent foramen ovale is present in 35% of the population. Very high PA pressures may cause mixed venous blood to pass through it.
- **Severe left-sided heart failure** (mechanism unclear) causes hypotension.
- **Coagulopathy** (in up to 83%) is probably caused by tissue factor or trophoblasts in the amniotic fluid stimulating the clotting cascade.
- **Diagnosis** is based on clinical presentation and laboratory findings. Monoclonal antibody TKH-2 has been used to demonstrate fetal mucin in the pulmonary vasculature, but it may still not be specific for the syndrome.
- The intact infant survival rate is 70%. Neurological status of the infant is directly related to the time elapsed between maternal arrest and delivery.
- Risk of recurrence is unknown. Successful subsequent pregnancies have been reported. Recommending elective caesarean for future pregnancies in an attempt to avoid labour is controversial.

How would you manage this lady after delivery of the fetus?

- Intensive care
- Survivors of the initial event are at risk of:
  - ARDS
  - Circulatory failure
  - DIC
- Treatment is supportive:
  - Ventilation
  - Inotropic support
  - Clotting factors
  - Factor VIIa for massive haemorrhage
- Uterine atony may necessitate oxytocin and carboprost (Hemabate™) (PGF$_2$).
- No form of therapy has been found to improve outcome.
- Hydrocortisone and adrenaline have been recommended due to the similarity of the condition with anaphylaxis.

Bibliography

Kramer M, Rouleau J, Baskett T, Joseph KS. (2006). Amniotic-fluid embolism and medical induction of labour: a retrospective, population-based cohort study. *Lancet*, **368**, 1444–8.

Locksmith GJ. (1999). Amniotic fluid embolism. *Obstetrics and Gynaecology Clinics of North America*, **26**(3), 435–44.

Oh TE, Bersten A, Soni N. (2004). *Intensive Care Manual*, 5th edition. Philadelphia: Butterworth-Heinemann.

Tuffnell DJ. (2005). United Kingdom amniotic fluid embolism register. *British Journal of Obstetrics and Gynaecology*, **112**(12), 1625–9.

Analgesia for circumcision

I want you to imagine I am the mother of a 2-year-old boy due to come into hospital for circumcision. I am very worried that he will suffer with pain after the operation. Can you explain to me how you will prevent this?

> This is a 'fluffy jumper' question that can easily be tackled badly! However, you should try to role-play and act in an interested and compassionate way! Your explanation should be in layman's terms.

'I can appreciate your concern. We tend to use a combination of techniques for pain relief, which keep the children comfortable after the operation. The first thing we will do, once he is asleep, is to put an injection of **local anaesthetic** into the base of his penis. This usually provides good pain relief for up to 12 hours after the operation. In addition to this, we have a variety of other pain relief options available. We would start with simple **paracetamol** followed by the addition of something stronger like **ibuprofen** or **voltarol**.

Local **anaesthetic gel** (lignocaine) can also be smeared onto the wound regularly to cover the first 24–36 hours. These measures provide good pain relief and can be administered by you at home. It can be a bit sore at home for a few days, but the medicines I have mentioned will keep him comfortable. In the rare event that something stronger was needed, we may use **morphine liquid** to drink but we would keep him in hospital if that were the case.'

How can you assess post-operative pain in children?

An assessment of pain can be made by experienced staff with the use of routine monitoring (**HR, BP** and **respiratory rate**) together with **behavioural assessment techniques** (e.g. child withdrawn or lashing out). It is important to repeat the assessments and **listen to the parents**. In older children (>4 years), one can use **numerical pain-rating scales** or **visual scales** like the face self-reporting scale, providing they have been understood pre-operatively.

What is the nerve supply to the penis?

The nerve supply to the penis is derived from the **pudendal nerve** (S2–4) which gives off the **dorsal nerve of the penis** bilaterally. These run **deep to Buck's fascia** and are just lateral to the dorsal arteries and veins bilaterally. They supply the distal two-thirds of the penis. Ventral branches from the dorsal nerves supply the frenulum. The **genitofemoral and ilioinguinal nerves** may also provide some sensory supply at the base.

Once the child is asleep and being monitored by a second anaesthetist, how do you perform a penile block?

The dorsal nerves are blocked with injections of **0.5% plain bupivacaine** either side of the midline deep to Buck's fascia. The volume would be **1 ml + 0.1 ml/kg** (max dose 2 mg/kg). This ensures that the local anaesthetic passes posteriorly to block the ventral branches supplying the frenulum. **Bilateral blocks are necessary** because there is a midline septum, which may prevent spread from a single injection. The risk of vascular injury is also reduced.

Could you use a caudal?

Yes.
To estimate the volume and dose required, the **regime of Armitage** may be employed. Using 0.25% plain bupivacaine, the volume is based on the weight and the level to be blocked.

- Lumbo-sacral block up to L1 – 0.5 ml/kg
- Block up to T10 – 1 ml/kg
- Block up to T6 – 1.25 ml/kg

What problems might be associated with a caudal?

- Dural tap
- Failure
- IV injection
- Hypotension (rare in children)
- Urinary retention
- Motor weakness necessitating overnight stay in hospital

Bibliography

Brown TCK, Eyres RL, McDougall RJ. (1999). Local and regional anaesthesia in children. *British Journal of Anaesthesia*, **83**, 65–77.

Budic I, Marjanovic V, Novakovic D. (2004). Penile block and inhalation anesthetics as a combined anesthesia in surgery of the penis in children. *Regional Anesthesia and Pain Medicine*, **29**(suppl 2), 61.

Mather SJ, Hughes DG. (1996). *A Handbook of Paediatric Anaesthesia, 2nd edition*. Oxford, UK: Oxford Medical Publications.

Anaphylaxis

You are anaesthetising a young woman for a hysteroscopy. Shortly following the injection of thiopentone, her blood pressure becomes unrecordable, she is flushed and her lungs are very difficult to ventilate with a bag and mask.

What are your immediate *actions?*

> You should be grinning inside if you get this question!
> The anaphylaxis drill should require practically no thought.

Anaphylaxis drill: *Initial therapy*

- **Stop administration** of suspected agent.
- **Maintain airway: give 100% oxygen.**
- **Lay the patient flat** with feet elevated.
- **Give adrenaline: i.m.** at a dose of 0.5–1 mg (repeated every 10 min if required).
  i.v. at a dose of 50–100 mcg for hypotension or cardiovascular collapse titrated up to 0.5–1 mg as required.
- **Give i.v. fluids** (crystalloid or colloid).

What secondary therapies would you administer or consider?

- **Antihistamines** – give chlorpheniramine 10–20 mg by slow i.v. infusion.
- **Corticosteroids** – give hydrocortisone 200 mg i.v.
- **Catecholamine infusion** – if poor response to initial bolus.
- **Bronchodilators**
- **Consider bicarbonate (0.5–1 mmol/kg).**

How would you investigate this patient for suspected anaphylaxis?

Investigation can be divided into **immediate** and **late**.

The diagnosis of anaphylactic or anaphylactoid reaction hinges around the plasma tryptase concentration.

Immediate
Identification of an anaphylactic/anaphylactoid reaction:
Take **10 ml venous blood** into a plain tube to be spun down to separate the serum and **store at −20 °C**. Send to reference laboratory for **tryptase estimation**.

Take several samples:

- Immediately if the clinical situation allows.
- 1 hour after start of reaction.
- 6–24 hours after the reaction.

The rise in tryptase is transient and so timing is important. Tryptase concentration is thought to reach a peak at 1 hour after an anaphylactic reaction, but there is evidence to suggest that the rise is earlier in reactions with hypotension; if the 1 hour sample only is taken, the rise may be missed. It is essential to label the samples with the appropriate timings.

Later
Identification of suspected agent.

- The patient should be referred to a regional allergy specialist.
- Skin prick tests.
- Anaesthetist is responsible for ensuring they are performed (either by himself or, ideally, a specialist in interpretation of skin tests).

Tell me about plasma tryptase.

- Protein contained in mast cells – 99% of total body tryptase is within mast cells.
- Released (along with histamine and other amines) in anaphylactic/ anaphylactoid reactions.
- **Sensitive and specific** diagnostic test for anaphylactic/anaphylactoid reactions.
- Half-life 2.5 hours.
- Basal level = 0.8–1.5 ng/ml.
- **Level >20 ng/ml seen in anaphylactic reactions**

NB Urinary methylhistamine is the principal metabolite of histamine, but is difficult to interpret outside the normal range, although it will be detectable for longer than plasma tryptase.

How do you perform skin prick tests?

- Testing should occur 4–6 weeks after the reaction.
- Testing should include a wide range of anaesthetic drugs as well as the suspected agents to establish those drugs that are safe for future use.
- Performed with 'neat' drug and 1 in 10 dilution.
- Positive control (histamine) and negative control (phenol saline) should be included for each test.
- A drop of drug is applied to the volar aspect of the forearm and a lancet stabbed through it to break the skin but not draw blood.
- Sites are inspected over 15 minutes for wheal and flare.
- A wheal of >2 mm larger than the negative control is regarded as positive.
- **A positive skin-prick test to 1 in 10 solution is a true positive**. (True reactions may have positive tests at much greater dilutions, e.g. 1 in 100 or 1 in 1000.)
- A positive test to 'neat' drug may or may not be significant.

> **Reporting:**
> - Give full explanation to the patient (Medic-alert bracelet).
> - Record in the case notes.
> - Inform GP.
> - Complete a 'Yellow card' to notify the MHRA.

Bibliography

Brown S, Mullins R, Gold M. (2006). Anaphylaxis: diagnosis and management. *Medical Journal of Australia*, **185**(5), 283–9.

Suspected Anaphylactic Reactions Associated with Anaesthesia. (2003). revised edition. Published by the *Association of Anaesthetists of Great Britain and Ireland and The British Society of Allergy and Clinical Immunology (working party)*.

Antepartum haemorrhage

You are called to the labour ward to see a 25-year-old P$_{2+1}$ lady in labour who has lost 700 ml of blood PV in labour. She looks pale and sweaty, her pulse is 140, regular and thready and her BP is 105/55. What would you do?

- ABC.
- Administer 100% oxygen via a non-rebreathing reservoir face-mask.
- Establish intravenous access with two large-bore cannulae.

■ Commence fluid resuscitation with crystalloid/colloid (not dextrans).
■ O-negative blood initially (usually 2 units available on the ward) until group-specific/fully cross-matched blood available (group specific takes 15 minutes).
■ Pressure bags and fluid warmer.
■ Head-down, left lateral tilt.
■ Call obstetrician, midwives and another anaesthetist (consultant if possible).
■ Inform haematologist.
■ Send blood for FBC, cross-match at least 6 units, coagulation screen, urea, electrolytes and LFTs.
■ Regular repeated Hb, platelet and coagulation studies.
■ Consider FFP, cryoprecipitate and platelets.
■ There may be a major haemorrhage trolley on the delivery suite.
■ Joint assessment with obstetricians as to the urgency of surgery.
■ Adequate maternal monitoring (CVP and invasive BP useful if there is time).
■ Fetal monitoring.
■ Treat the cause.

How would you assess the degree of blood loss?

The losses into the bed and onto pads could be estimated and the degree of hypovolaemia estimated by using physical signs such as tachycardia, BP, capillary refill time, skin colour and level of consciousness.

There may be an underestimation of the degree of hypovolaemia due to hidden losses.

What are the likely causes of her bleeding?

■ **Placenta praevia**   **Most**
■ **Placental abruption**   **likely**
■ Uterine rupture
■ Cervical or vaginal tear
■ Uterine atony
■ Coagulation or platelet problem

Her previous pregnancy resulted in a caesarean section. Is this relevant?

Yes. This increases the possibility of **placenta praevia** overlying the old uterine scar and increases the risk of uterine rupture. There is also a higher incidence of placenta accreta (adheres to the surface), increta (invades uterine muscle) or percreta (penetrates through uterine muscle), all of which may lead to life-threatening haemorrhage, necessitating a hysterectomy to stop the bleeding.

How would you anaesthetise this lady?

■ Initial resuscitation as already outlined.

- Aspiration prophylaxis – sodium citrate.
- Rapid sequence induction with cricoid pressure and left lateral tilt on the operating table.
- Equipment for a difficult intubation should be available.
- Consultant anaesthetist ideally in attendance or at least two pairs of 'anaesthetic hands'.

What measures are available to influence the degree of blood loss on the table?

These can be divided into surgical (including radiological), medical and haematological:

Surgical	Bimanual uterine compression and packing
	Aortic compression
	Uterine or internal iliac artery ligation
	Hysterectomy
Radiological	Arterial embolisation
	Balloon occlusion of iliac vessels
	(Need to be stable enough for potentially long X-ray procedure.)
Medical	Keep anaesthetic vapour concentration down
	Ergometrine
	Oxytocin
	Carboprost (Hemabate(^{tm}))– PGF$_{2\alpha}$
Haematological	Correct coagulopathy – FFP, cryoprecipitate, platelets
	Factor VIIa
	Cell salvage

Bibliography

Banks A, Norris A. (2005). Massive haemorrhage in pregnancy. *Continuing Education in Anaesthesia, Critical Care and Pain*, **5**(6), 195–8.
Oh TE. (2003). *Intensive Care Manual*. Philadelphia: Butterworth-Heinemann.
Wise A, Clark V. (2007). Obstetric haemorrhage. *Anaesthesia and Intensive Care Medicine*, **8**(8), 326–30.

Anticoagulants and neuraxial blockade

What is the incidence of spinal haematoma in neuraxial blockade?

In an extensive review of the literature, Tryba identified 13 cases of spinal haematoma following 850 000 epidural anaesthetics and 7 cases among 650 000 spinal techniques. Based on these observations, the calculated incidence is approximated to be less than **1 in 150 000 epidurals** and less than **1 in 220 000 spinal anaesthetics**. Because these estimates represent the upper limit of the 95% confidence interval, the actual frequency may be much less. A

Royal College of Anaesthetists National audit is currently under way to determine the complications arising from neuraxial blockade. The rarity of spinal haematoma as a complication of neuraxial blockade makes performing any adequately powered randomised controlled trial virtually impossible. There is also no current laboratory model. The actual incidence of neurological dysfunction resulting from haemorrhagic complications associated with central neuraxial block is unknown.

What are recommendations for neuraxial blockade in the presence of anticoagulation based on?

They are based on case reports, clinical series, pharmacology, haematology, and risk factors for surgical bleeding.

All the above factors are taken into consideration by recognised experts in the field of neuraxial anaesthesia and anticoagulation.

How do you decide whether or not to perform a neuraxial block in a patient taking anticoagulants?

The decision to perform a neuraxial block and the timing of catheter removal in a patient receiving anti-thrombotic therapy should be made on an individual basis, weighing up the small, though definite risk of spinal haematoma with the benefits of regional analgesia for a specific patient.

Indwelling catheters should not be sited or removed in the presence of therapeutic anticoagulation, as this appears to significantly increase the risk of spinal haematoma.

Identification of risk factors and establishment of guidelines will not completely eliminate the complication of spinal haematoma.

Post-operative monitoring and a robust Pain Service are essential to allow early evaluation of neurological dysfunction and prompt intervention.

What are ticlopidine and clopidogrel?

Ticlopidine and clopidogrel are thienopyridine derivatives that inhibit adenosine diphosphate-induced platelet aggregation. They also interfere with platelet fibrinogen binding and platelet–platelet interactions. These drugs are used in the prevention of cerebrovascular and cardiac thromboembolic events.

How long prior to the insertion of an epidural should these drugs be stopped?

Based on labelling and surgical reviews, the suggested time interval between discontinuation of thienopyridine therapy and neuraxial blockade is 14 days for ticlopidine and 7 days for clopidogrel.

Would you perform an epidural on a patient who is taking platelet GPIIb/IIIa inhibitors?

No. Platelet GP IIb/IIIa inhibitors exert a profound effect on platelet aggregation. They interfere with platelet–fibrinogen binding and platelet–Von Willebrand factor binding. Their use is primarily in acute coronary syndromes. Following administration, the time to normal platelet aggregation is 24–48 hours for abciximab and 4–8 hours for eptifibatide and tirofiban. Neuraxial techniques should be avoided until platelet function has recovered. GP IIb/IIIa antagonists are contraindicated within 4 weeks of surgery. Should one be administered in the post-operative period (following a neuraxial technique), the patient should be carefully monitored neurologically.

Would you perform an epidural on a patient taking long term NSAIDs?

Yes. NSAIDs appear to represent no added significant risk for the development of spinal haematoma in patients having epidural or spinal analgesia. The use of NSAIDs alone does not create a level of risk that will interfere with the performance of neuraxial blocks.

What if your patient were taking ginseng or garlic?

Garlic has been shown in vivo to inhibit platelet aggregation with one of its constituents, ajoene, found to potentiate the effect of other platelet inhibitors. Ginseng and ginsenosides have been found to prolong APTT and thrombin time in rats and demonstrate in vitro inhibition of platelet aggregation. There does, however, not seem to be specific concerns as to the timing of neuraxial block in relationship to the dosing of herbal therapy, post-operative monitoring or the timing of neuraxial catheter removal with regards to present data.

How would your anaesthetic technique be influenced if the patient was prescribed Fondaparinux or had been treated with a hirudin derivative?

Recombinant hirudin derivatives, including desirudin, lepirudin and bivalirudin inhibit both free and clot-bound thrombin. These drugs are used for the treatment and prevention of thrombosis in patients with heparin-induced thrombocytopaenia Argatroban, an L-arginine derivative, has a similar mechanism of action. Although there are no case reports of spinal haematoma related to neuraxial anaesthesia among patients who have received a thrombin inhibitor, spontaneous intracranial bleeding has been reported. Due to the lack of information available, no statement regarding risk assessment and patient management can be made.

Fondaparinux produces its anti-thrombotic effect through factor Xa inhibition and has a single daily dosing schedule due to a half-life of 21 hours. The actual risk of spinal haematoma with fondaparinux is unknown. Consensus statements are based on the sustained and irreversible anti-thrombotic effect, early post-operative dosing and the spinal haematoma reported during initial clinical trials. Close monitoring of the surgical literature for risk factors associated with surgical bleeding may be helpful in risk assessment and patient management.

Until further clinical experience is available, performance of neuraxial techniques should occur under conditions utilised in clinical trials (single needle pass, atraumatic needle placement, avoidance of indwelling neuraxial catheters). If this is not feasible, an alternative method of thromboprophylaxis should be considered.

Bibliography

Horlocker TT, Benzon H, Brown DL et al. (2003). Regional anaesthesia in the anticoagulated patient: defining the risks (the Second ASRA Consensus Conference on Neuraxial Anesthesia and Anticoagulation). Reg Anesth Pain Medicine, 28, 172–97.

Aspiration with an LMA

You are anaesthetising a healthy young patient in the left lateral position for an incision and drainage of a peri-anal abscess. He is spontaneously breathing on a laryngeal mask. Near the end of the case, the ODP notices gastric contents in the LMA tubing. What is your immediate management?

Immediate management would be:

- 100% Oxygen.
- Head down tilt (patient already in left lateral).
- Remove LMA and clear airway with suction.
- Secure airway with the aid of cricoid pressure, suxamethonium and tracheal intubation (may be performed in lateral position or supine position, lateral having an advantage if further aspiration, but may be technically more difficult).
- Suction trachea immediately after intubation (before ventilation drives gastric contents deeper into the lungs).

Further management:

- Insert a naso-gastric tube to empty the stomach.
- If the patient is stable, surgery could be completed.
- A chest X-ray should be performed looking for oedema, collapse or consolidation.
- If oxygen saturation persistently low, consider fibre-optic or rigid bronchoscopy, particularly if aspiration of food matter is suspected.
- Extubate in left lateral position if oxygen requirements permit. If not, an intensive care bed should be requested.

■ After extubation, the patient should be observed in recovery or in high
dependency for 2–5 hours. If the patient is asymptomatic, they may be
discharged back to the ward and observed.
■ If symptomatic, the patient is best managed in critical care and may require
CPAP or re-intubation. Aspiration pneumonitis, pneumonia or ARDS may
develop.
■ Prophylactic antibiotics are not indicated but infection should be treated if
it occurs.
■ The patient should be informed about what has occurred.

You perform a chest X-ray.

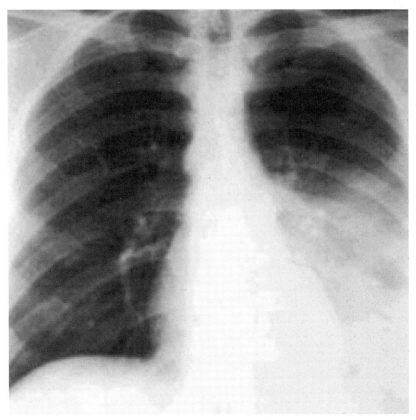

What does it show?

■ This is a PA film (not marked as AP) – (the authors accept that a PA film
would not be possible in this situation but the example was all we could
find!)
■ The alignment and penetration are good.
■ There is opacification of the left lower zone with loss of the left
hemidiaphragm consistent with left lower lobe consolidation.
■ The heart size is within normal limits (CTR <0.5).
■ The mediastinum is normal and there are no skeletal abnormalities.

Can you drawn the bronchial tree?

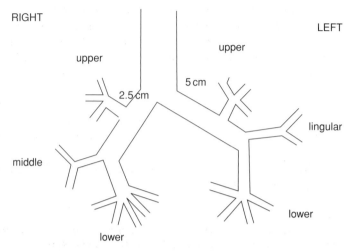

RIGHT

LEFT

upper

upper

5 cm

2.5 cm

lingular

middle

lower

lower

Branches:

- Right upper: Apical, anterior and posterior.
- Right middle: Medial and lateral.
- Right lower: Apical, anterior, posterior, medial and lateral.
- Left upper: Apical, anterior and posterior.
- Lingular: Superior and inferior.
- Left lower: Apical, anterior (with medial branch), posterior and lateral.

Where would the gastric contents go in the right lateral and supine position?

Aspiration in the supine position may distribute to both sides, but more frequently to the right side due to the position and size of the right main bronchus and particularly to the upper lobe. The right upper lobe will also be the most likely site in the right lateral position.

What is the pathogenesis and prognosis of aspiration-induced lung injury?

- Mendelson described his syndrome in 1946 in obstetric patients who had aspirated under general anaesthesia. He demonstrated the **role of acid** in its pathogenesis.
- Aspiration of acidic and **usually sterile** gastric contents into the lungs.
- pH <2.5 and volume > 0.3–0.4 ml/kg (~25 ml) thought to be required to produce aspiration pneumonitis from animal experiments. This has been disputed.
- First phase of injury begins in seconds and peaks in the first two hours and is due to **direct tissue damage** from gastric acid. Bronchospasm and pulmonary oedema may occur.

- Second phase peaks at 4 to 6 hours and is marked by infiltration of neutrophils, complement activation and acute inflammation.
- While normally sterile, gastric contents may become colonized with bacteria (often Gram-negative) in patients on antacid medications, in patients receiving enteral feeding or in those with gastro-paresis. In these patients early infections may contribute to lung injury.
- Secondary infection and progression to ARDS may occur.
- The majority of patients who aspirate under general anaesthesia remain asymptomatic (63% in one series). A minority will require ventilation (19%). Death occurred in ∼6% of patients in two series of aspiration pneumonitis cases occurring after anaesthesia and drug overdose.
- Aspiration pneumonitis occurs in 1 in 3000 anaesthetics and accounts for 10%–30% of anaesthetic deaths.

Bibliography
Christ A, Arranto CA, Schindler C et al. (2006). Incidence, risk factors, and outcome of aspiration pneumonitis in ICU overdose patients. *Intensive Care Medicine*, **32**(9), 1423–7.
Marik PE. (2001). Aspiration pneumonitis and aspiration pneumonia. *New England Journal of Medicine*, **344**(9), 665–71.
Warner MA, Warner ME, Weber JG. (1993). Clinical significance of pulmonary aspiration during the perioperative period. *Anesthesiology*, **78**, 56–62.

Atrial flutter

You are asked to assess a 57-year-old lady for total abdominal hysterectomy. She has a history of chronic asthma for which she is on long-term oral steroids and regular home nebulised salbutamol. An ECG has been performed.

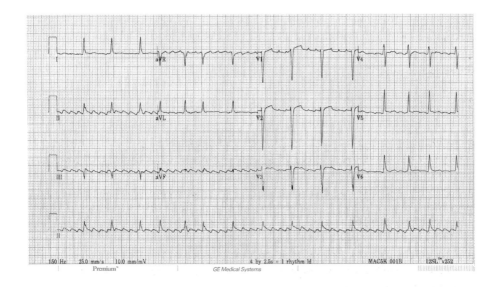

Tell me about the ECG?

Rate: 80–90 bpm
Rhythm: The rhythm is irregular and flutter waves are present. The rhythm is atrial flutter with a variable block, varying between a 2:1 and a 4:1 block.
Axis: The axis is at zero degrees.

How do you calculate the axis?

Normal cardiac axis is −30 to +90 degrees. Less than −30 degrees represents left axis deviation.

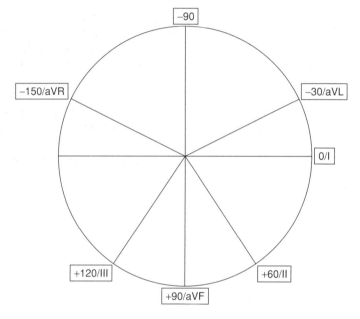

- **The simplest way to resolve cardiac axis is to use the net QRS deflection in leads I and aVF.**
- Lead I is at 0 degrees and lead aVF is at +90 degrees, i.e. they are perpendicular to each other; therefore, resolving the vectors in these two leads will give the axis.
- If lead I has a positive deflection and aVF a positive deflection, the axis has to lie between 0 and +90 degrees.
- In this case, lead I is very positive and aVF is isoelectric (i.e. one in which the R and S waves are of equal size) so the vector lies at 0 degrees. There is no contribution to the vector from aVF.
- **Another approach** is to first identify an isoelectric lead.
- Theoretically, the axis must lie perpendicular to this lead.

- In this example aVF is isoelectric; therefore, the axis lies either at zero degrees or 180 degrees.
- As lead I (counter clockwise to aVF) is positive and III (clockwise to aVF) is negative, the axis is zero degrees.
- **Another useful tip** – if lead **aVR** is positive, then the axis is abnormal because it has to lie between less than $-60°$ or greater than $120°$.

Why may the patient be in atrial flutter?

The atrial flutter may be due to her chronic respiratory disease, her treatment or due to other pathology.
Chronic respiratory diseases such as chronic asthma and COPD result in increased pulmonary vascular resistance and right ventricular strain. Increased right ventricular pressures lead to right atrial dilation, which may trigger atrial dysrhythmias. Furthermore, hypoxia and acidosis may increase the incidence of dysrhythmias.

Salbutamol is a beta-adrenergic agonist. It has a high degree of β_2 specificity. However, at higher doses significant β_1 effects occur. This produces tachycardia and reduces the threshold for atrial dysrhythmias. Furthermore, β-agonists and steroids may produce hypokalaemia.

Atrial flutter may also be caused by other disease processes such as:

- Ischaemic heart disease
- Hypertension
- Thyroid disease
- Cardiomyopathies or myocarditis
- Rheumatic/valvular heart disease
- Carcinoma of the bronchus
- Alcohol abuse.

How do β_2-agonists like salbutamol work?

β_2 **adrenergic receptors are G(s) protein coupled receptors**. They are found mainly on smooth muscle cells. These receptors consist of seven transmembrane domains and interact with G protein complexes on the intracellular surface. Binding of an agonist causes a conformational change in the β_2 receptor resulting in the Gs protein complex releasing GDP and binding GTP, thus activating the complex. The GTP/alpha complex dissociates from the beta/gamma subunit and activates adenyl cyclase to produce cAMP. The increase in cAMP activates protein kinases causing active calcium compartment shift resulting in smooth muscle relaxation and bronchial dilatation. Direct potassium channel activation by G proteins may also increase smooth muscle relaxation. The G-alpha subunit has intrinsic GTPase activity resulting in the hydrolysis of GTP to GDP returning the complex to its inactive state.

β_2-agonists also inhibit mast cell de-granulation and may inhibit vagal tone.

How would you manage her atrial flutter?

- A history should be taken to assess symptoms of cardiac insufficiency and an examination performed.
- Check electrolytes, thyroid function tests and a chest X-ray.
- Refer the patient to a cardiologist for further investigation and management.
- An echocardiogram can be performed to assess cardiac function and structure.
- Rate control does not appear to be an issue here but may be necessary in some cases. Suitable agents are beta-blockers (may not be appropriate in this case), verapamil or digoxin.
- Rhythm control with electrical or chemical cardioversion may be considered after an echocardiogram and appropriate anticoagulation (>3 weeks with INR >2.0).
- Anti-thrombotic therapy with warfarin or aspirin may be considered after stroke risk categorisation in accordance with the NICE guidelines. The annual risk of stroke in chronic AF is 3%–7%.
- Patients with recurrent atrial flutter may be considered for tricuspid isthmus ablation.

When would you anaesthetise her?

Consult with the surgeon regarding the urgency of the surgery. Ideally the procedure should be delayed until the management of her atrial flutter and asthma have been optimised.

Bibliography

Bajpai A, Rowland E. (2006). Atrial fibrillation. *CEPD British Journal of Anaesthesia*, **6**(6), 219–24.
Bovill JG, Howie MB. (1999). *Clinical Pharmacology for Anaesthetists*. London: Harcourt Publishers.
Kumar P, Clark M. (1994). *Clinical Medicine*. London: Baillière Tindall.
NICE. (2006). Atrial fibrillation. The management of atrial fibrillation. *NICE Guidelines*. June.
Sasada M, Smith S. (1997). *Drugs in Anaesthesia and Intensive Care* 1997. Oxford, UK: Oxford Medical Publications.

Awareness

You are called to see a patient on the surgical ward by the Sister because a patient describes being aware during surgery (you did not anaesthetise the patient).

How do you deal with the situation?

- **Inform the anaesthetist involved** and the head of the department – there may be a departmental policy or someone with a special interest in awareness.
- Interview the patient with a senior colleague – (Ideally the anaesthetist involved should do this.) Always have a witness present.

- Establish the events surrounding the time of alleged awareness by reviewing the anaesthetic charts, discussing with the anaesthetist involved and the patient.
- Establish whether it is true recall or dreaming. Recall may be further divided into explicit (patient can recall conversations which took place in theatre) or implicit (behavioural changes post-operatively due to intra-operative subconscious learning).
- Establish whether the patient was in pain – this has implications for long-term psychological sequelae such as nightmares and flashbacks.
- If there was a clear lapse in the standard of anaesthetic care, then honesty with an admission of fault and an apology is appropriate.
- Document all conversations and assessments in the case notes.
- Hospital management including the legal department may need to be informed in order that the events can be documented for future reference in case of legal action.
- Offer counselling for the patient.

What do you tell the patient?

It is important to acknowledge the patient's feelings and let them know you believe what they are saying. This helps with the well-recognised psychological sequelae following an episode of awareness. These include anxiety, insomnia, nightmares, depression, a morbid fear of hospitals and doctors and a preoccupation with death. It is helpful to explain why awareness might have occurred through no particular fault but instead because of the need to minimise the doses of anaesthetic agents given. If there is clear fault on the part of the anaesthetist, then it may still be wise to admit it. Although this is an admission of negligence, some say it may help to reduce anxiety for future anaesthetics if there was a definite reason for the awareness.

In summary, a full explanation of the events and an apology are recommended.

What is the legal situation regarding awareness?

An anaesthetist has a duty of care towards a patient. A patient who is going to have a general anaesthetic expects to be asleep and unaware. To decide whether there is a breach in the duty of care, the Bolam test is applied.

In the 1950s Bolam's leg was broken during a course of ECT. Bolam's expert witnesses claimed that the omission of a muscle relaxant was negligent. The experts called by the hospital were of the opinion that muscle relaxants were not essential. The judge ruled that:

> 'A doctor is not guilty of negligence if acting in accordance with a practice accepted as proper by a responsible body of medical opinion even though a body of adverse opinion also exists amongst medical men'.

An anaesthetist must therefore prove that the technique he used is one that is considered to be reasonable by his peers. This is done through review of the anaesthetic records by expert witnesses. If there is evidence of a shortfall in the standard of anaesthetic care, then the anaesthetist is guilty of negligence.

If the awareness can be clearly linked to the poor anaesthetic technique ('causation'), then compensation is payable.

When is awareness most likely?

- At induction and intubation.
- On transfer from the anaesthetic room to theatre.
- During procedures involving the use of muscle relaxants.
- TIVA.
- During procedures where low concentrations of volatile are used deliberately, e.g. LSCS or hypotensive patient.
- At emergence.

Awareness with explicit recall has a reported incidence of approximately 1/500 and is most common during obstetric GA (especially at intubation). Awareness with pain is far less common.

What are the causes of awareness?

- **Induction**   Low doses of drugs as above
                   Intubation too early or delayed due to difficulty or waiting for relaxant to work
- **Transfer**   Induction agent levels fall before adequate partial pressure of volatile builds up
- **During surgery** Equipment failure, e.g. breathing system leak/disconnection, vaporiser, malfunction or exhaustion, TIVA line tissued

How do you monitor depth of anaesthesia?

- **Simple clinical signs**   BP, HR, sweating, lacrimation, pupils
- **MAC**   Based on population studies
- **Isolated forearm technique**
- **Spontaneous skeletal muscle activity** Frontalis, lost with relaxants
- **Oesophageal contractility**   Depth of anaesthesia related to frequency of contractions
- **Evoked potentials**   Visual, auditory, somatosensory (changes in latency and amplitude)
- **EEG**
- **Spectral edge frequency**   Frequency when significant EEG activity is seen
- **Cerebral function monitor**   Processed EEG makes interpretation easier

- **Bispectral index**
- **Heart rate variability**   'Fathom' monitor – loss of respiratory sinus arrhythmia

---

Guedel Classification of the Stages of Anaesthesia:
(Described in 1937, spontaneous respiration with ether)

- **Stage 1   Analgesia**   Start of induction to LOC
  Regular, small volume respiration
  Normal pupils
- **Stage 2   Excitement**   LOC to onset of automatic breathing
  Irregular respiration
  Dilated, divergent pupils
  Active airway reflexes
  Loss of eyelash reflex
- **Stage 3   Surgical anaesthesia**
  Plane 1:   Regular, large volume respiration
  Eye movements stop, pinpoint pupils
  Loss of eyelid reflex
  Plane 2:   Intercostal respiration reduced
  Loss of corneal reflex
  Plane 3:   Diaphragmatic respiration
  Laryngeal reflexes reduced
  Normal pupils
  Plane 4:   Diaphragmatic respiration reduced
  Carinal reflex depressed
  Dilated pupils
- **Stage 4   Coma**   Apnoea, hypotension

Reprinted with the permission of Scribner, a Division of Simon & Schuster, Inc., from *Inhalation Anesthesia*, 2nd edition by Dr Arthur E. Guedel. Copyright © 1937, 1951 by The Macmillan Company. Copyright renewed © 1965, 1979 by Marian Guedel Hart. All rights reserved.

Bibliography

Aitkinhead AR. (1990). Awareness during anaesthesia: what should the patient be told? *Anaesthesia*, **45**, 351–2.

Aitkinhead AR. (1994). The pattern of litigation against anaesthetists. *British Journal of Anaesthesia*, **73**, 10–21.

Guedel AE. (1937). *Inhalation Anesthesia, 2nd edition*. New York: Macmillan Publishing Ltd.

Myles PS, Leslie K, McNeil J, Forbes A, Chan MT. (2004). Bispectral index monitoring to prevent awareness during anaesthesia: the B-Aware randomised controlled trial. *Lancet*, **363**(9423), 1757–63.

Pollard RJ, Coyle JP, Gilbert RL, Beck JE. (2007). Intraoperative awareness in a regional medical system: a review of 3 years' data. *Anesthesiology*, **106**(2), 269–74.

Pomfrett CJD. (1996). Awareness. *Handbook of Clinical Anaesthesia*, 614–15. Churchill Livingstone.

Pomfrett CJD. (2000). Monitoring depth of anaesthesia. *Bulletin 4*, The Royal College of Anaesthetists.

Bariatric surgery and drugs for obesity

A 45-year-old woman presents at your pre-operative assessment clinic. She has been listed for bariatric surgery. Her weight is 150 kg and her height 168 cm.

Classify obesity

The commonest way to classify obesity is using the Body Mass Index (BMI). This is the weight in kg divided by the square of the patient's height in metres. This was recommended by the US National Institutes of Health in 1998 and has been widely adopted by many medical organisations.

Classification	BMI (kg/m^2)
Healthy weight	18.5–24.9
Overweight	25–29.9
Obesity I	30–34.9
Obesity II	35–39.9
Obesity III	40 or more

How does waist circumference factor into the classification of obesity?

Body fat distribution provides additional risk that is not given simply by the BMI. Two practical methods to localise body fat distribution that have a great degree of epidemiological correlates are:

■ The waist circumference is a convenient and simple measurement that correlates well with BMI and with risk factors for cardiovascular disease. It is measured in centimetres at the midpoint between the lower border of the rib cage and the upper border of the pelvis. A waist circumference of >102 cm (~40 inches) in men and >88 cm (~35 inches) in women is consistent with abdominal obesity and puts patients at increased risk for metabolic complications.
■ The waist to hip ratio (WHR). A WHR of >1.0 in men and >0.85 in women correlates with abdominal fat accumulation.

BMI classification	Waist circumference		
	Low	High	Very high
Overweight	No increased risk	Increased risk	High risk
Obesity I	Increased risk	High risk	Very high risk

For men, a waist circumference of less than 94 cm is low, 94–102 cm is high and more than 102 cm is very high.

For women, a waist circumference of less than 80 cm is low, 80–88 cm is high and more than 88 cm is very high.

What drug management is available for treating obesity?

These can be classified into those drugs that act locally in the gastrointestinal tract, such as Orlistat, and those that act centrally.

Orlistat

Orlistat should be prescribed only as part of an overall plan for managing obesity in adults who meet one of the following criteria:

- BMI of 28.0 kg/m^2 or more with associated risk factors.
- BMI of 30.0 kg/m^2 or more.
- Orlistat is the saturated derivative of lipstatin which is a potent natural inhibitor of pancreatic lipase. Orlistat is derived from *Streptomyces toxytricini*. It reduces weight by around 9% on average and decreases progression to diabetes in high-risk patients. Adverse gastrointestinal effects are common and there may be a link to aggravation of existing hypertension.

Sibutramine

Sibutramine, a monoamine-reuptake inhibitor, inhibits the reuptake of norepinephrine, serotonin and dopamine, causing anorexia. It should be prescribed only as part of an overall plan for managing obesity in adults who meet one of the following criteria:

- BMI of 27.0 kg/m^2 or more and other obesity-related risk factors such as type 2 diabetes or dyslipidaemia.
- BMI of 30.0 kg/m^2 or more. Side effects include: dry mouth, insomnia, anorexia and a stimulatory effect on heart rate and blood pressure.

Rimonabant

- Selective cannabinoid type1 (CB1) endocannabinoid receptor antagonist. Blocking endogenous cannabinoid binding to neuronal CB1 receptors, may aid appetite control and weight reduction.
- Licensed for use as an adjunct to diet and exercise for the treatment of:
  - Obese patients (BMI $\geq$ 30 kg/m^2)
  - Overweight patients (BMI > 27 kg/m^2) with associated risk factor(s) such as type 2 diabetes or dyslipidaemia.
  - NB: The European Medicines Agency has since recommended the suspension of marketing of rimonabant due to its psychological side effects.

What are the indications for bariatric surgery?

Bariatric surgery is recommended as a treatment option for adults with obesity if all of the following criteria are fulfilled (as per NICE Guidelines):

- BMI $\geq$ 40 kg/m^2 or
- Between 35 kg/m^2 and 40 kg/m^2 with other significant disease (for example, type II diabetes or high blood pressure) that could be improved if they lost weight.

- All appropriate non-surgical measures have been tried but have failed to achieve or maintain adequate, clinically beneficial weight loss for at least 6 months.
- The patient has been receiving or will receive intensive management in a specialist obesity service.
- The patient is generally fit for anaesthesia and surgery.
- The patient commits to the need for long-term follow-up.
- First-line option (instead of lifestyle interventions or drug treatment) for adults with a BMI of more than 50 kg/m^2 for whom surgical intervention is considered appropriate.

Surgical approaches	
Malabsorptive	Jejuno-ileal bypass
	Biliopancreatic bypass
Restrictive	Vertical banded gastroplasty
	Gastric banding
	Roux-en-Y gastric bypass

What are the anaesthetic considerations in bariatric surgery?

(See other question on obesity.)

Pre-operative evaluation – with particular focus on issues pertinent to the obese patient. These include:

- Airway evaluation and preparation for a potentially difficult intubation.
- Cardiovascular status: Systemic hypertension
Pulmonary hypertension
Cardiac failure
Ischaemic heart disease
- Investigations: ECG, CXR, echocardiography (tricuspid regurgitation may indicate pulmonary hypertension). Baseline ABG (will guide post-operative respiratory management in terms of assessing carbon dioxide retention and parameters for weaning).
- Antibiotic prophylaxis – laparoscopic bariatric surgery has an infection rate of 3%–11%).
- DVT prophylaxis – morbid obesity is an independent risk factor for sudden post-operative death due to PE.
- Prophylaxis against aspiration pneumonitis

What are the important intra-operative factors?

Positioning

- Specialised table to accommodate the patient
- Protection of pressure areas –ulnar neuropathy, brachial plexus and sciatic nerve palsies have been described.

Respiratory changes

■ Decrease in vital capacity and ventilation perfusion mismatch.
■ Potential complications include mediastinal emphysema, pneumothorax and gas embolism.

Cardiovascular changes

■ An increase in systemic vascular resistance as a result of an increase in intra-abdominal pressure (IAP).
■ Compression of the inferior vena cava by increased IAP will decrease venous return.
■ Renal blood flow and GFR are decreased by an increase in IAP.
■ Invasive arterial monitoring may be required due to difficulties with correct NIBP cuff sizes.

What post-operative analgesia would you recommend?

■ Multimodal analgesia
■ Local anaesthetic should be infiltrated into the port sites at the end of surgery.
■ Regular simple analgesics, e.g. paracetamol, codeine or dihydrocodeine, tramadol.
■ PCA morphine if required.
■ Post-operative opioids via PCA have not been found to cause morbidity in terms of cardiorespiratory compromise in these patients and provide adequate analgesia.
■ Caution is advised with regards to the use of NSAIDs because of the concern about gastric ulcers following bariatric surgery

---

Key recommendations from AAGBI 'Glossy'

■ All trained anaesthetists should be competent in the management of morbidly obese patients and familiar with equipment and local protocols.
■ All patients should have height, weight and BMI recorded.
■ Every hospital – named consultant anaesthetist and a named theatre team member to ensure appropriate equipment and processes.
■ Protocols including details of availability of equipment should be readily to hand in all locations where morbidly obese patients may be treated.
■ Mandatory manual handling courses should include the management of the morbidly obese.
■ Pre-op assessment is a key component of management.
■ Early communication between staff is essential and scheduling of surgery should include provision for sufficient additional time, resources and personnel.
■ Absolute BMI should not be used as the sole indicator of suitability for surgery.

Bibliography

NICE Clinical Guideline 43 www.nice.org.uk. (2006). Obesity: Guidance on the prevention, identification, assessment and management of overweight and obesity in adults and children.

Ogunnaike, BO, Jones SB, Jones DB, Provost D, Whitten CW. (2002). Anesthetic considerations for bariatric surgery. *Anesthesia and Analgesia*, **95**, 1793–805.

Peri-Operative Management of the Morbidly Obese Patient, Association of Anaesthetists of Great Britain and Ireland June 2007.

Bends

You are an anaesthetist in a seaside town and are asked to assess a 22-year-old man who has been scuba diving and brought into the accident department unconscious.

How would you manage this patient initially?

The initial management would be generalised as the diagnosis is not known at this stage. Any history of preceding events may direct further therapy at the most likely diagnosis:

- Airway   Attention should be given to the possibility of a head or neck injury and the C-spine immobilised.
- Breathing   Highest FiO$_2$ available.
- Circulation   Large bore cannulae and fluids.

Can you list some differential diagnoses?

- Decompression sickness
- Near-drowning
- Head injury
- Convulsion – oxygen-induced
- Hypoxia
- Hypothermia
- Coincidental pathology, e.g. intracranial haemorrhage, cerebral infarction, epilepsy, cardiac event, intoxication, overdose

What is decompression sickness?

Decompression 'illness' may be described in terms of two syndromes:

1. Decompression sickness
2. Pulmonary barotrauma and arterial gas embolism

Decompression sickness

During a dive, the increased ambient pressure causes nitrogen to dissolve into tissues. On ascent, the decrease in pressure causes the nitrogen that has been dissolved in the body tissues to come out of solution. If ascent is too rapid, then the partial pressure of nitrogen in the tissues will rise above tissue hydrostatic pressure and gas bubbles form. Symptoms range from pains in the tissues around joints (the classical '**Bends**') to neurological impairment such as visual disturbances, convulsions, paraparesis and loss of consciousness. Nitrogen bubbles may also migrate from tissues into the venous system to cause **venous gas embolism**. This is usually asymptomatic. However, high levels of venous gas embolism in the pulmonary circulation can cause pulmonary hypertension, pulmonary oedema, retrosternal discomfort, cough and dyspnoea ('**the chokes**').

Pulmonary barotrauma and arterial gas embolism

Pulmonary barotrauma results from a diver holding his breath during ascent. This may cause pneumothorax, pneumomediastinum or arterial gas embolism. Arterial bubbles occlude vessels after which platelets and fibrin may be deposited at the bubble–blood interface. There may also be bubble–endothelium interactions culminating in a delayed reduction in blood flow and capillary leak.

Note that pulmonary barotrauma and arterial gas embolism may occur after a breath-hold dive of only 1 metre, whereas decompression sickness requires a significant depth-time exposure.

How is it treated?

■ **ABC: Fluids**   Immersion diuresis and bubble-induced endothelial damage may result in severe dehydration.
Aggressive fluid administration may also improve the rate of nitrogen washout. Use isotonic fluids without glucose.

■ **Oxygen**   Improves delivery to underperfused tissues but also reduces the partial pressure of nitrogen in the blood and hence in the tissues surrounding the bubble. The increase in tissue–bubble partial pressure gradient facilitates diffusion of nitrogen from the bubble back into the tissues, thus shrinking it and reducing symptoms

■ **Recompression**
The idea is to force gas back into solution initially and then allow excretion at a more controlled rate. A commonly used treatment table is that used by the US Navy. It consists of recompression at 25 ft/min to a depth of 60 ft (2.8 atm) followed by hyperbaric oxygen therapy at two depths – 60 ft and 30 ft. The rate of ascent is typically 1 ft/min and the length of treatment is variable depending on the depth and length of dive. The inspired pressure of oxygen should not be greater than 3 atmospheres and is given typically in cycles of 20 minutes separated by breathing air for 5–15 minutes. If airborne transfer is required, the patient is transferred with 100% oxygen at sea-level cabin pressure.

■ **Position**   Supine

Head-down position has no proven role in preventing arterial bubbles entering the cerebral circulation and may increase cerebral oedema. There is similarly no benefit in massive venous gas embolism. Therefore, the head-down position is not routinely recommended except perhaps in severe hypotension.

However, placing the injured diver in the supine position has two advantages. It may help to prevent hypotension and the rate of nitrogen washout is greater than in the sitting position.

- **Avoid hyperglycaemia**
- **Avoid hyperthermia**

Bibliography

Moon RE. (1999). Treatment of diving emergencies. *Critical Care Clinics*, **15**(2), 429–56.

Tetzlaff K, Shank E, Muth C. (2003). Evaluation and management of decompression illness – an intensivist's perspective. *Intensive Care Medicine*, **29**(12), 2128–36.

Bleeding tonsil

You are called to see a 4-year-old boy on the paediatric ward. He had a tonsillectomy 4 hours ago and has been vomiting blood for the last hour. His heart rate is 150 and his blood pressure is 95/60.

What are the problems in managing this case?

Problems with primary post-tonsillectomy haemorrhage (<24 hours):

- **Frightened child** and anxious parents
- **Hypovolaemia**
- **Full stomach**
- **Residual effects of the anaesthetic** 4 hours earlier
- **Difficult intubation** – bleeding and possible upper airway oedema from the previous intubation and surgery

Review of the previous anaesthetic chart and history and examination are, of course, mandatory. The consultant anaesthetist should be informed.

It is vital to ensure he is adequately resuscitated before embarking on another anaesthetic. Intravenous access (or interosseous if needed) should be established and resuscitation commenced with crystalloid/colloid 20 ml/kg (APLS recommends crystalloid).

How would you estimate blood loss?

The most helpful indicators of hypovolaemia are:

- **Heart rate**
- **Pulse volume**

- **Capillary refill time** (pressure for 5 seconds then release, normal refill <2 seconds)
- **Skin colour** (mottling/pallor/peripheral cyanosis)
- **Blood pressure** (80 + (2 × age in years), hypotension is a late sign
- **Conscious level**

The **degree of blood loss is often under-estimated**. Looking at the amount of blood vomited will be inaccurate because much of it is likely to have been swallowed. Haemoglobin and haematocrit estimations may help. Postural hypotension suggests significant hypovolaemia but measuring this would not be practical in a frightened child. Core:peripheral temperature difference >2 °C is a sign of poor perfusion to skin. Respiratory rate may be high as a compensatory response to hypovolaemic metabolic acidosis.

He should have blood cross-matched and available in theatre. FBC and clotting should be checked pre-operatively.

What anaesthetic technique would you employ?

There are two schools of thought as to the method of induction:

- **Rapid sequence induction** with cricoid pressure
- **Gas induction** in the head-down, left lateral position

A **rapid sequence induction with cricoid pressure** in the supine position is likely to be the most familiar technique. Although it is recognised that cricoid pressure does not protect the airway from bleeding in the pharynx, it is the technique most likely to secure the airway quickly. (A gas induction in the head-down, left lateral position may be fraught with potential problems.) There should be **two suction devices** in case one becomes blocked with clot and a variety of tube sizes and laryngoscope blades. The **ENT surgeon needs to be scrubbed** and prepared to perform a tracheostomy should the need arise.

Following intubation, a **nasogastric tube** may be inserted to empty the stomach. This is then removed prior to extubation. Once haemostasis is achieved, the child is extubated awake and in the head-down, left-lateral position.

Bibliography

Deakin CD. (1998). *Clinical Notes for the FRCA*. Churchill Livingstone.
Mather SJ, Hughes DG. (1996). *A Handbook of Paediatric Anaesthesia*, 2nd edition. Oxford, UK: Oxford University Press.
Ravi R, Howell T. (2007). Anaesthesia for paediatric ear, nose, and throat surgery. *Continuing Education in Anaesthesia, Critical Care and Pain*, **7**(2), 33–7.

Bronchopleural fistula

Can you tell me what a bronchopleural fistula (BPF) is?

This is a communication between the pleural cavity and the trachea or a bronchus. Clinically, this is seen as a persistent air leak for greater than 24 hours after the development of a pneumothorax.

Why does it occur?

- **After lung resection.** Most commonly associated with dehiscence of a bronchial stump (usually 3–10 days post-op).
- **Tumour invasion** of a bronchus.
- **Blunt or penetrating trauma** with disruption of a major bronchus.
- **Spontaneous pneumothorax** may result in a BPF, seen as persistent bubbling through an underwater seal chest drain.
- **Necrotising infection** such as pneumonia, lung abscess, empyema or TB can cause BPF.
- **ARDS** or acute lung injury may be complicated by BPF

How does it usually present?

The presentation depends on the **size of the air leak** and the **underlying pathology**.

- **Persistent bubbling** from the chest drain.
- **Cough** which may be productive of **foul sputum**.
- **Dyspnoea** the degree of which will depend on the lung compromise and whether the pleural cavity has been drained with a chest drain.
- **Systemic features of sepsis** if the cause is infective.
- An acute BPF with a large leak causes severe dyspnoea and may cause a **tension pneumothorax if it is not drained** (especially if CPAP has been used to try and help with the dyspnoea).

> **Problems with a large bronchopleural fistula on ICU**
>
> - Difficult to wean from a ventilator.
> - Hypoxia and hypercapnia result from inability to maintain alveolar ventilation.
> - Inability to apply PEEP.
> - Failure of lung re-expansion.
> - May need dual ventilation (two ventilators).
> - May need high frequency ventilation.
> - High mortality.

What features would you particularly look for in the pre-operative assessment if a patient with a fistula needs to come to theatre?

Often, the patient will have undergone lung surgery in the previous few days and a review of the anaesthetic chart is essential.

- **Airway** – Information such as **laryngoscopy grade** and the size and ease of placement of the **double lumen tube** are invaluable.

- **Breathing** – An **arterial blood gas** would help assess respiratory compromise. A **chest X-ray** may show loss of pneumonectomy space fluid and often collapse or consolidation in the remaining lung.
- **Circulation** – Resuscitation is often required. The patient may be **septic.**
- Most of the patients needing surgery have had failed medical treatment with a chest drain and antibiotics.
- The patency of any chest drain should be established. A new drain may need to be inserted.
- Sometimes, the BPF will be amenable to treatment (glue) via bronchoscopy, which may avoid the need for anaesthetic. This should be discussed with the surgical team.

What are the principles in providing anaesthesia?

- Involve an **experienced thoracic anaesthetist** – these are difficult cases.
- **Protect the good lung** from becoming soiled by infected material 'spilling over' from the affected side. Sit the patient upright as much as can be tolerated.
- **Avoid ventilation until the good lung is isolated.**
- A **double lumen tube** will be required to ventilate both lungs independently and to protect the BPF from positive pressure, which will worsen the leak.
- The double lumen tube (DLT) should be inserted into the 'good' side, i.e. avoiding any surgical sutures.
- TIVA would avoid the potentially unreliable delivery of volatile agents on one lung anaesthesia with a large leak.
- Close co-operation with the thoracic surgeon is essential. If the airway is difficult, they may be able to ventilate the patient with the rigid bronchoscope down the good side. It is likely the patient will have had a previous rigid bronchoscopy.
- The patient should be extubated as soon as possible, as 'negative pressure' ventilation is preferable. A thoracic epidural along with short acting anaesthetic agents will help achieve a prompt wake-up with good analgesia.

How would you anaesthetise this patient?

- Establish appropriate **monitoring** (including an **arterial line**), **i.v. access** and site a **thoracic epidural** if thoracotomy is planned.
- **Pre-oxygenation** with the patient as **upright** as possible.
- If an easy intubation is anticipated, then following **i.v. induction** with alfentanil and propofol and muscle relaxation with **suxamethonium**, a double lumen tube **(DLT)** should be inserted into the 'good' lung. If time permits, the position should be verified immediately using a **fibre-optic bronchoscope**. Once the endobronchial cuff is inflated and the lungs isolated, IPPV can be commenced via the endobronchial lumen.
- TIVA as maintenance with intermittent boluses of non-depolarizing muscle relaxant.

■ In the presence of a difficult airway, other options would include endobronchial intubation with a normal ETT into the good lung with a fibre-optic scope or using a rigid bronchoscope to either jet ventilate the good side, endobronchially intubate the good side or place an endobronchial blocker into the affected side.

■ Anaesthesia for a BPF is classically described in textbooks with either awake endobroncial intubation with topical analgesia of the airway, or inhalational induction and intubation under deep volatile anaesthesia. Both of these methods are difficult (especially in a compromised patient) and when dealing with bulky DLTs.

How would you insert a DLT into a patient with a difficult airway?

■ You are doing very well if you get on to this question!

■ One technique that has been described firstly involves awake fibre-optic intubation with a single lumen tube through the topically anaesthetised nose and upper airway.

■ Once general anaesthesia is induced, the DLT is mounted on the fibre-optic scope which is then repassed via the mouth. Once the fibre-optic scope is in the trachea alongside the nasal ETT, then the nasal tube's cuff can be deflated and the tube withdrawn slightly to allow the DLT to be railroaded into the trachea. The final position can be checked with the fibre-optic scope.

Bibliography

Gothard J, Kelleher A, Haxby E. (2003). *Cardiovascular and Thoracic Anaesthesia*. Butterworth-Heinemann.

Satya-Krishna R, Popat M. (2006). Insertion of the double lumen tube in the difficult airway. *Anaesthesia*, **61**(9), 896–8.

Burns

A 35-year-old man is brought into the accident department having been rescued from a house fire. He has burns to his face, arms and trunk but does not seem to be in much pain.

How would you assess the severity of the burn?

This can be assessed in several ways:

■ **Surface area** of a burn may be calculated by:
  ■ **Wallace rule of 9s**
  ■ **Palmar surface.** Each of the patients palm areas correlates to ~0.8% BSA
  ■ **Lund and Browder charts**

■ **Age** and **% of body surface area burnt** are the two most important prognostic factors.

As a guide: **% mortality = BSA of burn + age**

Other factors influencing outcome (and therefore classifying the burn as more severe) are:

Associated inhalational injury (doubles mortality rate)

Co-existent medical problems

■ **Classified according to depth**

- Partial thickness Superficial Epidermal
  Painful
  Red and moist
  Blanches

  Superficial dermal Some superficial dermal damage
  Painful
  Pale
  Blanches

  Deep dermal Deep dermal damage
  Painless but some sensation
  Mottled
  None blanching
  Delayed bleeding on prick

- Full thickness Dermis destroyed
  Insensate
  Waxy, leathery
  None blanching
  Does not bleed
  Will need grafting

■ A burn can be assessed as a **major burn** if:

Full thickness burn >10% TBSA (total body surface area)

Partial thickness burn >25% TBSA (or 20% at extremes of age)

Burns to hands, feet or perineum

Inhalational, chemical or electrical burns

Burns in patients with serious pre-existing medical conditions

Severe burn is >40% TBSA

How would you initially treat this patient?

Resuscitate the patient according to the ATLS guidelines:

Airway   Administer **100% oxygen** via a reservoir mask; this would also help to treat any CO poisoning. The **upper airway** is particularly susceptible to **oedema** and subsequent **obstruction**. A high index of suspicion should be maintained with regard to inhalational injury and **early intubation** with an **uncut tube** is frequently needed. **Suxamethonium** can be used in the first 24 hours. It should then be avoided for 2 years because the increased number of post-junctional receptors causes prolonged depolarisation and marked release of potassium.

Breathing   Blood gases should be taken immediately while remembering that the arterial PO_2 is unreliable for predicting CO poisoning. Early **bronchoscopy** if there is a risk of inhalational injury. If there is evidence of this injury, then perform **broncho-alveolar lavage** with 20 ml aliquots of **1.4% bicarbonate** until the aspirate is clear. This should be followed by 10 ml instilled via the ET tube and 10 ml nebulised every hour until clear for 6 hours.

Circulation 2 large bore i.v. cannulae should be sited. These may be difficult to place and may need to be placed through a burn.

Evaluation of **volume status** and use of a blood pressure cuff may be difficult in a burned patient. A **urinary catheter** and possibly an **arterial line** will be needed. One should aim for a urine output of at least 50 ml/hour in this patient.

Early referral to a regional burns centre would be appropriate.

How would you guide your fluid management?

There are several **formulae** that can help guide fluid management. Amongst them are:

Parkland	CSL 4 ml/kg per %TBSA in 24 hours (first half given in 8 hours)
Muir and Barclay (Mount Vernon)	0.5 ml PPF/albumin/kg per %TBSA every 4 hours for 12 hours, then 6-hourly for 12 hours
Brook	0.5 ml colloid/kg + 1.5 ml crystalloid/%TBSA Half over first 8 hours

The time of injury is the starting point for these calculations. It should be emphasized that these are only a **guide** and that assessment of resuscitation should be based clinically on **heart rate, BP, capillary refill, CVP, urine output**, peripheral and core **temperature** and the **mental state** of the patient. However, a PAFC is used in many centres as there is evidence of poor correlation between simple clinical parameters (heart rate and urine output) and the haemodynamics in severe burns.

What would make you suspicious of an inhalation injury?

- Points in the history: Explosion
  Fire in an enclosed space
  Inhalation of toxic fumes
  Alcohol intoxication
- On examination: Burnt face
  Raised carboxyhaemoglobin levels
  Stridor
  Soot in the sputum
  Burnt eyebrows or nasal hair.
  Respiratory distress

Is pain management a problem with burns patients?

Yes. Apart from the initial injury, they are subjected to multiple dressing changes and various operations. They develop **tolerance to opioids** very rapidly and therefore may require large doses of opioids and the use of **ketamine, entonox, paracetamol** and also **anti-depressants**.

Other problems you could be asked about:	
Early feeding	High catabolic state. Establishing N/G feeding in the first 4 hours improves outcome
Heat loss	Impaired homeostatic control and heat loss through burns
Sepsis	Impaired immune function
ARDS	Effects of burn wound mediators/↓plasma oncotic pressure/↑PAP → Multiple organ failure
Resistance to NMBs	May last 18 months (↑Ach receptors)
Arrhythmias and rhabdomyolysis	Occur with electrical burns
Burn wound excision	Limit to 20% per operation (warm theatre 28–32 °C/ big drips/warm fluids/potential for large blood loss)
Haematological	↑Hct for 48 hours – unreliable measure of resuscitation.
Effects	↓rbc $t_{1/2}$. ↓ Platelets due to microaggregation. Degree of consumption coagulopathy. DIC possible. Later thrombogenicity (↓Protein C, S and anti-Th III) → PE

Bibliography

Black R, Kinsella J. (2001). Anaesthetic management for burns patients. *British Journal of Anaesthesia*, Continuing Education and Professional Development, **1**(6), 177–80.

Haji-Michael P. *Intensive Care Unit Guidelines for the Care of the Patient with Burns* (Version III, 8/99). Withington Hospital ICU, Manchester.

MacLennan N, Heimbach DM, Cullen MD. (1998). Anaesthesia for major thermal injury. *Anesthesiology*, **89**, 749–70.

Morgan GE, Mikhail MS. (1996). *Clinical Anaesthesiology*, 2nd edition. Appleton and Lange.

Hettiaratchy S, Papini R. (2004). Initial management of a major burn: II – assessment and resuscitation. *British Medical Journal*, **329**, 101–3.

Carbon monoxide poisoning

You are asked to see a male patient who has been found in his garage with the engine of his car running. His face is cherry red.

What is the likely diagnosis?

The patient is likely to be suffering from **carbon monoxide poisoning**. It must not be forgotten that there could be co-existent problems such as self-poisoning with tablets.

What is carbon monoxide poisoning?

The usual definition is a **level of greater than 20% carboxyhaemoglobin** in the blood. Co-oximetry is needed to make the diagnosis.
Symptoms are:

20–30%	Throbbing headache
	Irritability
	Fatiguability
	Poor judgement
	Nausea and vomiting
30–40%	Confusion
	Syncope on exertion
>50%	Coma
	Convulsions
	Death

How does carbon monoxide poisoning affect O_2 delivery at tissue level?

CO and O_2 both bind to the α-chain of the haemoglobin molecule, but CO has about 250 times the affinity for the ferrous iron complex compared with O_2. This is a competitive and reversible effect.

Tissue oxygen delivery is affected in two ways:

1. There is a reduction in the availability of oxygen-binding sites and therefore a **reduction in oxygen carrying capacity.**
2. CO interacts with the remaining haemoglobin molecule to increase the affinity for the oxygen it carries. This results in a **left shift of the oxyhaemoglobin dissociation curve** such that haemoglobin is less keen to give up oxygen at tissue level. Thus, oxygen delivery is further reduced.

How would you manage carbon monoxide poisoning?

Resuscitation should always follow the ABC approach. The primary objective is to reverse tissue hypoxia. Removal of CO is of secondary importance. Oxygen is the treatment that accomplishes both of these goals. The patient should be given 100% oxygen. In severe cases hyperbaric oxygen therapy has been used (but is still controversial). Hyperbaric oxygen therapy (HBO) can provide nearly all the body's oxygen needs purely from the dissolved oxygen.

Poor prognostic indicators are:

- Increased duration of exposure
- Increasing age
- Low GCS at time of admission.

Current criteria for HBO therapy are:

- Carboxyhaemoglobin >20%
- Loss of consciousness at any stage
- Cognitive impairment
- Neurological signs and symptoms (except headache)
- Myocardial ischaemia/arrhythmia
- Pregnancy
- Difficulty assessing (e.g. concurrent drug over dose).

Co-existent problems such as other forms of self-poisoning or burns should also be addressed. The decision to transfer a patient to a hyperbaric chamber (usually in a different hospital) must take into account the carboxyhaemoblobin level, the time needed to transfer the patient and the patient's fitness for transfer.

What is the half-life of COHb in air, 100% O_2 and hyperbaric O_2?

Air (21% O_2)	240–300	minutes
100% O_2 (1 atm)	40–80	minutes
100% O_2 (3 atm)	23–25	minutes

As can be seen from these figures, simply administering 100% oxygen will significantly expedite the removal of carbon monoxide.

Bibliography

Brenner BE. (1995). *Comprehensive Management of Respiratory Emergencies*. Maryland, USA: Aspen Systems Corp.

Hawkins M, Harrison J, Charters P. (2000). Severe carbon monoxide poisoning: outcome after hyperbaric oxygen therapy. *British Journal of Anaesthesia*, **84**(5), 584–6.

Pitkin A. (2001). Hyperbaric oxygen therapy. *British Journal of Anaesthesia*, Continuing Education in Anaesthesia, Critical Care and Pain, **1**, 150–6.

Cauda equina syndrome

A 50-year-old woman presents 4 weeks after receiving an epidural steroid injection for chronic back pain. She is now experiencing severe back pain and perineal numbness.

What is the differential diagnosis?

- **Cauda equina syndrome**
- Chronic mechanical lower back pain

- Lumbar disc pathology
- Spinal cord compression from infection, neoplasm or haematoma
- Guillain–Barré syndrome
- Peripheral nerve disorder
- Conus medullaris syndrome
- Lumbosacral plexopathy

What are the causes of cauda equina syndrome?

- Vertebral disc herniation
  - Central disc prolapse – incidence of 1%–15%
- Neoplasm
  - Metastatic prostate cancer, ependymomas, schwannomas
- Inflammatory
  - Infective   e.g. spinal abscess
  - Non-infective   Diseases which predispose to developing vertebral fractures or spinal stenosis, e.g. Paget's disease
- Lumbar spinal stenosis
- Trauma
  - Violent Injuries to the lower back (gunshots, falls and road traffic accidents)
- Congenital
- Vascular
  - Spinal haemorrhages (subarachnoid, subdural, epidural)
  - Spinal arteriovenous malformations (AVMs)
- Iatrogenic
- Post-operative lumbar spine surgery complications
- Spinal and epidural anaesthesia resulting in an abscess or haematoma
- Epidural steroid injection

What further history would you seek from her?

- A history of severe low back pain
- Weakness of her legs
- Pain in one or, more commonly, both legs
- Saddle anaesthesia – Does wet toilet paper feel wet?
- A recent onset of bladder dysfunction, which may manifest as an inability to initiate or stop a stream of urine or as overflow incontinence
- Recent onset of faecal incontinence
- Sensory abnormalities in the bladder or rectum
- Recent onset of sexual dysfunction
- Severe recent trauma to her back
- Recent lumbar spine surgery
- A history of cancer
- Recent severe infection
- Spinal or epidural analgesia

What are the signs of the cauda equina syndrome?

- Saddle anaesthesia.
- Residual urine on bladder catheterization indicative of a neurogenic bladder.
- Lower motor neuron weakness is found in the plantar flexors and evertors.
- Lower limb reflexes are absent or impaired.
- Loss of anal tone.

What are the markers of infection?

- ESR and CRP

What further investigations would you carry out?

- Haematology   FBC, INR, APTT
- Biochemistry   Urea, electrolytes and LFT's
- Radiology
  - Plain X-ray may reveal vertebral fractures, tumour or infection
  - CT scan
  - An urgent MRI scan is probably the gold standard investigation to confirm and localise the lesion.

Anatomy relating to the cauda equina

The anatomy of the distal spinal cord and the cauda equina is responsible for the inconsistency in presenting signs and symptoms.

The conus medullaris is narrower than the more cephalad spinal cord and overlies the body of L1. It represents the termination of the spinal cord in the proximal lumbar spine. The conus medullaris continues to taper to form the filum terminale. The bridle of lumbar and sacral nerves descends below the conus medullaris to form the cauda equina or horse's tail.

The lumbar and sacral nerve roots contain:

- Sensory and motor function for the lower limbs
- Sensation to the perineum and genitals
- Voluntary and involuntary functions: micturition, defaecation and sexual function.

Compression of the cauda equina may involve all of the above functions, sensory only, motor only, or only those roots responsible for bowel and bladder function.

Bibliography

Bell DA, Collie D, Statham PF. (2007). Cauda equina syndrome: what is the correlation between clinical assessment and MRI scanning? *British Journal of Neurosurgery*, **21**, 201–3.

Gleave JR, Macfarlane R. (2002). Cauda equina syndrome: what is the relationship between timing of surgery and outcome? *British Journal of Neurosurgery*, **16**(4), 325–8.

Gosling J, Willian PLT, Whitmore I, Harris PF. (1966). *Human Anatomy Colour Atlas and Text*. London: Times Mirror International Publishers.

Lindsay KW, Bone I. (2004). *Neurology and Neurosurgery Illustrated*. Churchill Livingstone.

Cervical spine injury

What are the problems of anaesthetising a patient with a C6 transection 6 weeks after the accident?

Airway and breathing

■ **Cervical spine**	Difficult intubation — metalwork, reduced neck movement
■ **Respiratory insufficiency**	History of ICU admission
	Lower RTI's
	Impaired ability to cough
	Tracheostomy
	Atelectasis and V/Q mismatch

Circulation

■ **Cardiovascular problems**	**Autonomic hyperreflexia**
	Postural hypotension (may need pre-loading prior to induction)
	Bradycardia (especially with intubation, pre-treat with atropine)
■ **Venous access**	Cannulation can be difficult with decreased skin blood flow
■ **Anaemia**	Especially with chronic sepsis

Renal

■ **Renal impairment**	Due to recurrent UTIs (catheters and vesico-ureteric reflux)

Drugs

■ **Altered response to drugs**	**Suxamethonium** — denervation hypersensitivity Receptors spread from the end-plate to cover the whole muscle. Avoid between 3 days and 9 months. Decreased blood volume and decreased lean tissue mass result in decreased volumes of distribution for many drugs.
■ **Medication**	Anticoagulants, dantrolene, baclofen

Other

- **Positioning intra-operatively** Pressure sores, contractures and spasms
- **Decreased gastric emptying** Risk of aspiration
- **Temperature** Patients can become partially poikilothermic as normal mechanisms of thermoregulation are impaired.
- **Chronic pain problems**

Tell me about autonomic hyperreflexia.

- It is characterized by a grossly disordered autonomic response to certain stimuli below the level of the lesion.
- Occurs in about 85% of patients with a lesion higher than T7.
- Onset is from 3 weeks to 12 years post-injury.
- Results in hypertension (may be severe with diastolic >170 mmHg), sweating and headache. Reflex bradycardia and skin changes (pallor or flushing) above the level of the lesion are common.
- Neurophysiologically, there is loss of descending inhibition from higher centres and deranged alterations in connections within the distal spinal cord. This results in inappropriate sympathetic reflexes causing profound vasoconstriction.

What are the triggers of autonomic hyperreflexia?

- Pelvic visceral stimulation (especially bladder distension) is very commonly implicated.
- Bowel distension (including constipation)
- Uterine contractions
- Urinary tract infections
- Pressure sores

How is it treated?

- Removal of the cause (exclude bladder distension)
- Sit upright
- Drugs need to be of rapid onset: Sublingual nifedipine 10 mg
  GTN
  α-adrenergic blocking agents
  Hydralazine
  Clonidine
  Increasing depth of general anaesthesia
- Use of spinal anaesthesia
- Epidural anaesthesia is used to prevent autonomic hyperreflexia in parturients.

Bibliography

Hambly PR, Martin B. (1998). Anaesthesia for chronic spinal cord lesions. *Anaesthesia*, **53**(3), 273–89.

Chronic obstructive pulmonary disease

A 64-year-old man presents to A & E extremely short of breath, initially unable to give a history. He is recognised by one of the nursing staff as a man known to have chronic obstructive pulmonary disease and was ventilated on ICU during his last admission.

How can we classify this disease?

There are some traditional definitions of chronic bronchitis and emphysema that have been linked clinically with the classical 'blue bloater' and 'pink puffer', respectively. There is, of course, a spectrum of disease and most patients will have elements of both.

- **Chronic bronchitis**   Defined as daily cough with sputum production for at least 3 months a year for at least 2 consecutive years.
- **Emphysema**   A histological diagnosis defined as enlargement of the air spaces distal to the terminal bronchioles with destructive changes in the alveolar wall.
- **'Blue bloater'**   This clinically represents the bronchitic group. They are typically hypoxaemic and cyanosed with cor pulmonale (peripheral oedema, raised JVP, hepatomegaly) but with little dyspnoea.
- **'Pink puffers'**   Representing the emphysematous group. These patients have severe dyspnoea but relatively normal gas exchange.

Can you tell me a little about the pathophysiology?

There is a combination of:

- Mucosal inflammation
- Excessive secretions
- Bronchoconstriction.

There is a **reduction in lung elasticity** with a consequent fall in the maximum expiratory flow rate. With increasing alveolar destruction, the pulmonary vasculature may be damaged which, along with hypoxic pulmonary vasoconstriction, contributes to **pulmonary hypertension**. The overall effect is that of V/Q mismatch.

Lung function tests show an obstructive picture:

- Reduced FEV_1
- Reduced FVC
- Reduced FEV_1/FVC ratio
- Increased residual volume
- Increased FRC
- Increased total lung capacity
- Reduced diffusing capacity

What signs might you elicit in this man?

- Tachypnoea
- Cyanosis
- Accessory muscle use
- Intercostal recession
- Hyperinflated lungs
- Pulsus paradoxus
- Wheeze
- Prolonged expiratory time
- Cor pulmonale   Raised JVP, peripheral oedema, loud P2
- Signs of hypercapnia   Warm peripheries, bounding pulse, confusion, tremor, convulsions

What would be your initial management of this man?

- **Sit the patient up**
- **Oxygen** — **Oxygen therapy should be used to prevent hypoxia but should not worsen acidosis.**
  Oxygen should be started at ~40% and titrated up if O_2 saturation <90% and down if sats >93% or patient drowsy. ABGs should be done to assess pH and PCO_2
- **Bronchodilators** — A proportion of these patients will have an element of reversibility to their bronchoconstriction. Use a β-agonist (salbutamol or terbutaline) with an anticholinergic (ipratropium bromide).
- **Methylxanthines** — Intravenous theophylline may be considered if inadequate response to inhaled bronchodilators. Caution should be taken with patients on oral theophylline and levels should be taken in all patients.
- **Steroids** — Prednisolone 30 mg should be prescribed for 7–14 days.
- **Antibiotics** — Aminopenicillin or marcolide if increased purulent sputum.
- **NIV** — NIV should be considered in patients with pH <7.35.
- **Physiotherapy** — Should be considered in some patients.
- **Regular monitoring** — Clinical state and blood gases
- **Heart failure Rx** — If indicated, e.g. diuretics.

BTS advocate the use of antibiotics if two or more of:

- Increased breathlessness
- Increased sputum volume

Development of purulent sputum

This man deteriorates despite all this treatment. What further interventions are available to you?

■ **Doxapram** — Sometimes considered if NIV unavailable.
■ **Non-invasive ventilation** — Needs specialist equipment.
Needs co-operation from the patient.
Most valuable when used early.
Reduces requirement for IPPV and length of hospital stay.
■ **IPPV** — Ventilatory support considered in patients:
With a pH <7.26
A rising $PaCO_2$
Failing to respond to supportive treatment.

Favourable factors for IPPV:

■ Remediable cause for acute decline
■ First episode
■ Good quality of life

Less favourable factors:

■ Documented severe COPD unresponsive to therapy
■ Poor quality of life, e.g. housebound on maximal therapy
■ Severe co-morbidities

Bibliography

Girou E. Schortgen F, Delclaux C. (2000). Association of noninvasive ventilation with nosocomial infection and survival in critically ill patients. *Journal of the American Medical Association,* **284**(18), 2361–7.

Ikeda A, Nishimurak, Izumi T. (1997). Management of acute exacerbations of COPD. *Thorax,* **52** (Suppl. 5), S16–21.

(2004). *NICE Guidelines COPD.*

Chronic renal failure

You are asked to anaesthetise a 40-year-old patient with chronic renal failure on haemodialysis for repair of a recurrent left inguinal hernia.

What anaesthetic problems do these patients present?

Renal patients have multiple medical problems that impact on anaesthesia. These include anaemia, coagulation disorders, cardiovascular pathology and disorders of other body systems. They also have altered drug handling.

Anaemia
- **Normochromic, normocytic** (usually)
  Multifactorial causes: Iron deficiency due to repeated blood loss with haemodialysis and associated peptic ulcer disease.
  B_{12} and folate deficiency due to poor diet.
  Uraemia depresses erythropoietin production.
  Uraemia reduces red cell life span.
- Enquire about symptoms associated with anaemia, e.g. angina.
- Transfusion at Hb<5 g/dl, or if symptoms are present, has been recommended.
- Low haemoglobins are tolerated because of the shift of the oxygen dissociation curve to the right ($\uparrow$ 2,3DPG and uraemic acidosis).
- NB: Blood transfusion has effects on the immune system that may influence outcome after future transplantation.

Blood clotting
- Patients with end-stage renal failure have abnormalities of platelet function due to alterations in arachidonic acid metabolism and increased NO production. Defective endothelial release of von Willebrand/Factor VIII complex is thought to contribute and may be treated with cryoprecipitate or DDAVP intra-operatively.
- Bleeding time is prolonged.
- May have residual heparin from haemodialysis.
- Risks and benefits of neuroaxial blocks need to be carefully assessed.
- i.m. injections may be unwise.

Cardiovascular system
- **Hypertension** Present in 80% of patients – usually on medication. Volatiles may exacerbate hypotensive effect. Exaggerated changes in BP and heart rate with induction and laryngoscopy.
- **IHD**
- **CCF**
- Pre-operative ECG, CXR and echocardiogram are necessary.
- Carotid bruits – doppler studies may be necessary.
- Pericarditis – rare.
- Endocarditis – especially if vascular access site is infected.
- **Vascular access** – avoid forearm of non-dominant hand which should be preserved for a potential shunt.
- AV fistulas should be kept warm and protected intra-operatively.

Respiratory system
- SOB due to anaemia and acidosis.
- Pulmonary oedema.
- Pulmonary fibrosis associated with medical conditions.
- Infection.

Nervous system

- Neuropathy – autonomic (especially diabetics)/sensory/motor.
- Myopathy due to uraemia causes an exaggerated response to muscle relaxants.

Gastrointestinal system

- Delayed gastric emptying makes reflux and aspiration more likely.
- **Rapid sequence induction** may be needed (?modified).
- Peptic ulceration.
- Pre-medication should include an H_2 antagonist.

Endocrine/biochemical

- Hypocalcaemia and hypermagnesaemia (antacid consumption) potentiate relaxants.
- Blood sugar should be monitored and controlled as many renal patients have diabetes.
- Potassium rises in renal failure. Caution with suxamethonium and potassium containing intravenous fluids (e.g. Hartmann's).

Renal system

- Ideal weight should be known.
- A knowledge of daily urine volume normally passed and the dose of diuretic taken.
- **CVP** monitoring may be needed to guide fluid management.
- **Pre-operative dialysis** and knowledge of potassium level post-dialysis.
- **Intra-operative fluid**: Avoid large volumes of crystalloid.
- **Post-operative fluid**: Previous hours urine output plus insensible loss/hr.

How is drug handling altered in renal failure?

Many anaesthetic agents are potentiated in renal failure.
This may be due to:

- Decreased protein binding.
- Greater penetration of the blood–brain barrier.
- Systemic effect of uraemia.
- Elimination half-lives are prolonged.

  With respect to commonly used drugs:

- **Propofol** pharmacokinetics are unchanged.
- **Thiopentone** and **benzodiazepines** can de reduced due to reduced protein binding.
- **Morphine**, if used, must be carefully titrated as the metabolite morphine-6-glucuronide is active and accumulates.
- **Atracurium** is the muscle relaxant of choice (Hofmann degradation).
- **NSAIDs** – avoid.
- **Isoflurane** – safe.
- **Enflurane** – avoid due to potential for nephrotoxicity from fluoride ions.

> **Conduct of general anaesthesia:**
>
> **Pre-op:**   Medical assessment, dialysis, transfuse
>   Pre-med – antacid.
> **Intra-op:** Monitoring - including CMV5, consider A-line and CVP
>   Vascular access
>   Induction – RSI
>   Attention to pressor response.
>   Maintenance- IPPV, $\uparrow FiO_2$, N_2O safe.
>   Attention to fluid balance.
> **Post-op:** Consider HDU/ICU.
>   Oxygen should be mandatory.

> **Types of surgery common in renal patients:**
>
> ■ Vascular access procedures
> ■ Peritoneal dialysis access
> ■ Nephrectomy
> ■ Renal transplant
> ■ Parathyroidectomy

Bibliography

Holland DE, Old S. (1992). Anaesthesia for patients with impaired renal function. *Current Anaesthesia and Critical Care*, **3**, 140–5.
Milner Q. (2003). Pathophysiology of acute renal failure. *BJA CEACCP*, **3**, 130–3.
Morgan GE, Mikhail MS. (1996). *Clinical Anaesthesiology*, 2nd edition. Appleton and Lange.

Clearing the cervical spine in the unconscious polytrauma victim

A 24-year-old man was admitted to the accident and emergency department having been found at the side of the road. He is haemodynamically stable and appears to have sustained only facial and head injuries following a primary survey. His GCS is 3/15 and so you decide to intubate him.

Would you take any special precautions?

■ **ATLS protocol** dictates airway management with cervical spine control.
■ This is an emergency anaesthetic in a trauma victim.
■ Assume a **full stomach** so RSI is indicated.
■ Assume a **fractured C-spine** until this is proven otherwise.
■ **Difficult airway** suspected in facial trauma and so equipment and expertise should be immediately available to deal with this.

What would you do to protect his neck?

Following ATLS guidelines, he should be fully immobilised with:

- Spinal board.
- Appropriate hard collar.
- Head blocks or sandbags either side of his head.
- Tape across his chin and forehead.

For intubation:

- Remove the tape, blocks and collar.
- Manual in-line immobilisation is maintained by a dedicated person who ensures that the head and neck remain neutral, whilst allowing access to the face and neck.
- Once the airway is secured, the cervical spine must be fully immobilised again.

What imaging is required in this patient?

- 'Trauma series' films of lateral C-spine, CXR and AP pelvis.
- CT head as he has an altered conscious level.
- The UK Intensive Care Society advocates CT scanning of the cervical spine for any patient who is unconscious and having a CT scan of the head.
- When time permits, an AP of the C-spine and an open mouth view of the odontoid peg are required. An adequate film must be ensured, and this should show down to the C7/T1 junction.
- Further C-spine views such as a swimmer's view may sometimes be required.

Let's say the patient needs to be ventilated on the ITU for several days owing to his head injury. What are the problems with leaving him fully immobilised?

- **Pressure sores** are common after the prolonged use of hard collars, particularly after 48–72 hours.
- These can complicate spinal surgery as well as becoming a source for sepsis and may even require skin grafting.
- Hard collars have been demonstrated to **raise ICP**, which will obviously disadvantage the significant group of patients who have a co-existing head injury
- **Airway problems** are more common.
- Insertion of **neck lines** is more problematic.
- **Physiotherapy** is more difficult.
- **Thromboembolic disease** is more common.
- In patients who are nursed supine and immobilised, there are higher rates of enteral feeding failure associated with **gastric stasis, aspiration** and higher rates of **pneumonia**.
- Increased risk of bacteraemia and **sepsis** due to impaired basic hygiene (care of central venous catheters, oral care) and the need for at least four staff to log roll (cross-contamination).

Would you leave the full immobilisation in place then or remove it?

- ATLS guidelines traditionally require:
  - Normal plain X-rays
  - Normal skeletal and neurological examination
  - Carried out in a sober, conscious patient with no distracting injuries.
- Obviously, this is not possible in a sedated patient.
- One has to weigh the risks of an **undiagnosed unstable ligamentous injury** or a **missed unstable fracture** against the risks of prolonged immobilisation.

What would you do then? Do you know of any guidelines in this area?

Published guidelines exist, but from different sources. This may contribute to the non-standardized care. Some recommendations were published in a review article in 2004 in *Anaesthesia*, and the EAST group (www.east.org) also have a guideline.

Essentially, patients can be put into one of two groups depending on their clinical condition and expected progress.

Group 1 patients

- Likely to co-operate with a valid clinical examination at 48–72 hours.
- These patients are typically the intoxicated, those with no head injury and those undergoing a short period of post-operative ventilation.
- Three-view plain radiographs plus clinical examination is both sensitive and specific.

Group 2 patients

- Those who will not be clinically assessable inside 48–72 hours.
- Typically have severe head injuries, multiple injuries or organ failures.
- Prolonged immobilization places the patient at risk and 90%–95% of these will not have a cervical spine injury.
- These patients should have their necks cleared using combinations of plain films and CT scanning. Greater than 99.5% of cervical spine injuries would then be detected after expert interpretation.

Cervical spine injury

- There are approximately 1000 cases of cervical spine injury in the UK each year.
- These injuries complicate 2%–5% of all blunt polytrauma cases.
- The presence of a severe head injury increases the relative risk of a C-spine injury by up to 8.5 times.
- A missed or delayed diagnosis of cervical spine injury may increase the rate of severe neurological injury by up to 10%.
- Ligamentous injuries can occur in those whose bony cervical vertebrae are not fractured, but excess movement could potentially allow for damage to the cervical cord.
- A review of various studies and surveys tried to quantify the risks of isolated ligamentous injury and found this risk to be consistently under 1%, typically 0.1%–0.7%.

Bibliography

American College of Surgeons Committee on Trauma. (1997). *Advanced Trauma Life Support Manual for Doctors Student Course Manual*. Chicago: American College of Surgeons.

EAST. (1998). Practice management guidelines for identifying cervical spine injuries following trauma. http://www.east.org.

Morris C, McCoy E. (2004). Clearing the cervical spine in unconscious polytrauma victims, balancing risks and effective screening. *Anaesthesia*, **59**, 464–82.

Coeliac plexus block

What are the indications for a coeliac plexus block?

■ It is indicated in the management of malignant and non-malignant chronic pain.
■ In the non-malignant setting it has been used successfully in patients with acute and chronic pancreatitis.

In patients with cancer it is used particularly with upper abdominal tumours that have a significant visceral component to their pain, e.g.

■ Pancreatic carcinoma
■ Retroperitoneal metastasis
■ Colon or stomach cancer
■ Capsular distension of the liver or spleen.

What are the benefits of coeliac plexus block in malignant pain?

■ Reduction in systemic opiate consumption resulting in decreased nausea, constipation, sedation and increased appetite.
■ There is evidence that the use of high-dose opioids may have a negative effect on immunity and that utilising neurolytic blocks may have a survival advantage.

How would you perform this procedure?

■ Take **informed consent** and, as with all major nerve blocks, secure **intravenous access** and the help of a **skilled assistant**.
■ There are three approaches:

  1. The **retrocrural (classic)** approach
  2. The **anterocrural** approach
  3. Neurolysis of the splanchnic nerves

■ The needle is inserted at the level of the first lumbar vertebra, 5–7 cm from the midline.
■ The tip of the needle is then directed toward the body of L1 for the retrocrural and anterocrural approaches and to the body of T12 for neurolysis of the splanchnic nerves.
■ CT and ultrasound facilitate a transabdominal approach in patients who are unable to tolerate either the prone or lateral decubitus position or if the liver is so enlarged that a posterior approach is not feasible.

What are the complications of a coeliac plexus block?

- **Orthostatic hypotension** is described in 1%–3% of patients and may occur for up to 5 days post-procedure.
  Treatment consists of bed rest, fluid replacement and avoidance of sudden changes in position. This side effect disappears when compensatory vascular changes are fully activated.
- Other less common side effects include transient **diarrhoea** (treated with hydration and antidiarrhoeal agents, e.g. oral loperamide), **dysaesthesia, interscapular pain, reactive pleurisy, hiccoughing and haematuria.**
- Rare but important complications are **paraplegia** (due to spasm of the lumbar segmental arteries or direct vascular/neurological injury) and **bowel dysfunction,** occurring in 1:683 neurolytic coeliac plexus blocks.

What substances would you inject and at what doses?

- For neurolytic blocks 20 ml of 50%–100% **alcohol** per side is utilised.
- Bupivacaine 0.25% (5–10 ml) is injected prior to the alcohol, which can result in severe pain on injection.
- Phenol as a 10% formulation may be used and has the advantage of being painless on injection.

Agents used for neurolytic blocks

	Alcohol	Phenol	Glycerol
Concentration	50%–100%	4%–15%	50%–100%
Diluents	Nil	Glycerine (acts as a base from which phenol is slowly released) Saline Water	Nil
Baricity in CSF	Hypobaric	Hyperbaric	Not used in CSF
Pain on injection	+++	Nil	+
Onset	Immediate Painful side up	15–20 minutes Painful side down	15–20 minutes Not applicable
Use	Coeliac plexus Block Intrathecal Peripheral	Intrathecal Peripheral	Trigeminal neuralgia Facial pain
Complications	Neuritis (common)	Neuritis is uncommon Volume dependent toxicity	
Mechanism of action	Extracts fatty acids from myelin sheath and precipitates proteins	Non-specific nerve destruction	

Bibliography

Breivik H, Campbell W, Eccleston C. (2003). *Clinical Pain management: Practical Applications and Procedures*. London: Arnold.

Wedley J, Gauci C. (1994). *Handbook of Clinical Techniques in the Management of Chronic Pain*. Swizerland: Harwood Academic Publishers.

Complex regional pain syndrome

What do you understand by the term 'complex regional pain syndrome'?

There are two types of complex regional pain syndrome (CRPS) with defined diagnostic criteria.

Diagnostic criteria for CRPS I

1. An initiating noxious stimulus or cause of immobilisation.
2. Continuing symptoms (pain, allodynia, hyperalgesia) disproportionate to the initial event.
3. Evidence (at some time) of oedema, changes in skin blood flow or abnormal sudomotor (sweating) activity in the region of the pain. (trophic and vasomotor changes).
4. Exclusion of other diagnoses.

Criteria 2, 3 and 4 must be present.

Diagnostic criteria for CRPS II

1. Continuing pain, allodynia or hyperalgesia **following a nerve injury**, not necessarily limited to the distribution of the nerve.
2. Evidence (at some time) of oedema, changes in skin blood flow or abnormal sudomotor activity in the region of the pain.
3. Exclusion of other diagnoses.

> CRPS may be sympathetically maintained or sympathetically independent, which can be differentiated with diagnostic sympathetic block.

What are the clinical features?

■ Pain	A deep, burning pain localised to the limb
■ Allodynia	
■ Hyperalgesia	
■ Trophic changes	Loss of hair
	Changes to the nails
	Swelling and shininess
■ Vasomotor changes	The affected limb may be warm or cold.
■ Motor dysfunction	May present in affected limbs.
■ Localised osteoporosis	May or may not be present.

> **Some chronic pain terminology:**
>
> **Allodynia**   Pain from a stimulus that does not normally cause pain.
> **Hyperalgesia** A heightened response to a stimulus, which is normally painful.
> **Hyperpathia**   Severe pain in an area of numbness.

How might you manage this condition?

- Physical   Graded goal-directed exercise and physiotherapy to improve function as part of a multi-disciplinary approach.
- Pharmacological   Multiple agents are used for CRPS:
  - NSAIDS
  - Gabapentin
  - Pregabalin
  - Corticosteroids in some patients
  - Antidepressant
  - Anticonvulsants
  - NMDA blockers
  - Capsaicin cream
  - Opioids

  Sympathetic block   Will help differentiate sympathetically mediated pain and allow mobilisation. May be performed by ganglion block or intravenous regional anaesthesia with agents such as lidocaine or guanethadine. Long-term block may be performed by surgical or radio ablation.
- TENS   Some evidence to support use
- Psychotherapy   Cognitive behavioural therapy

Bibliography

Grady KM, Severn AM. (1997). *Key Topics in Chronic Pain*. Bios Scientific Publishers.

Wilson J, Serpell M. (2007). Complex regional pain syndrome. *British Journal of Anaesthesia*, Continuing Education in Anaesthesia Critical Care and Pain, **7**, 51–4.

Diabetes: peri-operative management

An elderly patient with IDDM is scheduled for an axillo-femoral bypass graft. What are the important features of a pre-operative assessment in diabetic patients?

■ **Glycaemic control**
It is important to get a feel for the patient's recent diabetic control, assessing glucose control as well as hydration and acid–base balance. Current hypoglycaemic agents should be reviewed. The patient will undergo a period of starvation as well as a surge of catabolic hormone secretion associated with the stress response to surgery.

Tight control of blood glucose has both short- and long-term advantages. In the **acute setting** inadequately treated diabetes can cause symptomatic hypoglycaemic episodes or severe dehydration with acidosis (lactic and/or ketoacids). Raised blood sugar levels peri-operatively have been linked with wound infection and poor neurological outcome in cardiac surgery.

In the **longer term**, improved glucose control can reduce the microvascular and neuropathic complications of this disease.

■ **Assessment of diabetic complications**
 Coronary artery disease
 Autonomic neuropathy
 Diabetic nephropathy
 Respiratory changes/airway assessment
 Associated endocrine disorders

Are these complications of diabetes of concern to you as an anaesthetist?

■ Diabetics are four to five times as likely to have **coronary heart disease** as non-diabetics and a proportion of these are asymptomatic.
■ **Autonomic neuropathy** occurs in up to 40% of type 1 diabetics and can take the form of postural hypotension, gastroparesis, diarrhoea and bladder paresis. There can be **unexpected tachycardia, arrhythmias and hypotension** (often unresponsive to atropine and ephedrine). Diabetics with autonomic neuropathy show **increased QT variability** (i.e. regional variations in ventricular recovery) and this may be a major factor in the 'sudden death syndrome' recognized in this group. **Gastroparesis** causes an increase in the volume of gastric contents with increased risk of aspiration. The degree of autonomic neuropathy is difficult to quantify pre-operatively, but the Valsalva manoeuvre and assessment of heart rate variability may be of benefit.
■ **Diabetic nephropathy** increases the risk of peri-operative renal failure and infection. Appropriate fluid and haemodynamic monitoring is essential.
■ **Respiratory**: diabetes is associated with a reduced FEV_1 and FVC. It has been estimated that 30%–40% of long-standing diabetics develop the **'stiff joint syndrome'** in which chronically raised blood sugar levels cause protein glycosylation and reduced elasticity of connective tissues. This is associated

with poor neck extension and mouth opening and a higher incidence of difficult intubation.

How would you manage this man's glucose control peri-operatively?

This is an elderly man who is insulin dependent undergoing a major surgical procedure. The main principles are:

■ Regular blood glucose monitoring.
■ Insulin and glucose infusions during the period of starvation.

There are many methods of providing continuous insulin/glucose infusions and hospital policy may dictate the regimen chosen. The two main regimens are:

1. Separate infusions of insulin and glucose – the insulin rate is adjusted according to the blood glucose level.
2. The Alberti regimen provides glucose, insulin and potassium in the same solution, thus eliminating the potential for giving insulin without glucose or vice versa.

As indicated above, these regimens should be commenced and stabilised pre-operatively and continued until the patient has resumed eating/drinking and their normal hypoglycaemic agents.

What is your preferred anaesthetic technique in this man?

This man requires a general anaesthetic and, if gastric stasis is suspected, then a rapid sequence induction is the technique of choice. In an elderly man with known vascular disease, an arterial line inserted pre-induction would be prudent, especially if there is a question of autonomic neuropathy. A high-dose opiate anaesthetic technique will reduce the sympathetic and hormonal response to surgery, providing both metabolic and haemodynamic stability.

Bibliography
McAnulty GR, Robertshaw HJ, Hall GM. (2000). Anaesthetic management of patients with diabetes mellitus. *British Journal of Anaesthesia*, **85**(1), 80–90.

Diabetic ketoacidosis

What is the mechanism of ketone production in diabetes?

Ketones are **produced from acetyl-CoA in the liver mitochondria** and are used as fuel by the brain and muscle. Acetyl-CoA is the end product of β-**oxidation** of fatty acids. If there is **excess fatty acid breakdown** (as in diabetes and starvation), then there will not be enough oxaloacetate to join with all the acetyl-CoA in order for it to enter the citric acid cycle. In this situation the **excess acetyl-CoA is diverted into ketone production**. The accumulation of ketoacids (β-**hydroxybutyrate and aceto-acetate**) cause a **metabolic acidosis** when levels reach about 10 mmol/l. The rate of production is usually slow, but can be as fast as 1 mmol/min.

Conditions required for ketone production

- **Insulin deficiency**. However, only a very low level of insulin is required to *inhibit* hepatic ketogenesis.
- **Counter-regulatory hormone excess** (an increase in glucagon, catecholamines and glucocorticoids)

Further pathophysiology . . .
Insulin lack accelerates glycogenolysis and gluconeogenesis. An **osmotic diuresis** results from the high blood glucose and causes uncontrolled urinary loss of K^+, Na^+ and water. This **decreased ECF volume** leads to pre-renal failure. Renal excretion of glucose is then inhibited, which leads to a further increase in plasma glucose level. Hyperglycaemia moves water out of cells into the ECF. This can decrease the serum $[Na^+]$. Nausea and vomiting frequently complicate the biochemical picture.

What are the actions of insulin?

Insulin prevents proteolysis, glycogenolysis and lipolysis and promotes uptake and storage of fuel. It is an anabolic hormone. Insulin binds to a specific membrane-bound receptor and alters intracellular cAMP levels.

Carbohydrate
- **Increases glycogen synthesis** (phosphofructokinase and glycogen synthase).
- **Inhibits glycogenolysis and gluconeogenesis**.
- **The increased uptake of glucose** into cells (such as adipose tissue and muscles) by increased glucokinase activity is now considered much less important.

Fat
- **Decreases triglyceride breakdown** in adipocytes (triglyceride–lipase).
- **Increases fatty acid synthesis** in the liver due to activation of acetyl CoA carboxylase.
- **Activates lipoprotein lipase**, which splits triglycerides enabling the fatty acids to enter adipose tissue for storage.
- **Increases esterification** of fatty acids with glycerol in adipose tissue.

Protein
- **Decreases proteolysis**.
- **Increases uptake of amino acids** into cells.
- **Increases mRNA translation**.

Increased K^+ and Mg^{2+} transport into cells

How would you manage a diabetic with ketoacidosis?

> **Treatment of DKA needs to address:**
>
> ■ **Fluid deficit/shock**
> ■ **Insulin deficiency**
> ■ **Hypokalaemia**
> ■ **Acidosis**
> ■ **Underlying/precipitating cause**

History

Examination   Sunken eyes
Reduced skin turgor
Acetone smell on breath
Kussmaul's breathing
Low BP
Decreased conscious level

Investigations

■ **Arterial blood gases** for acid–base balance
■ **Anion gap**
■ **Plasma glucose**
■ **Plasma Na$^+$ concentration** is usually low as an osmolar compensation for the high glucose. If the sodium is high, this represents severe water loss.
■ **Plasma K$^+$ concentration** may be high on presentation, but the total body potassium is low due to the absence of insulin allowing it to drift out of the cells.
■ **Urea and creatinine** Pre-renal failure from ECF depletion
                               Diabetic nephropathy
■ **Osmolality** of serum
■ **Serum/urinary ketones** (aceto-acetate). The ratio of β-hydroxybutyrate to aceto-acetate is governed by pH. As the pH decreases, the ratio increases. Conventional bedside tests for ketones only react with acetoacetic acid and therefore it is possible to have a very high β-hydroxybutyrate concentration and have the test only show a trace of ketones.
■ **PO$_4$** levels tend to follow K$^+$.
■ **CXR, ECG, FBC, blood cultures, urine culture and sputum culture** to look for underlying cause.

Monitoring   ECG/heart rate/BP/temp./resp. rate/urine output/NG tube
Regular blood glucose monitoring
HDU/ICU

Treatment

■ **ECF volume** should be replaced with **normal saline** (CVP line may be needed).
■ Start with 1–2 litres in the first hour. More than 6 litres may be needed.

- **Insulin** (actrapid) at 0.1 unit/kg bolus and then 0.1 unit/kg per hour.
- **Potassium** replacement should begin when serum [K^+] becomes less than 4.5 mmol/l. 20 mmol/hour if K^+ is 4–5 mmol/l, 40 mmol/hour if 3–4 and 40–60 mmol/hour if <3 mmol/l.
- **5% or 10% Dextrose** should be started when the plasma glucose falls below 14 mmol/l.
- **Bicarbonate therapy** is controversial. Several centres use it if pH<7.0 or if the [HCO_3^-] is <5.0 mmol/l.

The problems with it are: Large Na^+ load
Increased CO_2 production (may easily enter cells and cause a paradoxical intracellular acidosis)
Hypokalaemia
Metabolic alkalosis as ketoacids disappear
Left-shift of oxyhaemoglobin dissociation curve

- **Phosphate therapy** has no proven benefit.
- **The underlying cause** must be treated (myocardial infarction, infection, etc.).

Anion gap

$$= (Na^+ + K^+) - (HCO_3^- + Cl^-)$$

- Normal value = 10 – 18 mmol/l.
- Represents unmeasured anions, e.g. albumin, sulphate and phosphate.
- An increase is due to an unmeasured anion that is balanced by H^+ causing an acidosis, e.g. lactate or ketoacids.

Complications

- Shock and lactic acidosis
- Coma
- Cerebral oedema
- Hypothermia
- DVT
- Iatrogenic electrolyte imbalance

Bibliography

Goguen JM, Josse RG. (1993). Management of diabetic ketoacidosis. *Medicine International*, **21**(7), 275–8.

Kumar PJ, Clark ML. (1994). *Clinical Medicine*, 3rd edition. Baillière Tindall.

Sonksen P, Sonsken J. (2000). Insulin: understanding its action in health and disease. *British Journal of Anaesthesia*, **85**(1), 69–79.

Viallon A, Zeni F, Lafond P et al. (1999). Does bicarbonate therapy improve the management of severe diabetic ketoacidosis? *Critical Care Medicine*, **27**(12), 2690–3.

Weatherall DJ, Ledingham JGG, Warrell DA. (1996). *The Oxford Textbook of Medicine*, 3rd Edition. Oxford University Press.

Down's syndrome

A 7-year-old boy with Down's syndrome is scheduled to undergo a 90-minute dental conservation procedure.

What is Down's syndrome?

Down's syndrome (Trisomy 21) occurs in approximately 1:700 births (the commonest congenital abnormality). The incidence increases with increasing maternal age and the majority (95%) have an extra chromosome 21 because of non-disjunction at the time of gamete formation. It less commonly results from translocation (4%) and it is these parents who are at great risk of having further affected children.

What are the features of Down's syndrome?

No single feature is pathognomonic of the syndrome, but the association of several signs can usually lead to a clinical diagnosis. These include:

■ Skull	Flattened face and occiput
	Third fontanelle
	Brachycephaly
	Small mouth and ears
■ Eyes	Prominent epicanthic folds
	Oblique palpebral fissure
	Brushfield spots
	Squint, nystagmus
	Cataracts
■ Hands	Single palmar (Simian) crease
	Short fingers
	Wide gap between first and second toes
■ Respiratory	Macroglossia (50%)
	Micrognathia
	High arched palate (70%)
	Subglottic stenosis (2%–6%)
	OSA (50%–75%)
	Increased susceptibility to respiratory infections
	Atlantoaxial instability (15%)
	Short, broad neck
	Adenotonsillar hypertrophy
■ Heart	16%–60% have some sort of cardiac abnormality
■ CNS	Developmental delay
	Epilepsy (10%)
	Early onset Alzheimer's
■ Endocrine	Hypothyroidism (40%)
■ GIT	Gastro-oesophageal reflux
■ Immune	Leukaemia (risk increased by 20 times)
	Immunosuppression and increased infections

> **Cardiac abnormalities associated with Down's syndrome:**
>
> ■ Endocardial cushion defects   40%
> ■ VSD   27%
> ■ PDA   12%
> ■ Fallot's tetralogy   8%
> ■ Others   13%

What abnormalities are relevant to anaesthesia?

Airway management

Patients with Down's syndrome have a large, protruding tongue, a small mandible and an increased incidence of subglottic stenosis leading to difficult intubation and the need for a smaller tracheal tube than expected.

Atlantoaxial instability occurs in about 15% and is due to laxity of the transverse atlantal ligament. It is asymptomatic in most cases, particularly if the atlantoaxial distance is less than 6 mm. Care must be taken when manipulating the head and neck during laryngoscopy/intubation and during anaesthesia in general because of reduced muscle tone. There is still debate as to whether all Down's patients should have cervical spine X-rays prior to anaesthesia. The current consensus seems to be that those who are symptomatic should be X-rayed.

Careful assessment of the airway and review of previous anaesthesia records may give some indication as to the expected ease of laryngoscopy.

Post-extubation stridor, post-operative chest infections and pulmonary oedema are more common than in the normal population.

Cardiac

The cardiac abnormalities associated with Down's syndrome are outlined above. The main clinical problem is pulmonary hypertension, which may also be present in the absence of an anatomical lesion (? related to chronic anaemia). Anaesthesia is based around controlling the balance between pulmonary and systemic vascular resistance.

■ **Intellectual impairment**

May cause difficulties with co-operation at induction.

■ **Associated epilepsy**
■ **Higher incidence of hepatitis B** in institutionalised patients

Bibliography

Allt J, Howell C. (2003). Down's syndrome. *British Journal of Anaesthesia*, Continuing Education in Anaesthesia, Critical Care and Pain, **3**, 83–6.

Mitchell V, Howard R, Facer E. (1995). Down's syndrome and anaesthesia. *Paediatric Anaesthesia*, **5**, 379–84.

Dural tap

You are performing an epidural on a 23-year-old primigravida in labour. As you advance your Tuohy needle, you notice clear fluid coming out.

What are you going to do?

There are two alternative strategies in this situation:

- **Resite the epidural** – the commonest approach involves resiting the epidural in an adjacent space. The obvious anxiety is that some of the solution may subsequently pass into the subarachnoid space. To avoid a high block, the local anaesthetic doses should be given in smaller and divided doses (and by an anaesthetist). Post-delivery, an infusion of crystalloid may be continued epidurally to try to reduce the incidence of headache.
- **Use a subarachnoid catheter** – some anaesthetists will insert an end-hole catheter and give increments of local anaesthetic (0.5–1 ml of 0.5% heavy or plain bupivacaine) to achieve analgesia. CSF catheters may reduce the incidence of headache by causing a fibroblast reaction and sealing the tear.

What will you tell the obstetricians?

Traditionally, there was a view that these women should not be allowed to have an active second stage and were often delivered with forceps. This, however, does not seem to reduce the incidence of post-dural puncture headache and current practice allows **normal delivery providing the second stage is not prolonged**. For this reason, the obstetrician should be informed.

Tell me about the pathophysiology of post-dural puncture headache.

Inadvertent spinal tap is a well-recognized complication of epidural analgesia and the incidence is around 1% in obstetric practice. Headache occurs in around 80%, typically from 2–24 hours post-puncture. The headache is thought to be due to **loss of CSF via the tear resulting in traction on the intracranial contents**. A reduction in CSF pressure may lead to cerebral vasodilatation and headache and some therapies, e.g. sumatriptan assume this to be part of the problem.

What are the signs and symptoms of post-dural puncture headache?

- Severe postural headache with a temporal relationship to a dural puncture
- Typically bilateral and occipital/frontal
- Neck ache
- Nausea and vomiting
- Photophobia
- Rarely there can be cranial nerve palsies.

It is usually self-limiting, but can last for months and is associated with significant morbidity.

What would your initial management be?

- Full explanation to the mother
- Bed rest (as far as is practical)
- Adequate hydration
- Simple analgesics
- Stool softeners
- (Epidural saline could be considered)
- (Others – i.v. caffeine, sumatriptan)

When and how would you perform an epidural blood patch?

- **When** **After 24 hrs**

  It has been demonstrated (Loeser et al., 1978) that a patch performed within 24 hours has a 70% failure rate, while a patch after 24 hours has a failure rate of 4%. The initial 24 hours are generally managed conservatively and, if the headache persists, blood patching is discussed with the patient. Magnetic resonance imaging (Beards et al., 1993) has shown that the dural tear is indeed patched by the injected blood and, together with a mass effect, acts to increase CSF pressure. A single blood patch leads to resolution of symptoms in 80%–90% of patients with a success rate of 95% after a second patch.

- **How** Two anaesthetists (one a consultant).
  Aseptic technique performed in theatre.
  Locate epidural space at, or just below, site of dural tap.
  20 ml of patient's blood taken aseptically.
  Slow injection of blood into epidural space.
  Stop injecting if pain or paraesthesia (otherwise 20 ml injected)
  Place patient supine.

Bibliography

Beards SC, Jackson A, Griffiths AG, Horsman EL. (1993). Magnetic resonance imaging of extradural blood patches: appearances from 30 min to 18 h. *British Journal of Anaesthesia*, **71**(2), 182–8.

Loeser EA, Hill GE, Bennett GM, Sederberg JH. (1978). Time versus success rate for epidural blood patch. *Anesthesiology*, **49**, 147–9.

Eisenmenger's syndrome

You are asked to anaesthetise a 16-year-old male patient who has Down's syndrome and Eisenmenger's syndrome. The patient has a mental age of 6 years. He presents for emergency surgery with a cold, white, pulseless and painful left leg.

This is obviously a complicated case!

What is Eisenmenger's syndrome?

This exists in any condition in which communication between the systemic and pulmonary circulations gives rise to pulmonary hypertension ultimately resulting in right-to-left shunt. This functional reversal causes cyanosis.
   Eisenmenger's syndrome may be associated with:

- ASD
- VSD
- PDA
- Other complex anomalies

What are the general principles of anaesthetising this patient?

When anaesthetising this patient, there will be problems related to:

- Down's syndrome (see question on Down's syndrome)
- Eisenmenger's syndrome
- Emergency anaesthesia.

What are the principles of anaesthetising a patient with Eisenmenger's syndrome?

The key points are:

- **Managing the balance between SVR and PVR**. A drop in SVR (or a rise in PVR) will increase the right-to-left shunt. PVR is fairly fixed in these patients and therefore difficult to manipulate.

Factors that increase PVR are: Hypoxia
                                 Hypercarbia
                                 N_2O
                                 Histamine
                                 Low lung volumes

Under anaesthesia, the **SVR is far more prone to change**. Most induction agents decrease SVR and therefore would result in an increase in cyanosis.

   Ketamine has been used for induction (although it increases PVR as well).

   Noradrenaline and metaraminol have been used to maintain SVR.

   Atropine may be needed to prevent reflex bradycardia.

- **Care with i.v. injections to avoid paradoxical air embolus**
- **Maintenance of adequate circulating volume**
- **Avoid myocardial depressants.**
- **NB: SBE prophylaxis – would no longer be recommended.**

How is the speed of both gas and intravenous induction affected by the presence of a right-to left shunt?

- **Gas induction**   This is slower because the blood from the lungs (that has equilibrated with alveolar anaesthetic gases) is 'diluted' by the blood, with a low partial pressure, which has by-passed the lungs. The resulting brain partial pressure of agent is therefore slower to equilibrate with alveolar gas.
- **Intravenous induction**   This is quicker because some of the agent will behave like a 'paradoxical embolus' and enter the systemic circulation, by-passing the lungs, causing a rapid rise in brain concentration.

What may be the cause of the ischaemic leg?

It may be due to a paradoxical embolus, for example, from a deep vein thrombosis passing through the defect in the heart.
   It could also be thrombus from the atria if the patient is in atrial fibrillation.

Eisenmenger's complex:	Original description in 1897 at post-mortem. Pulmonary vascular disease in the presence of VSD and right ventricular hypertrophy.
Eisenmenger's syndrome:	Redefined in 1958 by Wood. Pulmonary hypertension at the systemic level caused by high pulmonary vascular resistance with reversed or bidirectional shunt via a large VSD.

Although both definitions refer to a VSD, the site of the communication is not important.

Bibliography

Bird TM, Strunin L. (1984). Anaesthesia for a patient with Down's syndrome and Eisenmenger's complex. *Anaesthesia*, **39**, 48–50.

Goldstone JC, Pollard BJ. (1996). Adult congenital heart disease: specific examples. *Handbook of Clinical Anaesthesia*, Edinburgh, UK: Churchill Livingstone.

Mather SJ, Hughes DG. (1996). *A handbook of Paediatric Anaesthesia*, 2nd edition. Oxford, UK: Oxford Medical Publications.

Sammut MS, Paes ML. (1997). Anaesthesia for laparoscopic cholecystectomy in a patient with Eisenmenger's syndrome. *British Journal of Anaesthesia*, **79**, 810–12.

Electro-convulsive therapy

A 52-year-old male with a long history of manic depression is scheduled for electro-convulsive therapy. He is a heavy smoker and a recently diagnosed hypertensive. He is taking a tricyclic antidepressant and an anti-hypertensive.

Tell me what you know about ECT

- ECT involves direct stimulation of the brain with an electrical current applied via transcutaneous electrodes.
- The resultant spike and wave activity seen on the EEG is accompanied by a **generalized motor seizure** and **an acute cardiovascular response**.
- **CNS effects** include a marked increase in both cerebral blood flow and intracranial pressure.
- The long-term benefits are improvement in the symptoms of depression, mania and some types of schizophrenia, particularly drug-resistant conditions.
- The typical cardiovascular response to ECT is a **biphasic autonomic nervous system stimulation**.
- Initial **parasympathetic** response
  - Transient bradycardia lasting 10 to 15 seconds
  - Increased salivation
  - Occasionally, asystole, especially with repeated stimuli.
- Followed immediately by a more prominent **sympathetic** response
  - Transient tachycardia and hypertension lasting 5 min or longer
  - Occasionally myocardial ischaemia and infarction.

Do you routinely do anything to attenuate these cardiovascular responses?

- Parasympathetic effects can be attenuated with an **anticholinergic** drug
  - Glycopyrrolate is more appropriate than atropine
  - It does not cross the blood–brain barrier and is effective in treating bradycardias and as an antisialogogue.
  - Atropine can cause confusion in this susceptible population.
- The sympathetic responses can be blunted by administration of:
  - Short-acting **opioids** such as alfentanyl or fentanyl
  - Short-acting β-**blockers** such as esmolol or labetalol.

Bearing this in mind, what pre-operative assessment should be undertaken in this patient?

- Standard anaesthetic and medical history and assessment should be performed.
- His history of smoking and hypertension puts him at risk of **ischaemic heart disease** and this should be looked for carefully.
  - History of exercise tolerance, chest pains, cardiac failure

- Clinical examination looking for signs of **heart failure** or **end-organ damage**
- 12-lead ECG as baseline
- Dynamic testing if appropriate (Exercise ECG, stress echo)
- U&Es and urine dipstick to look for evidence of renal impairment
- Transthoracic echocardiogram if concerns about ventricular function.

If this patient had ischaemic heart disease, is it safe to proceed with ECT?

- Treatment can be undertaken in those with co-existing medical problems, but their cases should be considered carefully by the multi-disciplinary team, led by consultant psychiatrist and anaesthetist.
- If the patient has a condition refractory to conventional treatment, then ECT may be in his best interests, balancing the risks of the treatment against the potential benefit.
- Stable ischaemic heart disease is not an absolute contra-indication to ECT.
- Appropriate precautions would include:
  - Cardiology review to ensure optimisation
  - Availability on-site of senior anaesthetic and critical care facilities (i.e. not suitable for isolated-site ECT)
  - Controlling the pressor response with opioids and alpha or β-blockers
  - Invasive arterial monitoring may be required.

When we give anaesthetics for ECT, we cause attenuation of the seizures with anaesthetic drugs. Is this important?

- EEG seizure activity lasting 25–50 seconds is associated with the optimal antidepressant response.
- Induction agents have anticonvulsant properties and would be expected to reduce seizure activity in a dose-dependent manner.
- Delicate balance between achieving adequate anaesthesia and optimal duration of EEG seizure.
- Often need relatively larger doses of induction agents though, as patients are often on chronic medications, such as benzodiazepines, or take enzyme-inducing drugs (including alcohol).

Which induction agent would you use?

- **Propofol** has been shown to limit the ECT-induced seizure activity and there have been concerns that its routine use may limit the effectiveness of the therapy. However, it is commonly used in reduced doses of 0.75 mg/kg. Its cardiovascular effects blunt the sympathetic responses well and it has a rapid recovery profile.
- **Methohexitone** was considered the gold standard for ECT, but is no longer available.
- **Thiopentone** can be used, but has marked anti-epileptiform properties.

Why do you give muscle relaxants during ECT?

▨ Tonic–clonic seizure activity can cause injury and severe myalgias so patients would require physical restraint.
▨ Use of muscle relaxants reduce myalgias and can prevent serious injuries such as fractures and dislocations.
▨ A reduced dose of suxamethonium is recommended by the Royal College of Anaesthetists −0.5 mg/kg.

What potential problems are there with using suxamethonium

▨ **Bradyarrhythmias** can occur especially when associated with the parasympathetic phase of the seizure.
▨ **Myalgias**
▨ **Hyperkalaemia**
▨ **Suxamethonium apnoea**
▨ **Malignant hyperpyrexia** in those susceptible.

What alternatives are there to suxamethonium?

▨ Mivacurium is the only practical alternative.
▨ Other NDMRs have been used, but they have a prolonged action.

ECT – further information

▨ ECT to provoke a generalized epileptic seizure was first described in 1938 and was performed without anaesthesia for almost 30 years subsequently.
▨ ECT is most useful for the treatment of severe and medication-resistant depression and mania.
▨ It has also been used more recently in the treatment of schizophrenic patients with affective disorders, suicidal drive, delusional symptoms and catatonic symptoms.
▨ Typically, the acute phase of ECT is performed three times a week for 6 to 12 treatments.
▨ In successful cases, initial clinical improvement is usually evident after 3 to 5 treatments.
▨ Maintenance ECT can be performed at progressively increasing intervals from once a week to once a month to prevent relapses.
▨ Short-term memory loss is common after ECT and more serious cognitive dysfunction has been described.

Bibliography

Ding Z, White P. (2002). Anesthesia for electro-convulsive therapy [review article] *Anesthesia and Analgesia*, **94**, 1351–64.

Interim statement from The Royal College of Anaesthetists on electro-convulsive therapy (ECT) provided in 'remote' sites. http://www.rcoa.ac.uk/index.

Setting standards for ECT use in England and Wales. *NICE Clinical Guidance.* May 2003. www.nice.org

Epidural abscess

You are asked to see a patient 5 days post-spinal anaesthesia. The surgical team is concerned regarding the presence of an epidural abscess. What are the symptoms and signs of an epidural abscess?

The classic triad of symptoms and signs are:

- Fever
- Back pain
- Neurological deficit.

However, all three are present in only 13% at presentation. Presentation is often vague with fever and back pain appearing before neurological deficit. Some patients may complain of headache. Examination may reveal tenderness over the spine and neck stiffness.

When would you expect symptoms to start?

Symptoms tend to begin >4 days after central nerve blockade.

What is the incidence of epidural abscess?

Spontaneous epidural abscess is rare, occurring in 0.2–1.2 cases in 10 000 hospital admissions.

The incidence following central nerve blockade is difficult to estimate, but may be as frequent as 1:1000 or as rare as 1:100 000.

What are the risk factors for developing an epidural abscess?

- Compromised immunity: diabetes, immunosuppressant therapy, HIV infection and liver cirrhosis.
- Source of infection: haematological spread from distant sources of infection such as respiratory, soft tissue or urinary tract infection can occur.
- Disruption of the spinal column: central nerve blockade and spinal surgery can lead to the introduction of infection from the skin or the accumulation of haematoma, which may then become infected.
- Difficult insertion of central nerve blockade: multiple attempts at insertion may increase the risk of haematoma formation and lead to breakdown of aseptic technique.

- Disordered clotting: anti-thrombotic and anti-platelet treatments, and intrinsic coagulopathies may increase the risk of haematoma formation, which may then become infected.
- Prolonged use of central catheters: infection is rare when catheters are used for less than 2 days but may become significant with more prolonged use.

What is the cause of the neurological deficit?

Direct compression of the spinal cord may cause neurological injury, although significant deficit can occur without evidence of compression and deficit is often worse than the degree of compression would suggest. It has been suggested that leptomeningeal thrombosis or spinal artery compression may result in cord ischaemia.

How would you investigate a suspected epidural abscess?

- FBC, ESR and CRP
- Raised white cell count occurs in the majority of patients.
- Raised ESR occurs more frequently even with early presentation. Thrombocytopaenia may be present.
- Imaging: plain X-rays are usually unhelpful.
- CT is more reliable, but the greatest sensitivity is from myelography and MRI.
- MRI has a sensitivity of ~90%, is non-invasive and is the investigation of choice.
- Myelography with high resolution CT has been used in some cases with non-diagnostic MRI.
- Lumbar puncture: analysis of CSF may show leukocytosis and raised protein. LP in the context of spinal compression and local infection carries considerable risk and is probably inappropriate with the advent of reliable imaging techniques.
- Cultures: blood culture and pus culture from radiological aspiration may identify the causative organism.

Causative organism in epidural abscess secondary to epidural catheter
- *Staphylococcus aureus*
- *Staphylococcus epidermidis*
- *Pseudomonas aeruginosa*
- Coagulase-negative Staphylococci
- Pyocyaneus

How would you manage an epidural abscess?

- ABC: Patients may develop septic shock and require resuscitation.
- Antibiotics: Microbiological advice should be sought. Staphylococcal infections account for the majority of epidural abscesses and therefore

empirical management should be with appropriate agents such as intravenous flucloxacillin and/or a third-generation cephalosporin. Patients with known MRSA should be treated with vancomycin or teicoplanin. Treatment should then be guided by culture results. Intravenous antibiotics should be continued for at least 3–4 weeks after which oral antibiotics may be introduced. Antibiotics should be continued for 6–12 weeks.

■ Surgical drainage: posterior or occasionally anterior laminectomy should be performed early to limit neurological damage.
■ Percutaneous drainage: radiological percutaneous drainage may be possible for dorsal abscesses.
■ Steroids: there is no evidence for the use of corticosteroids to treat an epidural abscess and the use of steroids in infection is contentious.

What is the prognosis?

Mortality rates of 13%–16% are still quoted. Permanent neurological deficit is more common in patients developing epidural abscess secondary to central nerve blockade with 62% having permanent deficit. 27% will be left with severe deficit. Early identification and treatment improves outcome.

Whose responsibility is it to check?

All surgical and nursing staff caring for patients after central nerve blockade should be aware of the symptoms of epidural abscess and early referral should occur. Persistent or increasing motor block should be identified by the anaesthetist at the post-operative visit or by nursing staff. Bowel or bladder function disruption is particularly ominous. Some centres have given patients information at discharge, as symptoms may appear after discharge.

Bibliography
Grewal S, Hocking G, Wildsmith JAW. (2006). Epidural abscesses. *British Journal of Anaesthesia*, **96**(3), 292–302.

Epilepsy

You are asked to anaesthetise a 50-year-old male for an elective open cholecystectomy. On your pre-operative visit, you discover he is a known epileptic.

Tell me about epilepsy?

Epilepsy is defined as two or more unprovoked epileptic seizures. The quoted incidence of active epilepsy in the community varies but in the US it is quoted as 0.8% (8 per 1000). Approximately 9% of people will have at least one seizure in their lifetime and 3% will be given the diagnosis of epilepsy at some point. Males have a greater incidence of epilepsy than females.

Do you know any classification syndromes for epilepsy? Has this changed recently?

The International League Against Epilepsy (ILAE) first published their classification of epilepsy in 1981 and then updated it in 1989. They have recently proposed a revised diagnostic approach and classification syndrome. Description of epilepsy is based on five parts or 'axes':

1. Ictal phenomenology.
2. Seizure type, e.g. self-limiting or continuous, generalised or focal.
3. Syndrome. Diagnosis of known epilepsy syndromes if possible.
4. Aetiology (if known).
5. Impairment.

What side effects are associated with anti-epileptic drugs?

Common side effects to most of these drugs include sedation, somnolence, fatigue and weight changes. There are more specific blood dyscrasias and abnormalities associated with certain agents.

Blood abnormality	Drugs
Hyponatraemia	Carbamazepine
Abnormal LFTs	Carbamazepine
	Sodium valproate
Anaemia	Phenytoin
	Phenobarbitone
	Vigabatrin
Thrombocytopaenia	Carbamazepine
	Sodium valproate
	Primidone
	Ethosuximide
Leukopaenia	Carbamazepine
	Primidone

What are the implications of anaesthetic drugs in this patient?

There are two major implications of the use of various anaesthetic agents:

■ **Pro-convulsant and anti-convulsant properties of anaesthetic agents**
Many agents have both pro and anti-convulsant properties.

Intravenous induction agents may cause excitatory phenomena, while also having anti-convulsant properties. Etomidate may produce EEG changes and prolong the seizure duration during ECT compared to propofol. Case reports of seizures after etomidate have been published. Propofol may cause excitatory movements, but is thought to be safe in epilepsy. Some anaesthetists still avoid its use in epilepsy, especially if driving restrictions may result from possible seizures. Thiopentone is a potent anti-convulsant despite excitatory phenomena at induction.

Regarding volatile agents, seizures have been reported following enflurane and EEG changes may be seen many hours after administration.

Neuromuscular blocking drugs have theoretical implications as the breakdown product of atracurium, laudanosine, is pro-convulsant in high concentrations in dogs, but does not appear to be a clinical problem in humans.

Other agents include ketamine, which may cause excitatory phenomena, but produces EEG suppression and has been used to treat status epilepticus, and benzodiazepines have clear anti-convulsant properties.

■ **Interaction between anaesthetic agents and anti-epileptic medication**
Many of the anti-epileptic medications have a sedative action on patients. Some of the drugs cause enzyme induction (phenytoin, carbamazepine, primidone, and barbiturates), while others may cause enzyme inhibition.

How would you anaesthetise this patient?

The key consideration is the limitation of seizure activity in the peri-operative period.

■ **Pre-operative:** Ensure epilepsy is well controlled pre-operatively (if not, then referral to a neurologist may be appropriate) and that anti-epileptic medication is continued peri-operatively. This may involve changing from oral to parenteral preparation to ensure the patient does not miss a dose of their medication. Urea and electrolyte levels should be measured and corrected. Full blood count is indicated if haemopoetic side effects of medications are possible. Some anaesthetists would advocate benzodiazepine pre-medication for this patient.

■ **Induction:** Full anaesthetic monitoring and pre-oxygenation. Intravenous induction with opioid (fentanyl), induction agent (thiopentone would seem most appropriate), and neuromuscular blockade (atracurium), followed by endotracheal intubation and ventilation.

■ **Maintenance:** Volatile agent maintenance (not enflurane) in oxygen and air with positive pressure ventilation **ensuring normocapnoea.** Close observation for signs of seizure activity (movement, pupil changes, autonomic activity). This should be managed with intravenous benzodiazepines as first line and with intravenous sodium valproate or phenytoin as second line. Systemic opioids such as morphine are suitable for analgesia. Normothermia and normoglycaemia should be maintained.

■ **Emergence:** Reversal of neuromuscular blockade and 'awake' extubation should be performed. Delay in emergence may be due to unidentified seizures or interactions of anti-epileptic medication and anaesthetics.

■ **Post-operative:** Early re-introduction of anti-epileptic medication. Sodium valproate and phenytoin are available as intravenous preparations if the enteral route is unavailable. Patients with recurrent post-operative seizures are best nursed on a high dependency unit. A patient-controlled morphine infusion is suitable for post-operative pain relief if the patient is able to comply.

Bibliography

Bovill JG, Howie MB. (1999). *Clinical Pharmacology for Anaesthetists*. Harcourt Publishers.

Gratrix AP, Enright SM. (2005). Epilepsy in anaesthesia and intensive care. *British Journal of Anaesthesia, CEPD Reviews*, **5**(4), 118–21.

Hutton P, Cooper GM, James FM. (2002). *Fundamental Principles and Practice of Anaesthesia*. Informa Health Care.

ILAE taskforce website. www.ilae-epilepsy.org.

NICE. (2004). The epilepsies. The diagnosis and management of the epilepsies in adult and children in primary and secondary care. *NICE Guidelines*. Oct.

Guillain–Barré syndrome

You are called to see a 25-year-old man on a medical ward with a 10-day history of progressive weakness.

What is the differential diagnosis?

- Guillain–Barré syndrome
- Motor neurone disease
- Multiple sclerosis
- Polyneuropathy – polio, HIV
- Hypo/hyperkalaemic periodic paralysis (or iatrogenic).

What is the clinical picture of Guillain–Barré syndrome?

This syndrome is characterised by:

- **Progressive, symmetrical, ascending flaccid motor weakness**.
- Around 80% have **sensory symptoms** (pain is very common).
- Around 65% have **autonomic dysfunction**.
- It is often preceded by an infective illness.

The age-specific curve shows a bimodal distribution with peaks in young adults and the elderly. Males are more commonly affected. The main problems in the acute situation are:

- **Respiratory failure** requiring assisted ventilation due to progression of the paralysis to involve respiratory muscles.
- **Autonomic neuropathy** which can be severe causing orthostatic hypotension and cardiac arrhythmias.

> Disease named after two case reports by Guillain, Barré and Strohl in 1916
> The full spectrum of GBS ranges from acute inflammatory demyelinating polyneuropathy to the pure motor variants and the Miller–Fisher syndrome.
> Miller–Fisher syndrome (1956) describes the association of ophthalmoplegia, ataxia and areflexia.

What are the causes of this syndrome ?

The syndrome may be an immune reaction triggered by either infection or vaccination.

Antecedent *infections* include:

| ■ **Campylobacter** | *Campylobacter jejuni*, a major cause of bacterial gastroenteritis worldwide, is the most frequent antecedent pathogen (up to 45% in some studies) |
| ■ **Cytomegalovirus** | The second commonest associated infection which particularly affects young females |

- ■ **Epstein–Barr virus**
- ■ **Mycoplasma**
- ■ **Association with HIV**

It is likely that immune responses directed towards the infecting organisms are involved in the pathogenesis by cross-reaction with neural tissues.

Possible associated *vaccinations* include influenza, polio, rabies and rubella. Most large-scale epidemiological studies have failed to find a cause–effect relationship. In up to 30% of cases no cause is found.

There is **widespread segmental demyelination of peripheral nerves**. Cerebrospinal fluid typically shows few cells with a high protein content (in 90% of cases), though the diagnosis remains a clinical one.

Why or when might you intubate these patients?

Around 25% of patients require mechanical ventilation, so close monitoring must be ensured should a deterioration in respiratory function occur. Forced vital capacity (FVC) should be measured regularly. There are no 'rules' regarding mechanical ventilation. However:

- ■ Some recommend ventilation if the FVC < 1L (others < 10–15 ml/kg)
- ■ The speed of deterioration will also influence any decisions
- ■ Other factors, e.g. aspiration, bulbar weakness should be taken into account

Early tracheostomy is recommended.

Do you know of any specific treatments?

■ **Plasma exchange**	Involves the removal of about 200 ml/kg of plasma over 4–6 sessions and replacement with colloid or crystalloid Thought to work by removal of a humoral demyelinating factor. This treatment does not influence mortality but reduces the ventilation and complication rate.
■ **Immunoglobulin**	Intravenously for 5 days Much more convenient than plasma exchange Randomized control trials show that immunoglobulin and plasma exchange are equally effective in reducing the time to functional recovery.
■ **Immunosuppressants**	Steroids and other immunosuppressants are no longer recommended.

What other problems might they encounter on ICU?

- Pneumonia
- Line infections
- DVT
- Nutritional deficits
- Psychological — There should be early and active psychological support for the patient and relatives.
- Autonomic neuropathy — Ensure adequate circulating volume and sedation. β-blockers, atropine and pacemakers have all been used to manage autonomic disturbances.
- Pain — Pain is common (especially in the back and lower limbs) and can be a major problem. Opiates are often required. A randomized, double-blind cross-over trial showed that carbamazepine is a useful adjuvant for pain control, reducing narcotic requirements. Intensive physiotherapy is essential.
- GI haemorrhage

Do you know the prognosis?

Around 80% make a near complete recovery, although the speed of recovery is variable. At least 10% will have a significant permanent disability and the mortality rate is 5–10%.

Poorer prognosis is associated with:

- Older patients
- Preceding *Campylobacter jejuni* infection
- Need for mechanical ventilation
- Rapid progression of symptoms
- Extensive disease.

Bibliography
Hinds CJ, Watson D. (1996). Neurological disorders, *Intensive Care, A Concise Textbook*. 2nd edition. London, UK: Saunders.

Seneviratne U. (2000). Guillain–Barré syndrome. *Postgraduate Medical Journal*, **76**, 774–82.

Tripathi M, Kaushik S. (2000). Carbamazapine for pain management in Guillain–Barré syndrome patients in the intensive care unit. *Critical Care Medicine*, **28**(3), 655–8.

Heart block and temporary pacing

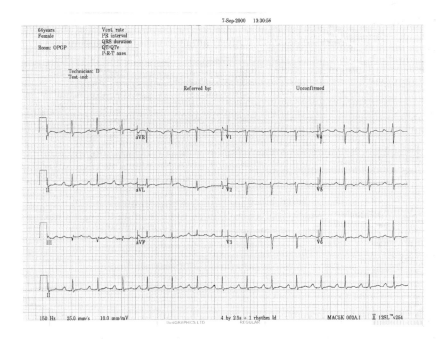

Have a look at this ECG. What does it show?

The ECG shows sinus rhythm at a rate of 87 beats per minute. The axis is normal. The PR interval is prolonged. There are no other abnormalities. The diagnosis is first-degree heart block.

How do you know it is first-degree heart block?

The normal PR interval is 120–210 milliseconds (some books say 200 ms!). The PR interval is measured from the start of the P wave to the start of the ventricular complex, whether that is a Q or an R wave. At a standard paper speed of 25 mm/s, each small square is equivalent to 40 ms. The normal PR interval is therefore 3–5(ish) small squares.

What types of heart block are there?

The term 'heart block' usually refers to atrio-ventricular block as distinct from 'bundle-branch' block.

Atrio-ventricular heart block is classified into first-, second- or third-degree depending on the effect on atrio-ventricular conduction.

First-degree   As described above.
Second-degree **Mobitz type I** (or Wenkebach)
                              Mobitz type II

In **Mobitz type I** block the PR interval increases successively with each beat until a QRS complex is 'dropped'. When seen in young, fit people (often nocturnally) with high vagal tone, it may be benign. When it cannot be attributed to high vagal tone it may have a similar prognosis to Mobitz type II.

In **Mobitz type II** block there is intermittent failure of A-V conduction. This results in 2:1 or 3:1 A-V block, for example. The block is usually below the A-V node and is associated with an increased incidence of Stokes-Adams attacks, slow ventricular rates and sudden death.

Third-degree There is total interruption of A-V conduction such that the ventricular 'escape' rate bears no relation to the atrial rate. The ventricular rate is determined by the site of the block, which may be nodal or infra-nodal. A nodal block resulting in a His-bundle pacemaker may have a fairly 'normal' rate and narrow QRS complexes. An infra-nodal block resulting in a pacemaker from the left or right bundle-branch will have a slow rate with broad QRS complexes.

What are the indications for pacing pre-operatively?

Suggested indications include:

- Acute anterior myocardial infarction (MI)
- Acute MI with Mobitz type II or third degree block (?also new BBB)
- First-degree heart block with bifascicular block
- Any symptomatic brady-arrhythmia
- Refractory supra-ventricular tachy-arrhythmia

How may peri-operative pacing be achieved?

- **Transthoracic non-invasive** The anterior patch must be negative and placed just to the left of the xiphoid process to avoid the pectoral muscle-mass. The posterior patch is placed inferior to the left scapula.
- **Epicardial** Usually performed by surgeons during cardiac surgery.
- **Transvenous** May or may not be balloon-tipped to help with insertion. Requires X-ray control to check its position in the apex of the right ventricle (pointing down). A pacing wire that is pointing towards the left shoulder may be in the coronary sinus.
- **Transoesophageal** Used when slow atrial rhythm. Left atrium lies anterior to the oesophagus. The pacer is switched on and advanced until capture occurs (usually at 30–35cm from teeth).

Bibliography
Bennett DH. (1994). *Cardiac Arrythmias*, 4th Edition. BH Publishing.
Bourke ME. (1996). The patient with a pacemaker or related device. *Canadian Journal of Anaesthesia*, **43**, 5(2), R24–32.
Deakin CD. (1998). *Clinical Notes for the FRCA*. Churchill Livingstone.
Morgan GE, Mikhail MS. (1996). *Clinical Anaesthesiology*, 2nd edition. Appleton and Lange.

Heparin-induced thrombocytopaenia

You are asked to see a 60-year-old woman on the High Dependency Unit who is 6 days post-open abdominal aortic aneurysm repair. She is acutely short of breath and complaining of pain on inspiration. How would you approach this situation?

- **ABC** approach adding supplemental oxygen to achieve adequate oxygen saturation.
- In the absence of immediate life-threatening conditions, ascertain the history and examine the patient.
- Review the notes and order appropriate investigations such as an arterial blood gas, FBC, chest X-ray and an ECG.

What is your differential diagnosis?

- Pleuritic pain may indicate a **pulmonary embolism, infarct, infection** or **effusion**. DVT should be looked for, although it is common to have a PE without clinical evidence of a DVT.
- Cardiac causes would include an **acute coronary syndrome** or **pulmonary oedema** from ventricular failure.
- There may be abdominal pathology such as **viscus perforation** or ischaemia causing acidosis and peritonitis.
- **ARDS** is a possibility.
- **Pneumothorax**

The drug chart shows that the patient has been on LMW heparin post-operatively as prophylaxis against thromboembolism. The full blood count is given to you.

RBC	5.11	x10^{12}/l	(3.80–5.80)
Hb	10.1	g/dl	(11.5–16.5)
PCV	0.33		(0.37–0.47)
MCV	89.5	fL	(79–97)
MCH	33.2	pg	(27.0–32.0)
RDW	15.4		(11.5–16.0)

```
PLT    45    x10⁹/l   (150–400)
WCC   10.5   x10⁹/l   (4.0–11.0)
```

Does the FBC concern you?

Yes. There is **thrombocytopaenia** and mild anaemia. This patient has been exposed to, and treated with, heparin, which in combination with a possible PE would make me suspect a diagnosis of **heparin-induced thrombocytopaenia** syndrome or HIT.

What do you mean by thrombocytopaenia?

- Platelet count below the reference range.
- It can broadly be defined as an abnormal fall in platelet count as this can be more relevant.
- A decline in platelet count of >50% occurring between 4–14 days after heparin therapy is suspicious of HIT irrespective of the actual value.

What can you tell me about heparin-induced thrombocytopaenia?

- HIT is an acquired disorder of hypercoagulability caused by administration of heparin.
- Heparin can cause one of **two recognisable conditions.**
  HIT Type I   Clinically less significant. It is non-immune-mediated platelet aggregation and occurs in about 10% of patients on heparin. The platelet count usually stays above 100 and recovers spontaneously.
  HIT Type II   Underlying process is **antibody-mediated platelet activation** resulting in thrombocytopaenia. There is an associated increase in **thrombin generation**, which overall leads to a high-risk of arterial and venous thrombosis.

Heparin-induced thrombocytopaenia – thrombotic (HITT) or Type II

- Type II – **Autoimmune disorder.** After heparin administration, an **immune complex** can form between **heparin** and **platelet factor 4** (PF4) that is released by platelets. This heparin–PF4 complex is seen as 'foreign' and **IgG antibodies** are formed against the complex. The heparin/PF4/IgG complexes cross-link and **activate platelets.** More PF4 is released (creating a vicious circle of more complexes) and **thrombin generation** occurs via the clotting cascade.
- Paradoxical high risk of thrombosis (with a low platelet count)
- **'White clots'** form as they are platelet rich.
- **50%** of patients develop heparin-dependent antibodies post-cardiopulmonary by-pass (within 5–10 days). Only a proportion will get platelet activation.

- **Antibodies** seem to be **transient** and last **40–100 days**. Re-exposure to heparin before that time can cause **rapid onset of HIT**.
- Likelihood of developing HIT according to **heparin type:** bovine lung UFH > porcine intestinal mucosal UFH > LMWH.
- **Patient type:** post-surgical > medical > obstetric patient.
- Female > male.

How does HIT present?

- The **fall in platelet count** typically begins 5–10 days after starting a heparin course, but in about one-third of patients an abrupt fall in platelets occurs on giving heparin. This group has usually received heparin within the past 100 days and these patients already have clinically significant levels of HIT antibodies.
- **Venous thrombosis** such as DVT and PE are more common than **arterial thrombosis**, although lower limb arterial thromboses are often seen if looked for.
- **Skin lesions** at heparin injection sites can occur and range from erythematous plaques to skin necrosis.
- A quarter of patients who receive an intravenous heparin bolus in the presence of circulating HIT antibodies will have an **acute systemic reaction**, often with fever, chills, respiratory distress and hypertension.
- Circulatory collapse and cardio-respiratory arrest have been reported. The reaction occurs 5–30 minutes following the bolus injection and is accompanied by a fall in platelets.
- **Decompensated DIC** can occur, but only in about 10% of cases.
- NB: Other causes of thrombocytopaenia are common on intensive care – especially after cardiac surgery, e.g. intra-aortic balloon pumps, sepsis and haemofiltration.

How is it diagnosed?

HIT is a **clinical** syndrome. The diagnosis is based on one or more of the classical clinical features such as:

- Thrombosis
- Thrombocytopaenia
- The systemic reaction
- DIC

The **'4Ts' scoring system** is frequently used to gauge the clinical likelihood of HIT.

Laboratory diagnosis with **enzyme-linked immunosorbent assays** that look at platelet activation are sensitive but not specific. Their **negative predictive value is high** but their positive predictive value is not so good. For this reason, testing in the absence of a high clinical suspicion (or worse – **screening) is not helpful**.

Probability of HIT 6–8 = High 4–5 = Intermediate 0–3 = Low	Points (2, 1 or 0)–Maximum score = 8		
	2	**1**	**0**
Thrombocytopaenia	>50% fall or platelet nadir 20-100 × 10^9/l	30%–50% fall or platelet nadir 10-19 × 10^9/l	Fall <30% or platelet nadir <10 × 10^9/l
Timing of platelet count fall or other sequelae	Clear onset from days 5–10; or less than 1 day (if heparin exposure within past 100 days)	Consistent with immunization but not clear (e.g. missing platelet counts) or onset of thrombocy-topaenia after day 10	Platelet count fall too early (without recent heparin exposure)
Thrombosis or other sequelae (e.g. skin lesions)	New thrombosis; skin necrosis; post heparin bolus acute systemic reaction	Progressive or recurrent thrombosis; erythematous skin lesions; suspected thrombosis not yet proven	None
Other causes for thrombocytopaenia are not evident	No other cause for platelet count fall is evident	Probable other cause is evident	Definite other cause is present

From Lo *et al.*, 2006. © 2006 International Society on Thrombosis and Haemostasis. Reproduced with permission.

Does it matter which type of heparin you use?

Type II HIT occurs more frequently with unfractionated heparin, in approximately 1% of all patients treated. Approximately 0.1% of patients treated with low-molecular weight heparin will develop HIT.

How would you manage this lady on the HDU if she were diagnosed with HIT? Do you need to continue her tinzaparin?

- **All heparin should be stopped immediately** when the diagnosis of HIT is suspected or confirmed, including the heparin in pressure-monitoring lines and intravenous flushes. The patient was probably on LMWH as prophylaxis against DVT in the post-operative period and the risk of this occurring increases once the heparin is stopped.

■ There is also a high risk of thrombosis with established HIT (50% over 30 days if not anticoagulated by other means) and so immediate substitution with an **alternative non-heparin anticoagulant** is required.

■ **Platelet transfusions** should be **avoided** – this may 'fuel the fire'.

What alternative anticoagulants are there to heparin in this situation?

There are currently two alternatives available in the UK.

■ **Danaparoid sodium** (Orgaran) is a mixture of heparin sulphate (83%), dermatan sulphate (12%) and chondroitin sulphate (5%). It exerts its anticoagulant effect by **catalysing the inactivation of factor Xa by antithrombin**. There has been some cross-reactivity reported in patients with HIT antibodies, but this is rare. Monitoring is with Factor Xa assays.

■ **Lepirudin** is a recombinant hirudin derived from leeches, and forms an irreversible 1:1 complex with thrombin. There is no cross-reactivity with the HIT antibodies, but there have been reports of immune reactions to the drug itself. Monitoring is via APTT.

The risks of thrombotic complications remain for approximately 5–6 weeks due to the presence of HIT antibodies. Specialist haematology advice should be sought, but the patient usually remains anticoagulated during this time.

Can you use warfarin?

Coumarins including warfarin are contraindicated in acute HIT because they increase the risk of microvascular thrombosis causing venous limb gangrene and skin necrosis. Warfarin induces an **acquired Protein C deficiency** – Protein C being a natural anticoagulant.

Bibliography
BNF. 53 (March, 2007). Section 2.8.1 Heparin.
de Maistre E, Gruel Y, Lasne D. (2006). Diagnosis and management of heparin-induced thrombocytopenia. *Canadian Journal of Anesthesia*, **53**(6), S123–S134.
Klein A, Vuylsteke A, Nashef SAM. (2008). *Core Topics in Cardiothoracic Critical Care*, Cambridge, UK: Cambridge University Press.
Lo G, Juhl D, Warkentin T et al. (2006). Evaluation of pretest clinical score (4 Ts) for the diagnosis of heparin-induced thrombocytopenia in two clinical settings. *Journal of Thrombosis and Haemostasis*, **4**, 759–65.
Warkentin TE, Greinacher A. (2004). *Heparin-Induced Thrombocytopenia*, 3rd edition, USA: Marcel Dekker.
www.frca.co.uk/resources/clinical anaesthesia/HITS.

Hypertension and ischaemic heart disease

You are presented with an 80-year-old woman with hypertension, diabetes mellitus and a touch of indigestion on climbing stairs.

Describe her pre-operative assessment for cataract surgery.

A standard pre-operative assessment should be undertaken with particular attention to the impact of her medical conditions.

- Hypertension and diabetes are risk factors for ischaemic heart disease and the 'indigestion' on exertion may reflect undiagnosed angina.
- A history of similar pains at rest or associated with other precipitants should be sought.
- Other features should be looked for in the history pointing to end-organ damage such as orthopnoea, SOBOE or ankle swelling from ventricular failure, renal disease or CVAs.
- An assessment of exercise tolerance should be made, and if all she can manage is a flight of stairs before getting angina, this warrants further investigation as it is a predictor of mortality.

Control of the diabetes and hypertension may be evident from the notes, the GP's letters or from the patient. A medication history is important with regard to the diabetes and hypertension.

Other routine enquiries such as previous anaesthetics, last meal and reflux, airway assessment and an explanation of the procedure are, of course, mandatory.

If you are concerned about her having IHD, how would you investigate her?

- Clinical assessment may reveal evidence of ventricular failure or peripheral vascular disease, for example, and help guide your assessment.
- Simple tests such as the ECG can provide evidence of previous infarcts, ischaemia, ventricular hypertrophy and the state of the conducting system.
- CXR can assess the cardiac size and show evidence of LVF with lung congestion.
- Simple tests for end-organ damage include measurement of urea and electrolytes and dipstick urine analysis. A lipid profile should be checked.
- An echocardiogram is useful if there is a history or clinical findings suggestive of failure or of valvular heart disease to quantify the resting function.
- Dynamic assessment can be difficult in this group as mobility may be a problem, but the simplest test is an exercise ECG which may prove diagnostic as her pain seems to be brought on with minimal effort.
- More formal dynamic functional testing may be appropriate as may coronary angiography if her first-line tests show ischaemia.
- She may also have a GI cause for her pain and, after excluding a cardiac cause, USS of the abdomen or endoscopy may be necessary.

How would you assess control of her diabetes?

Motivated patients often keep records of their blood sugars and isolated BMs can often be found in the medical records.

- Hba1c is the commonest method of assessing control over about the previous 6 weeks.
- An Hba1c of 7% represents an average blood sugar of 8.3 mmol/l during this time.
- Good control is usually considered to be a value less than 7%.

> **'BM'** originally stood for Boehringer Mannheim, a German pharmaceutical company (now called Roche) – they developed blood glucose testing strips!

With regard to control of her blood pressure, what drugs is she likely to be on?

There are various classes of drugs used to treat hypertension:

- ACE inhibitors are particularly useful in the diabetic as they can delay progression of renovascular disease and protect against left ventricular dysfunction.
- Angiotensin II antagonists may be used if there is intolerance to ACEIs.
- Thiazide diuretics are advocated as first-line therapy for isolated hypertension and in the treatment of heart failure, particularly in the elderly.
- β-blockers can be used, particularly if there is associated ischaemic heart disease but these should be used with caution in diabetics.
- Alpha-blockers are used to treat hypertension, but they can cause hypotension in the elderly.
- Calcium channel blockers are appropriate especially if there is associated ischaemic heart disease.

Her BP is 190/105 mmHg after three measurements both at pre-op assessment and today. What would you do?

She has poorly controlled hypertension.

- Assess what investigations and treatment she has received so far along with compliance with her current drug regimen.
- 'White coat' hypertension is a possibility and blood pressures from the primary care physician may be available.
- As she is having non-urgent surgery, her operation should be postponed while her blood pressure is controlled and her cardiac symptoms investigated.

What are the risks in anaesthetising her?

The biggest risks are of peri-operative cardiac events.
The commonest problems are:

■ Haemodynamic instability (particularly profound hypotension on induction)
■ Myocardial ischaemia
■ Cardiac arrhythmias.

> ■ Isolated hypertension itself, with no evidence of end-organ damage, is probably not directly linked to an increase in peri-operative morbidity and mortality.
> ■ Hypertension though can be associated with cardiovascular, renal, endocrine and cerebrovascular disease, which may be underlying or as a consequence of the hypertension.
> ■ Careful pre-operative assessment should identify these patients and they should be investigated further and treated as appropriate.

Describe the control of blood pressure in this lady, both in the immediate and long term.

■ Her blood pressure is not dangerously elevated and so I would discuss this with her primary care physician and leave the choice of drug to them.
■ In the elderly, small doses of short-acting drugs are generally best to start with and depending on her current therapy, the addition of a thiazide diuretic, calcium channel blocker or ACE inhibitor may be appropriate.
■ Causes of **secondary hypertension** (which is usually endocrine or renal in origin) should always be excluded.
■ These may be indicated by history and examination, but usually occurs in younger patients.
■ Obesity, salt intake, hypercholesterolaemia and diabetes should also be addressed.
■ Acute control of severe hypertension can usually be gained by intravenous infusions of nitrates or β-blockers, including labetalol or calcium channel blockers such as nifedipine. A cardiologist should be involved.
■ Oral therapy with β-blockers, ACE inhibitors and diuretics can usually be started once the acute crisis is controlled.

If she comes back with her cardiovascular problems under control and she is scheduled to have her cataract done under a local anaesthetic block, how would you manage her diabetes peri-operatively?

The Royal College of Anaesthetists and The Royal College of Ophthalmologists have produced guidance for the management of patients having cataract surgery under local anaesthesia and these state that fasting is not required, assuming that there are no anticipated peri-operative problems and that the patient is not going to have any sedation.

- The patient should take their usual insulin or anti-hypoglycaemic tablets and eat and drink as normal.
- Diabetic patients should still be done early on the list to allow them the maximum time to recover, but the emphasis is on minimising disruption both to their physiology and to their normal routine.
- Regular BMs should be taken.

White coat hypertension

So-called white coat hypertension is relevant to anaesthetic practice and can be defined as a persistently elevated clinic arterial pressure in combination with a normal ambulatory arterial pressure. Values currently accepted are a BP of 140/90 mm Hg or greater in the presence of an average daytime reading of less than 135/85 mm Hg. (This can obviously be difficult to measure.)

The majority of the studies in this area show a benign prognosis for white coat hypertension. Data suggests that patients who present for elective surgery with admission hypertension that then settles to normotensive levels are probably at less risk of cardiovascular complications than patients with sustained hypertension.

Bibliography

Howell S, Sear J, Foëx P. (2004). Hypertension, hypertensive heart disease and perioperative cardiac risk. [Review] *British Journal of Anaesthesia*, **92**, 570–83.

Spahn D, Priebe H-J. (2004). Preoperative hypertension: remain wary? 'Yes' – cancel surgery? 'No'. *British Medical Journal*, **92**, 461–4.

The Royal College of Anaesthetists and The Royal College of Ophthalmologists. (2001). Local Anaesthesia for Intraocular Surgery. www.rcoa.ac.uk/docs/rcarcoguidelines.pdf.

Williams B, Poulter N, Morris J *et al.* (2004). British Hypertension Society guidelines for hypertension management 2004 (BHS-IV): summary. *British Medical Journal*, **328**, 634–40.

ICU neuropathy

What are the causes of muscle weakness in critically ill patients?

> This could bring up an enormous list of the various causes and it helps to think for a few moments to try and categorize the main areas for discussion. The examiners will use this opening question to close down in more detail on one or two subjects they wish to discuss.

A suitable classification might be:

- **Pre-existing medical conditions**
  - Guillain–Barré syndrome
  - Myasthenia gravis
  - CNS lesions, e.g. trauma, polio, MND
- **Drug related** Muscle relaxants
  - Aminoglycosides (may interfere with neuromuscular transmission)
  - Magnesium (in pre-eclampsia)
  - Steroids (typically proximal weakness/wasting)
  - Poisoning, e.g. botulinum toxin, organophosphates
- **Metabolic** Hypokalaemia
  - Hypophosphataemia
- **Myopathy** (acquired)
  - Immobilization, disuse atrophy
  - Malnutrition, leading to muscle wasting and weakness. A paper in the *BMJ* in 1994 showed that up to 40% of patients (not ICU) are undernourished at presentation and that there is an average loss of 5.4% body weight in hospital. Therefore, ICU patients are often malnourished and catabolic.
  - Protein turnover is increased secondary to surgery, trauma and critical illness.
  - Necrotising myopathy
  - Critical illness myopathy (CIM)
- **Critical illness neuropathy**

Tell me a bit more about critical illness neuropathy.

- This is an acquired neuropathy **commonly** found in association with severe sepsis and multiple organ failure, increasing in frequency with prolonged ICU stay and sepsis.
- The problem affects more than half of adult patients admitted to general ICUs for more than 1 week and more than 70% of those with sepsis and multiorgan failure.
- It has been recognized as a clinical entity since 1983 when described by Bolton *et al.*
- The cause remains unknown and there is no specific treatment.
- Clinically, there is a flaccid weakness with absent/reduced tendon reflexes and muscle wasting.

- The condition has various names:
  - Critical illness polyneuropathy (CIP)
  - Critical illness myopathy (CIM)
  - Acute necrotizing myopathy of intensive care
  - Acute quadriplegic myopathy
  - Critical illness neuromuscular disease
  - Critical illness neuromyopathy
  - Critical illness polyneuromyopathy,
  - ICU-acquired paresis
  - Quadriplegic and areflexic ICU illness.
- Neuromuscular weakness typically presents when attempting to wean the patient from the ventilator. Earlier diagnostic clues may be a relative lack of movement after regaining consciousness and/or the loss of deep tendon reflexes.
- Other diagnoses should be considered, although most cases will be due to **critical illness polyneuromyopathy**.
  - Spinal cord disease should be excluded, West Nile virus infection, acute disseminated encephalomyelitis, etc.
  - A neuromuscular transmission defect (e.g. NMBs, unrecognized myasthenia gravis).
  - Porphyria and recurrent chronic inflammatory demyelinating polyneuropathy.
- Differentiating the most common causes of ICU-acquired generalized weakness (myopathy, neuropathy, or a combination of the two), is useful because they have differing prognoses. Electromyography is helpful in differentiating CIP from CIM. An elevated serum creatine kinase may help to identify CIM. Muscle biopsy can address the relative contribution of myopathy to the picture because the neuropathy can be adequately assessed electrophysiologically (nerve conduction studies). CSF protein levels are normal (cf. Guillain–Barré).
- The prognosis for recovery from a **CIM** is more favourable, most patients recovering fully within 1–3 months.
- Patients with widespread muscle necrosis may recover incompletely.
- Patients with **CIP** recover slowly because the axons regenerate at 1 mm/day. This takes many months and recovery is often incomplete Evidence of polyneuropathy is apparent after 5 years in over 90% of CIP patients.

Bibliography
Bolton CF, Brown JD, Sibbald WJ. (1983). The electrophysiological investigation of respiratory paralysis in critically ill patients. *Neurology*, **33**(suppl), 186.

Young GB, Hammond RR. (2004). A stronger approach to weakness in the intensive care unit. *Critical Care*, **8**(6), 416–18.

ICU nutrition

Why is nutritional support important in ICU patients?

A significant number of patients admitted to hospital are malnourished, up to 40% according to McWhirter. The majority of patients that are admitted to intensive care are catabolic and will have had a preceding period of starvation due to their surgery or underlying pathology.

> **Complications of poor nutritional support**
>
> ■ Impaired wound healing
> ■ Reduced muscle bulk/strength and delayed mobilisation
> ■ Increased incidence of respiratory infection
> ■ Problems with weaning from mechanical ventilation

How can you make an assessment of a patient's nutritional status on ICU?

There are **objective markers** that can be used in the assessment of *malnutrition*, but many of these are flawed when faced with a patient with multiorgan failure on intensive care. There are **other methods** that are more clinically orientated.

Traditional objective assessment tools
■ Triceps skinfold thickness
■ Hand grip tests
■ Serum albumin ($t_{1/2}$ 14–20 days)
■ Serum prealbumin ($t_{1/2}$ 24–48 hours)
■ Serum transferrin
■ Total iron-binding capacity
■ Lymphocyte count

These are relatively insensitive and non-specific markers, e.g. albumin affected by trauma, sepsis and excess extracellular water.

Other methods
■ Subjective global assessment (SGA) – history and physical factors
■ Hill and Windsor (bedside nutritional assessment)

Lean body mass assessment – experimental methods
■ Bioimpedence
■ Measuring total body water or potassium
■ Neutron activation
■ Muscle biopsy to measure muscle fibre area

These methods are similarly difficult to interpret in a critical care setting. A nutritional history should be elicited (including normal weight and recent food intake) and there are formulae to derive ideal body mass and daily calorific requirements.

This question initially seems difficult to answer (as rarely formally done on ICU).

Your answer should emphasise that a detailed history and examination are still the mainstay of nutritional assessment.

However, you will need to be aware of the tests available.

Be wary of starting your answer with a negative comment about how difficult it is to assess nutritional status on ICU – perhaps mention this at the end, with the reasons why.

What routes can be used for nutritional support?

Nutrition can be provided either by:

- **Enteral feeding** Can be given by **nasogastric, nasojejunal or percutaneous gastrostomy/jejunostomy** tubes. Post-pyloric feeding is becoming more popular as gastric atony can be a problem in critically ill patients Side effects: diarrhoea, aspiration.
- **Parenteral feeding** Often through a dedicated central venous catheter, although peripheral polyurethane catheters or peripherally inserted central catheters (PICC) can be used.

Some enteral feeding guidance

- 'Underfeeding' may provide a protective safety barrier (33%–65% of calculated feed received led to less mortality than >65% of feed received).
- NICE recommend that, for the first 48 hours, parental nutrition should be <50% of calculated requirement.
- Nurse head-up 45%.
- Accept gastric residual volumes of 200–250 ml.
- Early use of prokinetics

What problems are associated with parenteral nutrition?

- Central venous catheter Complications related to insertion
  Catheter-related sepsis
  Displacement
  Occlusion / thrombosis
- Metabolic Hypo/**hyper**glycaemia
  Metabolic acidosis
  Potassium, sodium and phosphate imbalance
  Excess CO_2 production
  Hypercholesterolaemia/hypertriglyceridaemia

	Essential fatty acid/vitamins / trace element deficiencies
■ Intestinal	TPN fails to reverse intestinal villous atrophy and bacterial translocation can occur
■ Hepatobiliary	Abnormal liver function tests. This is multifactorial
■ Refeeding syndrome	↑Glu, ↓MgSO$_4$, ↓K$^+$, ↓PO$_4$ seen when refeeding malnourished patients

What are the advantages of enteral nutrition?

■ More physiological route for digestion and absorption
■ Prevents mucosal atrophy – intestinal enterocytes receive a proportion of their own nutrition directly from the gut lumen and enteral nutrition helps maintain mucosal blood flow
■ Supports the normal gut flora
■ Reduction of bacterial translocation → ↓ **risk of sepsis**
■ Fewer metabolic complications
■ No catheter-associated complications of TPN – in particular, the risk of central line sepsis.

What can you tell me about immunomodulation and feeding?

Critically ill patients have impaired gastrointestinal function (↓motility, ↓secretions, mucosal atrophy, altered flora → ↑ bacterial translocation) secondary to an acute phase response. Increased bacterial translocation is associated with an increased risk of sepsis. To reduce this, there has been interest in dietary components with immunomodulatory properties. Caution should be used in extrapolating the results of studies in particular groups of patients (e.g. head injuries) to other ICU patient groups.

■ **Glutamine**	The most abundant amino acid in the body. Fuel for enterocytes and some lymphoid cells. Precursor of glutathione (anti-oxidant). Becomes a *conditionally* essential amino acid in critical illness. **Can significantly reduce mortality and length of stay.**
■ **Arginine**	Promotes T-cell proliferation, macrophage and natural killer cell function. Beneficial in cancer patients and elective general surgical patients. Role in nitric oxide formation. May actually cause harm in the critically ill.
■ **Taurine**	Becomes a *conditionally* essential amino acid in critical illness. Anti-oxidant Modulates inflammatory cytokines.

- ▪ **Omega-3 fatty acids**   Anti-inflammatory activity via prostaglandin.
- ▪ **Ribonucleotides**   Promote protein synthesis.
- ▪ **Anti-oxidants**   Selenium probably offers most benefit (if any).
- ▪ **Trace elements**

Typical daily nutritional requirements:

Water	30 ml/kg
Na+	1.2 mmol/kg
K+	0.8 mmol/kg
Calories	30 kcal/kg
Protein	0.25 g nitrogen/kg
	(10 g nitrogen ~ 60 g protein)
Fat	2 g/kg
Glucose	2 g/kg

Bibliography
Edmonson WC. (2007). Nutritional support in critical care: an update. *Continuing Education in Anaesthesia, Critical Care and Pain*, **7**(6), 199–202.
Lalwani K. (1997). Current aspects of parenteral nutrition. *Anaesthesia Review*, **13**, 201–21. Edinburgh, UK: Churchill Livingstone.

ICU stress ulceration

Can you tell me something about the pathophysiology of stress ulcers in intensive care patients.

Stress ulceration in intensive care patients is relatively common (approaching 90% by day 3 with no prophylaxis), although the incidence of clinically important gastrointestinal bleeding is less than 2%.

There are six major risk factors:

- ▪ Respiratory failure requiring ventilation for >48 hours
- ▪ Coagulopathy
- ▪ Sepsis
- ▪ Hypotension
- ▪ Hepatic failure
- ▪ Renal failure

The normal mechanisms that aim to ensure an intact mucosal barrier to protect the gastric epithelium come under attack in the critically ill patient.

- ▪ Mucus production is reduced from surface mucous cells.
- ▪ Mucosal blood flow is impaired.

■ Mucosal prostaglandin production is reduced and these (especially PGE2) are involved in the regulation of gastric acid secretion by parietal cells. Prostaglandins normally inhibit acid secretion by activating Gi, thereby reducing adenylyl cyclase activity and cAMP production. CyclicAMP in turn regulates H^+ transport via protein kinases and H^+K^+ATPase.

■ Other factors may include increased gastrin production, acid-base abnormalities and reflux of bile.

■ The result is an imbalance between acid secretion and normal protective mucus production. It should be noted that **impaired mucosal blood flow and resultant mucosal ischaemia seem to be a major factor in critically ill patients**.

Two types of ulcer are classically eponymised:

■ Curling's ulcers   associated with extensive burns
■ Cushing's ulcers   associated with intracranial pathology and gastric acid hypersecretion.

■ Ranitidine and sucralfate are the most effective agents. Ranitidine is associated with a lower incidence of clinically significant bleeding, sucralfate with a lower incidence of pneumonia.

■ Nosocomial pneumonia is the main complication of ulcer prophylaxis treatment.

What measures have been employed to try and reduce the incidence of stress ulcers?

Adequate resuscitation is the main priority with **maximal oxygen transport to the gastric mucosa**. Attention should be paid to optimising cardiovascular variables and ensuring adequate gas exchange.

Other methods are used for stress ulcer prophylaxis:

■ **Enteral feeding**

■ **Sulcralfate**	This is an aluminium salt of sulphated sucrose and is given in a dose of 1g by NG tube, 6-hourly. It forms a paste at low pH, which preferentially binds to areas of peptic ulceration, thereby providing a physical barrier to the effects of acid. Some investigators have demonstrated a reduction in the rate of nosocomial pneumonias in patients treated with sulcralfate.
■ **Antacids and H₂-antagonists**	These are the more traditional drugs used for stress ulcer prophylaxis and may effectively reduce the risk of bleeding. There is, however, some concern that, by increasing the pH of gastric contents, there is an increased risk of bacterial colonisation and subsequent nosocomial pneumonia.

Proton pump inhibitors Some recent studies suggest that PPIs are effective stress ulcer prophylaxis, but despite limited data they are becoming first-line in many ICUs.

The meta-analysis by Messori *et al.* suggests that ranitidine is **ineffective** in the prevention of gastrointestinal bleeding in ICU patients and may increase the risk of pneumonia. The evidence for the use of sucralfate remains inconclusive.

Bibliography

Cook DJ, Fuller HD, Guyatt GH. et al. (1994). Risk factors for gastrointestinal bleeding in critically ill patients. *New England Journal of Medicine*, **330**, 377–81.

Daley RJ. (2004). *Critical Care Medicine*, **32**(10), 2008–13.

Eddleston JM, Vohra A, Scott P. et al. (1991). A comparison of the frequency of stress ulceration and secondary pneumonia in sulcralfate- or ranitidine-treated intensive care unit patients. *Critical Care Medicine*, **19**, 1491–6.

Eddleston JM, Pearson RC, Holland J, Tooth JA, Vohra A, Doran BH. (1994). Prospective endoscopic study of stress erosions and ulcers in critically ill adult patients treated with either sucralfate or placebo. *Critical Care Medicine*, **22**, 1949–54.

Messori A, Trippoli S, Vaiani M, Gorini M, Corrado A. (2000). Bleeding and pneumonia in intensive care patients given ranitidine and sucralfate for prevention of stress ulcer: meta-analysis of randomised controlled trials. *British Medical Journal*, **321**(7269), 1103–6.

Tryba M, Cook D. (1996). Current guidelines on stress ulcer prophylaxis. *Drugs*, **54**(4), 581–96.

Infantile pyloric stenosis

You are asked to anaesthetise a 4 kg, 5-week-old boy for pyloromyotomy for pyloric stenosis. Blood gases reveal the following findings pH 7.53, PCO_2 5.3, BE +10, HCO_3^- 32.7

Tell me about this condition? What is the incidence and sex distribution?

- Infantile pyloric stenosis is the most common surgical condition presenting in the first 6 months of life.
- It has an incidence of approximately 3 per 1000.
- The aetiology is not fully understood. However, genetic factors are thought to be involved with a higher incidence seen in the offspring of affected individuals.
- Males are affected four times as frequently as females and Caucasians are more frequently affected than black or Asian infants.

Do you know anything about the pathology of this condition?

Yes. Hypertrophy of the circular pyloric muscle with spasm causes gastric outflow obstruction. There are multiple theories on the pathogenesis of pyloric stenosis but **reduced or immature innervation** (particularly cholinergic) and **reduced neuronal nitric oxide synthase activity** are thought to play a role in producing hypertrophy and spasm.

How does the condition present?

- Presentation usually occurs between the third and fourth week of life but may be earlier or later.
- Progressive, non-bilious, projectile vomiting is the classical presenting complaint.
- Associated hunger but failure to thrive.
- Dehydration will develop if the child is not treated and mild jaundice may be present (due to starvation).
- Examination may reveal a firm 'olive'-like tumour in the right hypochondrium, particularly after vomiting, though this is becoming less common with earlier diagnosis.
- Diagnosis is now most frequently confirmed with ultrasound.

6%–20% will have an additional abnormality. These may be gastrointestinal such as oesophageal atresia, Hirschprung's disease, malrotation, anorectal anomalies or cardiac abnormalities.

How would you assess the degree of dehydration?

Dehydration may be defined as mild (<5% dehydrated), moderate (5%–10%), or severe (>10%) based on the clinical findings.

Signs	Mild <5%	Moderate 5%–10%	Severe >10%
Decreased UO	+	+	+
Dry mucosa	+/−	+	+
Decreased skin turgor	−	+/−	+
Prolonged cap refill	−	+/−	+
Tachypneoa	−	+/−	+
Tachycardia	−	+/−	+

Fluid deficit in mls = Wt × % dehydration × 10

Tell me about the biochemical abnormalities you may expect in this baby.

The classic biochemical abnormality is **hypochloraemic alkalosis** with hyponatraemia and hypokalaemia. Gastric secretions consisting of gastric acid (HCl), water, sodium and potassium are lost through vomiting. HCO_3^- produced during gastric acid synthesis is retained and produces progressive alkalosis. Initially the rising HCO_3^- may overwhelm renal resorptive capacity and alkaline urine will be produced. However, as hyponatraemia and dehydration develop, **hydrogen ions are lost in exchange for sodium producing paradoxical aciduria**. Gastric potassium loss combined with renal exchange for sodium and intracellular shift caused by alkalosis produce hypokalaemia. Severe dehydration with lactic acidosis and ketosis from starvation may produce a degree of reversal of the alkalosis.

Would you anaesthetise this child now?

No! The case is urgent but not an emergency. Correction of dehydration and biochemical abnormalities should be performed before surgery. A nasogastric tube should be inserted and significant dehydration treated with i.v. fluid boluses (20 ml/kg normal saline or colloid). Multiple fluid correction regimens exist but must include sodium chloride, potassium, glucose and adequate water. The resuscitation goals should include restoration of circulating volume with urine output >1 ml/kg per hour and normalisation of biochemistry (i.e. Cl >106, Na >135, $HCO_3^- <26$, and normal pH and BE. The high-normal chloride is required to ensure correction of the alkalaemia).

What factors must be considered when anaesthetising this infant?

The anaesthetic issues may be divided into those specific to this condition and those general to anaesthetising neonates and infants.
In addition to the pre-operative measures above, the patient should be protected from aspiration. This may be achieved by aspiration of the NG tube with the patient in three or four positions (supine, lateral, and prone). A rapid sequence induction will offer the safest protection against aspiration.
However, inhalational induction, intravenous induction with non-depolarising neuromuscular blockade and awake intubation have all been described in the literature.
General issues for neonates include:

- Different airway anatomy.
- Use of uncuffed and correctly sized endotracheal tubes (3.5 mm ID with a size each side available).
- Meticulous calculation of correct fluid and drug doses.
- Limited cardio-respiratory reserve with rapid development of hypoxia (low FRC, high BMR).
- Risk of bradycardia (immature sympathetic innervation).
- Increased heat loss (high surface area to weight ratio).
- Increased susceptibility to induction agents and opioids.
- Post-operative risk of apnoeas and hypoglycaemia.

Bibliography
Buss PW, McCabe M, Evans RJ. (1997). *Advanced Paediatric Life Support*. London, UK: BMJ Books.
Fell D, Chelliah S. (2001). Infantile pyloric stenosis. *British Journal of Anaesthesia, CEPD Reviews*, 1(3), 85–8.
Hernanz-Schulman M. (2003). Infantile pyloric stenosis. *Radiology*, **227**(2), 319–31.
Hulka F, Campbell TJ, Campbell JR *et al*. (1997). Evolution in the recognition of infantile hypertrophic pyloric stenosis. *Pediatrics*, **100**(2), E9.
Ohshiro K, Puri P. (1998). Pathogenesis of infantile hypertrophic pyloric stenosis: recent progress. *Pediatric Surgery International*, **13**(4), 243–52.

Inhaled peanut

A 3-year-old boy has been admitted to casualty having inhaled a peanut 1 hour ago. You have been asked to assess him.

What are the symptoms of foreign body aspiration in a child?

There may be cough, choking, gagging and dyspnoea. If the obstruction persists, the airway reflexes become fatigued resulting in an 'asymptomatic period'. Presentation after this time may be associated with airway erosion or infection. Peanuts can cause problems related to obstruction of the airway or secondary to the oil causing an inflammatory reaction.

What clinical signs would you look for?

- **Non-specific** signs of distress – tachycardia, tachypnoea and sweating
- Use of **accessory muscles** of respiration, **'tripod'** position
- Audible wheeze and stridor
- Examination of the chest may reveal **unilateral signs** such as increased percussion due to air trapping, wheeze and mediastinal shift or signs of lobar collapse. There may also be bronchial breathing and crackles depending on the duration of obstruction.

How would you manage the case?

Immediate assessment and initial management would follow the ABC principle. The need to intervene immediately is then determined. Most foreign body aspirations can wait until a suitable starvation time has elapsed providing the child is not too distressed. Dried beans or peas may require early intervention as they will expand with time.

Nebulised adrenaline (1:1000 solution at 0.5 ml/kg, max 5 ml) could be used as a holding measure to help reduce airway oedema (α effect). Heliox is also an option.

How would you anaesthetise this child having starved him?

- Consultant help should be available.
- Calm environment
- Insertion of a cannula prior to induction would be ideal, but may be determined by likelihood of causing more distress to the child.
- An **inhalational induction** with **sevoflurane in 100% oxygen** followed by endotracheal intubation to secure the airway would be appropriate.
- The **surgeon should be on hand**
- ET tube may then be replaced with a **Storz ventilating bronchoscope**. A T-piece can then be connected to the side arm of the bronchoscope. A muscle relaxant may be used if necessary and lignocaine could be used to anaesthetise the airway.

- In principle, positive pressure ventilation should be avoided until the peanut has been removed but it may be necessary if the bronchoscope lumen is narrow and the procedure is long.

Why don't you want to use halothane?

Halothane has advantages and disadvantages over sevoflurane.

Advantages	More potent.
	Can achieve higher inhaled concentrations with halothane vaporiser (5 × MAC) compared with sevoflurane vaporiser (3 × MAC) – may make it easier to intubate without relaxant
	Less likely to lighten quickly resulting in laryngospasm.
Disadvantages	Longer time in stage two anaesthesia.
	Slower onset than sevoflurane and slower return of airway reflexes.
	Arrhythmias in children with hypoxaemia and hypercarbia.

Bibliography

Hagberg CA. (2000). *Handbook of Difficult Airway Management*, Churchill Livingstone.

Hatch DJ. (1999). New inhalation agents in paediatric anaesthesia, *British Journal of Anaesthesia*, 83(1), 42–9.

Mather S, Hughes D. (1996). *A Handbook of Paediatric Anaesthesia, 2nd Edition*. Oxford Medical Publications.

Morton NS. (1999). Large airway obstruction in children. Parts 1 and 2. *CME core topic, RCA Newsletter*.

Intracranial pressure

What is normal intracranial pressure?

- Around 10 mmHg or less
- Sustained pressure of >15 mmHg is termed 'intracranial hypertension'
- Areas of focal ischaemia if ICP > 20
- Global ischaemia if ICP > 50
- Treatment usually considered if ICP > 20

Cerebral perfusion pressure:

$$CPP = MAP - ICP (or\ CVP\ if\ greater)$$

- Normal CPP = 80–100 mmHg.
- Remember that adequate tissue perfusion is not just a function of CPP but depends on blood flow and oxygen content.

What are the causes of raised intracranial pressure?

According to the **Munro–Kelly hypothesis** (1852) the contents of the cranium are not compressible. Any significant increase in the volume of brain tissue, blood or CSF within the cranium will lead to a rapid rise in intracranial pressure (ICP).

The causes of raised ICP may therefore be divided into three broad categories:

- **Brain**   Tumours
  - Infection/abscess
  - Oedema – three types: vasogenic, cytotoxic, interstitial
- **Blood**   Extradural
  - Subdural
  - Intracerebral
  - Subarachnoid
  - Venous congestion (e.g. cavernous sinus thrombosis)
- **CSF**   Outflow obstruction, e.g. SAH, meningitis, tumours
  - Increased production – choroid plexus papilloma (extremely rare !)
  - Benign intracranial hypertension (usually young, obese women).

What are the symptoms and signs of raised intracranial pressure?

- **Symptoms** Headache
  - Vomiting
  - Drowsiness
  - Confusion
  - Neck stiffness
  - Seizures
- **Signs**   Depressed GCS
  - Papilloedema (late sign)
  - Cushing reflex (hypertension and bradycardia)
  - Irregular respirations
  - Seizures
  - Hemiparesis
  - IV cranial nerve palsy (false localising sign due to long intracranial course)
  - III cranial nerve palsy due to tentorial coning
- **Coning** Two major types:
  1. **Tentorial** – part of the temporal lobe compresses the brainstem on the contralateral side. This results in an ipsilateral IIIn palsy, decreased GCS, Cushing reflex and decerebrate rigidity.
  2. **Cerebellar**- the medulla is compressed by the cerebellar tonsils passing through the foramen magnum resulting in Cheyne–Stokes breathing, sudden apnoea and neck stiffness.

What are the indications for ICP monitoring following head injury?

Some suggested indications include:

■ **GCS<8 with an abnormal CT scan**
■ Normal CT scan but two or more of the following factors
    Age >40
    Hypotension
    Unilateral posturing
    Bilateral posturing

How can you measure intracranial pressure clinically?

There are four methods commonly used via the skull and a lumbar approach via a CSF catheter.

1. Epidural catheter	Strain gauge transducer at tip or fibre-optically supplied light reflecting off a pressure-sensitive membrane
2. Subdural bolt or catheter	Prone to blocking and leak but less risk of infection than ventricular catheter
3. Ventricular catheter	Gold standard, accurate, CSF can be drained but risk of infection
4. Intraparenchymal catheter	Light reflecting pressure-sensitive membrane

The appropriate monitor will display the ICP and a waveform.

Lundberg waves:

A-waves Sustained pressure waves (60–80 mmHg) every 5–20 minutes
Life-threatening and represent cerebral vasodilatation in response to ↓ CPP. Need urgent treatment.
B-waves Small and short lasting waves (10–20 mmHg) every 30–120 seconds. Caused by fluctuations in CBV.
C-waves Small oscillations (0–10 mmHg), reflect changes in systemic arterial pressure.

Bibliography
Deakin CD. (1998). *Clinical Notes for the FRCA*. Churchill Livingstone.
Hodgkinson V, Mahajan RP. (2000). The management of raised intracranial pressure. *RCA Bulletin 1*.
Morgan GE, Mikhail MS. (1996). *Clinical Anaesthesiology*, 2nd Edition. Appleton and Lange.
Stone DJ, Sperry RJ, Johnson JO, Spiekermann BF, Yemen TA. (1996). *The Neuroanaesthesia Handbook*. St Louis, USA: Mosby.

Ischaemic heart disease

Tell me about the principles of anaesthetising a patient with ischaemic heart disease (IHD).

> This is a question about myocardial oxygen supply and demand. You must relate the physiology to clinical practice.

The over-riding principle is to **avoid cardiac ischaemia** by ensuring that supply of oxygen to the myocardium always meets demand.

Supply

$$\text{Supply of oxygen} = \text{Blood flow} \times \text{Oxygen content}$$

Blood flow is determined by:

- **Heart rate** determines coronary blood flow because diastole shortens with increasing heart rate.
- **Aortic pressure** (particularly diastolic)
- **Extravascular compression** of the coronary arteries (by a contracting ventricle). Blood flow in the coronary arteries is therefore greater in diastole. Compression during systole is greatest at the endocardium and this explains why this area is particularly susceptible to ischaemia. Blood flow in the left coronary artery may be reversed during systole.
- **Neurohumoral factors.** These are not of great importance. Autonomic nerve stimulation causes coronary vasoconstriction but this is offset by the vasodilatation that accompanies an increase in the myocardial metabolism.
- **Metabolic factors.** Coronary blood flow closely parallels myocardial metabolic activity.

Oxygen content is determined by:

- Haemoglobin concentration (but this alters viscosity and therefore blood flow!).
- SaO_2
- PaO_2

$$\text{Oxygen content} = (1.34\,\text{ml of}\,O_2 \times \text{Hb}\,\text{g/dl} \times \%SaO_2) + (0.003 \times PaO_2)$$

Demand

Determinants of myocardial oxygen demand are:
- **Preload**, which determines LVEDP ⎤ Remember Laplace's law
- **Afterload** ⎦
- **Heart rate**
- **Contractility**
  In clinical practice this means avoiding:

- **Hypoxia!**
- **Hypotension** – especially diastolic
- **Hypertension** – because it causes increased myocardial wall tension and thus further extravascular compression. It should be noted that pressure work increases myocardial O_2 consumption much more than volume work (increasing cardiac output) so hypertension must be avoided.
- **Tachycardia** – shortened diastole
- **Stimulation of the autonomic nervous system**

A patient with ischaemic heart disease should be monitored for signs of ischaemia so that treatment can be instituted.

Monitoring options include:

■ **CMV5**   Leads II and V5 together detect 95% of ischaemic events.
■ **PAFC**
■ **TOE**
■ **Arterial line**   To detect hypotension quickly

What are the 'risk periods' during anaesthesia for patients with IHD?

The 'risk periods' are those times during the anaesthetic when the patient is more likely to develop **hypotension, hypertension and tachycardia.**

■ **Anxiety** pre-operatively causes hypertension and tachycardia.
■ **Induction** can cause hypotension.
■ **Laryngoscopy** and **intubation** can cause hypertension and tachycardia as can:
■ **Surgical incision**
■ **Extubation**
■ **Pain** post-operatively
■ **Hypoxia** is frequently responsible for ischaemic cardiac events post-operatively.

Do you know any ways of modifying these responses?

■ Pre-medication with anxiolytics, oxygen and usual cardiovascular medication
■ **Beta-blockers** – in the last couple of decades there has been huge interest in peri-operative beta-blockade and trying to reduce peri-operative cardiac events. Several papers in the late 1990s demonstrated a beneficial effect from beta-blockade, e.g. Wallace et al showed that peri-operative atenolol for 1 week in patients at high risk for coronary artery disease significantly reduced the incidence of post-operative myocardial ischaemia and this reduced risk of death lasted for as long as 2 years after surgery. More recent evidence, however, has given grounds for less enthusiasm.
■ Nitrates to induce coronary vasodilatation.
■ Caution with induction agents to avoid significant hypotension. An arterial line prior to induction ensures continuous monitoring of the blood pressure.
■ Opioid-based anaesthetic technique.
■ Lignocaine spray to the cords (prior to intubation and extubation)
■ Use of neuroaxial blocks (prevents stress response but beware hypotension)
■ Post-operative oxygen

> **β-Blockers – current evidence**
>
> ■ ***Recommendations for beta-blocker medical therapy*** **from ACC/AHA**

Class I

■ Beta-blockers should be continued in patients undergoing surgery who are receiving beta-blockers to treat angina, symptomatic arrhythmias, hypertension, or other ACC/AHA Class I guideline indications.

■ Beta-blockers should be given to patients undergoing vascular surgery who are at high cardiac risk owing to the finding of ischaemia on pre-operative testing.

Class IIa

■ Beta-blockers are probably recommended for patients undergoing vascular surgery in whom pre-operative assessment identifies coronary heart disease.

■ Beta-blockers are probably recommended for patients in whom pre-operative assessment for vascular surgery identifies high cardiac risk, as defined by the presence of more than one clinical risk factor.

■ Beta-blockers are probably recommended for patients in whom pre-operative assessment identifies coronary heart disease or high cardiac risk, as defined by the presence of more than one clinical risk factor, who are undergoing intermediate-risk or vascular surgery.

  ● *However...*

■ The large **POISE study** (2008) has added some caution in that, although the treatment arm (metoprolol) had less cardiac events, the overall mortality was significantly higher as a result of more strokes, probably due to hypotension.

■ Beta-blockers are no longer first-line treatment for hypertension unless it is associated with coronary heart disease.

How do you assess cardiac risk?

■ **History** and **examination** to identify risk factors.
■ Plan appropriate intervention to reduce risk and improve outcome.
■ **Investigations:** the history may dictate the need for some assessment of functional capacity

ECG	Arrhythmias predict peri-operative cardiac events
Exercise ECG	Negative test correlates with low-risk
Dobutamine stress echo	Can detect silent ischaemia
Ambulatory ECG	
Echocardiogram	Questionable value as a predictor of post-operative cardiac events
Thallium scan	(with dipyridamole)
	Behaves like K^+
	Shows 'cold' spots
	No predictive value in most studies

MUGA scan	Using technetium-99m
	Not of prognostic value
Coronary angiography	Expensive but useful
	Decrease in mortality rate afforded by
	CABG negated by risks of procedure itself

■ **Scoring systems**
- **Goldman** was one of the first (1977) nine factors. Max score = 53
- **Detsky** (1986) – additional factors to Goldman: MI at any time, unstable angina within 6 months, CCS angina Class III and IV, pulmonary oedema. Max score = 120.
- The **Revised Cardiac Risk Index** is now widely used

> Please see Long Case 20 'The one about pre-op assessment of IHD'

Goldman Index of Cardiac Risk in non-cardiac surgery

M.I. <6 months		10
Age >70 years		5
S3 or raised JVP		11
Important aortic stenosis		3
Rhythm other than sinus		7
>5 VPBs per minute pre-op		7
Poor general medical state		3
-pO$_2$	<8 kPa	
-pCO$_2$	>6.7 kPa	
K+	<3.0 mmol/l	
HCO$_3$-	<20 mmol/l	
Urea	>18 mmol/l	
Creatinine	>260 μmol/l	
Chronic liver disease		
Bedridden		
Intraperitoneal, intrathoracic		
Or aortic surgery		3
Emergency operation		4
Total		53

		Risk of cardiac death (%)
Class I	<5 points	0.2
Class IV	>25 points	56

Bibliography

Berne RM, Levy MN. (1997). *Cardiovascular Physiology*, 7th Edition. Mosby.

Deakin CD. (1998). *Clinical Notes for the FRCA*. Churchill Livingstone.

Fleisher LA, ACC/AHA. (2007). Guidelines on Perioperative Cardiovascular Evaluation and Care for Noncardiac Surgery. http://www.acc.org/clinical/perio/dirIndex.htm.

Juste RN, Lawson AD, Soni N. (1996). Minimising cardiac anaesthetic risk: the tortoise or the hare? *Anaesthesia*, **51**, 255–62.

Mangano DT. (1999). Assessment of the patient with cardiac disease – an anaesthesiologist's paradigm. *Anaesthesiology*, **91**, 1521–6.

Sear JW, Giles JW, Howard-Alpe G, Foëx P. (2008). Perioperative beta-blockade, What does POISE tell us, and was our earlier caution justified? *British Journal of Anaesthesia*, **101**(2), 135–7.

Wallace A, Layug B, Taleo I et al. (1998). Prophylactic atenolol reduces postoperative myocardial ischemia. *Anesthesiology*, **88**(1), 7–17.

IVRA for Dupuytrens contracture and LA toxicity

You are anaesthetising for a list that includes a 60-year-old man for superficial forearm surgery to be done under intravenous regional anaesthesia (Biers block).

How would you proceed?

- It is important to check with the patient and the surgeon the exact nature of the surgery as intravenous regional anaesthesia (IVRA) is mainly suitable for skin surface surgery and the **effect reliably lasts for about 30 minutes**.
- The patient should be assessed and prepared as for any other anaesthetic (although there is no evidence to suggest that the patient comes to any harm by not being fasted as the incidence of complications is so rare).
- Suitable IV access (usually 20G) is obtained both in the operative arm distal to the cuff and in the non-operative arm.
- Establish routine monitoring.
- A **double-cuffed tourniquet** is applied to the upper arm of the operative limb.
- An Eschmark bandage or elevation is used to **exsanguinate the limb**.
- The distal then the proximal cuffs are inflated to 100mmHg above the systolic BP.
- Inject a dilute solution of local anaesthetic and wait 10–15 minutes for the block to take effect.

What local anaesthetic would you use?

- Usually **prilocaine 0.5%**, 40–60 ml depending on the size of the arm (max dose 6 mg/kg).
- Prilocaine is an amide local anaesthetic, which has less protein binding than others and has the advantage that it is more rapidly metabolized (hepatic and extra-hepatic) and hence **less toxic**.
- Prilocaine is closely related to lidocaine and is very similar in its clinical action. It can cause **methaemoglobinaemia** when used in high dosage

(>600 mg) – this is usually benign and resolves within a couple of hours. The **treatment is methylene blue** 1 mg/kg i.v. over 5 minutes.

■ Lidocaine 0.5% up to a maximum dose of 3 mg/kg is an alternative.

What would you do if the patient complains of cuff pain?

■ It is possible to deflate the distal cuff for a few minutes leaving the upper proximal cuff inflated, and then inflate the distal cuff again over the now anaesthetised skin.

■ The upper proximal cuff can then be deflated.

■ This does remove the safety feature of the double cuff.

■ As some of the anaesthetic effects and discomfort are probably caused by ischaemic neuropraxia, this may not solve the problem of cuff discomfort.

What precautions do you take to avoid systemic toxicity?

■ The double cuff remains inflated for a minimum of 15 minutes for prilocaine or 20 minutes with lidocaine (which takes longer to metabolise and 'fix' to the tissues).

■ There are strict maximum doses which should not be exceeded. Secure i.v. access and monitoring is mandatory prior to the injection of large doses of local anaesthetic. Full resuscitation equipment must be immediately available.

If the cuff leaks, what symptoms and signs would you expect to see?

■ Systemic toxic effects due to local anaesthetic overdose primarily involve the central nervous and cardiovascular systems.

■ In general, the CNS is more sensitive to local anaesthetics than the CVS, so CNS manifestations tend to occur earlier.

■ Brain excitatory effects occur before the depressant effects.

■ Usually about 4–7 times the convulsant dose needs to be injected before cardiovascular collapse occurs.

■ **Bupivacaine is more cardiotoxic** than lidocaine, which is why it is not used for IVRA.

CNS symptoms and signs include the following:

■ Perioral + tongue paraesthesia
■ Metallic taste
■ Dizziness
■ Slurred speech
■ Diplopia
■ Tinnitus
■ Confusion
■ Restlessness
■ Muscle twitching
■ Convulsions/coma

CVS symptoms result from progressive sodium channel blockade with the eventual formation of re-enterant tachycardias:

- Bradycardia
- Prolonged PR interval
- Widened QRS
- Progressive conduction blockade
- Re-enterant tachycardias
- VF

Do you know of a specific antidote to LA toxicity?

Intralipid® has been used successfully to restore electrical activity after the failure of conventional resuscitation in cardiac arrests. It has been reported in case reports as a successful therapy during prolonged cardiac arrest following local anaesthetic blocks and toxicity. An initial bolus of 1.5 ml/kg of 20% intralipid is followed by an infusion of 0.25 ml/kg per minute with additional boluses if required. In 2007, The AAGBI published guidelines for the management of severe local anaesthetic toxicity. These include the possible use of cardiopulmonary bypass and lipid emulsion.

Bibliography

Ahmad M, Saynor G. (2005). Fasting before prilocaine Biers' block. *Emergency Medicine Journal*, **22**, 558–9.

Picard J, Meek T. (2006). Lipid emulsion to treat overdose of local anaesthetic: the gift of the glob. *Anaesthesia*, **61**(2), 107–9.

The Association of Anaesthetists of Great Britain and Ireland. (2007). *Guidelines for the Management of Severe Local Anaesthetic Toxicity.*

Jehovah's Witness

What is the basis for Jehovah's Witnesses not accepting blood?

Since 1945, following a discussion in *The Watchtower* of Psalm 16 verse 4 (**'Their drink offering of blood I will not offer nor take up their names into my lips'**), Jehovah's Witnesses have refused transfused blood or blood products. The acceptance of blood is considered to be a violation of God's laws. This belief is further based on Genesis, Leviticus and Acts, all of which describe the prohibition of the consumption of blood.

> 'But flesh with the life thereof, which is the blood thereof, shall ye not eat' (**Genesis** 9: 3–4)
> 'ye shall eat the blood of no manner of flesh: for the life of the flesh is the blood thereof: whoever eateth it shall be cut off' (**Leviticus** 17:10–16)
> 'That ye abstain from meats offered to idols, and from blood and from things strangled' (**Acts** 15: 28–29)

A reform movement now exists, called 'The Associated Jehovah's Witnesses for Reform on Blood', who are campaigning for the abolition of the blood transfusion policy.

What methods are available for minimising blood loss in a Jehovah's Witness?

Pre-operatively
- Discussion with the patient regarding which (if any) blood products they are prepared to accept. Patients are frequently highly informed. At the patient's request, a member of the Jehovah's Witness Hospital Liaison Committee may need to be involved. Similarly, the patient will need to be seen on his or her own as well.
- Full investigation of anaemia
- Involvement of a haematologist (consider pre-op erythropoietin or iron)
- Consultant involvement
- In obstetric cases, discuss the increased risk of hysterectomy (for PPH) and the use of an ultrasound scan to determine the placental site.

Intra-operatively
- Positioning (avoiding venous congestion)
- Staged procedures
- Use of local or regional anaesthesia means the patient can stay awake and retract their prohibition if they feel the need
- Hypotensive anaesthesia – of proven use but important to weigh risks against benefits
- Haemodilution techniques–both hypervolaemic and normovolaemic
- Tourniquets
- Meticulous surgical technique/experienced surgeon
- Vasoconstrictor use

■ Use of drugs that affect coagulation, e.g. tranexamic acid, aprotinin and desmopressin
■ Cell-saver use will need to be discussed with the individual patient (*Watchtower*, 1989)
■ Balloon occlusion/ligation of arteries that supply the bleeding area

Post-operatively
■ Minimal blood letting for laboratory testing
■ ICU
■ Erythropoietin
■ GI bleeding prophylaxis
■ Methods to decrease O_2 consumption: IPPV/barbiturates/neuromuscular blockers/hypothermia/hyperbaric oxygen therapy
■ Perfluorocarbons
■ Progesterone to decrease menstrual bleeding.

Tell us about the legal aspects of giving blood to adults and children and consent validity

■ It is **unlawful to administer blood to a patient who has refused it** by the provision of an Advanced Directive or by its exclusion in a consent form. To do so may lead to criminal proceedings.
■ Properly executed **Advance Directives must be respected** and special Jehovah's Witness consent forms should be widely available.
■ **A child's right to life is paramount and must be considered before the religious beliefs of his or her parents.**
■ If a child under 16 years old wishes to receive blood against their parents' wishes they must be shown to be **'Gillick competent'**.
■ In a **life-threatening emergency in a child** unable to give competent consent, **all life-saving treatment should be given**, irrespective of the patients' wishes.
■ In children of Jehovah's witnesses under the age of 16 years the well-being of the child is overriding. If the parents refuse to give permission for blood transfusion, it may be necessary to apply for a legal **'specific issue order'**. This is a serious step that should be taken by two consultants.
■ In the case of children, application to the high court for a 'specific issue order' should only be made when it is felt entirely necessary to save the child in an elective or semi-elective situation.
■ Except in an emergency, a doctor can decline to treat a patient if they feel pressurised to act against their own beliefs. The patient's management should be passed to a colleague.

Bibliography
Kaufman L, Ginsberg R. (1999). *Anaesthesia Review 15*. Churchill Livingstone.
Milligan LJ, Ballamy MC. (2004). Anaesthesia and critical care of Jehovah's Witnesses. *Continuing Education in Anaesthesia, Critical Care and Pain*, **4**, 35–9.
The Association of Anaesthetists of Great Britain and Ireland. (2005). *Management of Anaesthesia for Jehovah's Witnesses*, 2nd edition.

Laparoscopic cholecystectomy

What are the problems associated with anaesthetising a patient for laparoscopic cholecystectomy?

The problems associated with laparoscopy are caused by:

- **Pneumoperitoneum**
- CO_2 used as the insufflation gas
- **Positioning** on the table, i.e. reverse Trendelenberg
- **Surgical procedure** itself, i.e. cholecystectomy.

These can be discussed in terms of their **physiological effects on the cardiovascular and respiratory systems** in particular. Other, less important changes are also seen in renal, metabolic and neuro-endocrine physiology.

Effects on the cardiovascular system

Haemodynamic changes are secondary to pneumoperitoneum, reverse Trendelenberg, hypercarbia and the effects of the GA itself:

- **↓ Cardiac Index**   ↓ venous return by compression of IVC and reverse Trendelenberg position
  Paradoxically, CVP and PCWP ↑ – may be a result of central redistribution of blood or ↑ intrathoracic pressure
- **↑ SVR**   Aortic and splanchnic compression may also be due to humoral factors like catecholamines, PGs and vasopressin
- **↑ MAP**
- **Ischaemia**   Alterations in supply/demand
- **Arrhythmias**   Vagally mediated → A-V dissociation
                                           Nodal rhythm
                                           Sinus bradycardia
                                           Asystole
                  Ventricular – related to high CO_2
- **Cardiac failure**

Effects on the respiratory system

These effects are mainly due to pneumoperitoneum and the use of CO_2 as the insufflation gas. Reverse Trendelenberg position actually attenuates some of the adverse effects (cf. Trendelenberg for gynaecological surgery).

- **↓ FRC**   Diaphragmatic displacement cephalad
             ↓ chest wall dimension and muscular tone
             Changes in intrathoracic blood volume
             →   **Atelectasis**
                  Pulmonary shunting
                  Hypoxaemia
- **↑ Airway Pressures**   Peak airway pressure ↑ 6 cmH_2O
                        May result in **barotrauma** or **pneumothorax**
- **↑ Physiological dead space**
- **↓ Total lung compliance**

■ **CO_2 absorption** $ETCO_2$ rises by 8–10 mmHg then plateaus at new level after about 40 minutes
Respiratory acidosis with CVS consequences if not corrected
Usually need 25% ↑ in minute volume

■ **Endobronchial intubation**   The carina moves upwards during insufflation
May also manifest as bronchospasm

Effects on the renal system

As cardiac output reduces so too will renal blood flow and GFR. Renal vascular resistance will increase with the raised intra-abdominal pressure. These factors may lead to an overall reduction in urine output particularly with a prolonged procedure.

Additional potential problems

■ Acid aspiration
■ Trocar injuries
■ Venous gas embolism
■ Bleeding
■ Burns and explosions
■ DVT

Bibliography

Hacking R, Doyle P. (2006). Anaesthesia and minimally invasive procedures. *Anaesthesia and Intensive Care Medicine*, **7**(2), 43–6.

Latex allergy

A staff nurse presents for elective surgery and claims to have a history of possible latex allergy.

Who is at risk from developing latex allergy?

High-risk groups include:

■ Patients with previous documented reactions
■ Those exposed to repeated medical or surgical procedures involving the use of latex (especially bladder catheterisation)
■ Health-care workers
■ Patients with a history of atopy (may show cross-reactivity with certain foods especially banana, chestnuts and avocado)
■ In spina bifida patients the prevalence may be as high as 60%.

What types of allergy to latex do you know?

▪ Contact dermatitis   Type IV delayed hypersensitivity reaction to the chemical accelerators, anti-oxidants and stabilisers used in the manufacturing process
T-cell mediated

▪ Anaphylaxis   Type I immediate hypersensitivity reaction to latex proteins in previously sensitised patients
IgE mediated

How do you test for it?

Testing takes place 4–6 weeks after the reaction.

▪ **Skin-prick testing**   Involves puncturing the skin with a thin needle through a drop of dilute antigen. The concentration of solution is important to avoid false negatives. There is a smaller risk of anaphylaxis than with intra-dermal testing.

▪ **RAST**   Radioallergoabsorbent testing is **less sensitive and more expensive** than skin-prick testing, but **avoids the risk of anaphylaxis**.

As there are many different latex proteins that may be implicated in the allergic response, a negative response to one antigen does not imply that the patient is not latex sensitive. A strong clinical history suggestive of allergy is important.

How would you manage this case?

Having already been notified in advance, there is time to prepare the theatre environment and equipment necessary to undertake such a case. All theatre and ward staff should be aware of the necessary precautions to be taken. There should be a 'latex-free' box of equipment available and lists of equipment that are:

1. Latex-free
2. May be modified to be used.
3. Must not be used at all.

Pre-medication is controversial, but may be given to patients who are considered to be very sensitive.

A suggested protocol for adults would be

IV chlorpheniramine 10 mg 6 hourly
IV ranitidine 50 mg 8 hourly
IV hydrocortisone 100 mg 6 hourly
Salbutamol (inh/neb) for asthmatics

This would be given for 24 hours pre-operatively and at least 12 hours post-operatively. The patient should be first on the list and anaesthetised in a theatre unoccupied for at least 2 hours. The most important piece of equipment is latex-free gloves. All other equipment should be checked with the database in the 'latex-free' box.

> **Latex anaphylaxis:**
>
> ■ Reaction typically begins 30–60 minutes after the start of the procedure (cf. anaphylactic reaction to i.v. drugs).
> ■ Management as for anaphylaxis – think of latex-free environment as soon as is practical.

Bibliography

Dakin MJ, Yentis SM. (1998). Latex allergy: a strategy for management. *Anaesthesia*, **53**, 774–81.

Local anaesthesia for carotid endarterectomy

You are asked to anaesthetise a 76-year-old man for a carotid endarterectomy. What are the indications for this operation?

The indication for carotid endarterectomy is **symptomatic** carotid stenosis of >**70%**.

For these patients there is a 16% absolute risk reduction in the combined risk of post-operative death and stroke over more than 5 years giving a number needed to treat of 6.3 (Rothwell *et al.*). Evidence is weaker for lesser degrees of stenosis.

> **Complications of carotid endarterectomy**
>
> ■ **Peri-operative stroke.** The incidence of peri-operative stroke is approximately 2.2%, but is higher in those with a history of previous stroke (4.2%).
> ■ **Peri-operative myocardial infarction.** Co-existing ischaemic heart disease is a significant cause of peri-operative morbidity and mortality in patients undergoing carotid endarterectomy. The 30-day risk of MI is 2.2%. In one study 13% of patients had a 'silent' Troponin I rise, which has prognostic implications.
> ■ **Other co-morbidity.** Patients presenting for carotid endarterectomy are frequently elderly with significant co-morbidities such as chronic obstructive pulmonary disease, hypertension (~70%), and diabetes.
> ■ **Cranial nerve injury** – usually transient
> ■ **Airway compression**

Which nerves are blocked to perform carotid endarterectomy under local anaesthesia?

■ Lesser occipital nerve
■ Greater auricular nerve

- Transverse cervical nerve
- Supraclavicular nerve

All these nerves arise from the ventral rami of C2–4 and are sensory only, radiating from the posterior border of sternocleidomastoid just inferior to the accessory nerve.

C1 has no sensory nerve fibres.

These nerves lie on the transverse processes of their corresponding vertebra and may be blocked here (**deep cervical plexus block**). or at the level of their cutaneous branches (**superficial cervical plexus block**).

The accessory nerve is the 11th cranial nerve and, together with the ventral ramus of C2, supplies sternocleidomastoid and trapezius (together with ventral rami of C3–C4).

Branches of the trigeminal nerve supplying the submandibular area may also be required to block the discomfort of surgical retraction.

Local infiltration of the carotid sheath is needed because it has a cranial nerve supply.

How do you perform a deep cervical plexus block?

- Draw a line from the tip of the mastoid process to the anterior tubercle of C6 at the level of the cricoid cartilage.
- Intervals of 1.5 cm below the mastoid process on this line indicate the position of the transverse processes of C2–C4 (feel C2 tubercle just below mastoid; C6 tubercle is Chaissaignac's).
- Three injections are directed medially and downwards onto the transverse processes at these points.
- 5 ml of local anaesthetic is injected after the needle is directed laterally off the transverse processes through each.

What are the potential complications of this technique?

- Vertebral artery injection
- Phrenic nerve runs just below mastoid and is frequently blocked too
- Horner's syndrome
- Recurrent laryngeal nerve block
- Intrathecal injection
- Hypoglossal nerve block

How do you perform a superficial cervical plexus block?

- The injection point is given by drawing a line laterally from the cricoid cartilage to the point where it meets the posterior border of sternocleidomastoid.
- Insert a 22 g short bevelled 'block' needle perpendicular to the skin until it 'pops' through the cervical fascia.
- Inject 10 ml of local anaesthetic. It should track up and down if the needle is in the right plane.

■ An additional 10 ml of local anaesthetic may be infiltrated along the middle third of the posterior part of the sternocleidomastoid up and down the posterior border of the sternocleidomastoid between the skin and muscle.

■ Supplementation by the surgeon is often needed (this is also the case when the deep block is used). Patients are also less likely to require supplementary analgesia in the 24 hours after surgery with the deep cervical plexus block.

■ An intermediate plexus block is also described where the injecting needle pierces the investing fascia of the neck, deep to the S.C. layer, but superficial to the deep cervical (pre-vertebral) fascia.

What alternative regional technique may be used for carotid endarterectomy?

Cervical epidural is an alternative technique and does provide good operating conditions. However, it is associated with a significant risk of major anaesthetic complications including dural puncture, epidural venepuncture and respiratory muscle paralysis.

What are the advantages and disadvantages of local anaesthesia vs. general anaesthesia for carotid endarterectomy?

Advantages of local anaesthesia

There is preservation of autoregulation, the patient acts as his own cerebral monitor, there may be a lower incidence of BP variation and there is less need for drugs to control BP post-operatively.

■ A large-scale study of general anaesthesia vs. local anaesthesia (GALA), however, recently concluded that there is 'no reason to prefer LA or GA'.

■ A meta-analysis of the **non-randomised** studies showed that the use of local anaesthetic was associated with significant reductions in the odds of death from all causes, stroke, myocardial infarction and pulmonary embolism within 30 days of surgery.

■ A meta-analysis of the **randomised** studies showed that the use of local anaesthetic was associated with a reduction in the risk of local haemorrhage within 30 days of surgery, but there was no evidence of a reduction in the odds of operative stroke. However, the trials were small and in some studies intention-to-treat analyses were not possible.

Disadvantages of local anaesthesia

■ No fall in cerebral metabolic rate due to GA.
■ Discomfort due to a fixed posture held for a protracted period.
■ Need for co-operation.
■ Higher BP during the operation.
■ If there is cerebral ischaemia, the patient may not cooperate.

Bibliography
Breivik H, Campbell W, Eccleston C. (2003). *Clinical Pain Management: Practical Applications and Procedures*. London: Arnold.

Howell SJ. (2007). Carotid endarterectomy. *British Journal of Anaesthesia*, **99**, 119–31.

Pandit JJ, Satya-Krishna R , Gration P. (2007). Superficial or deep cervical plexus block for carotid endarterectomy: a systematic review of complications. *British Journal of Anaesthesia*, Advance Access June 18, 2007, DOI 10.1093/bja/aem160.

Lumbar sympathectomy

Where anatomically do the sympathetic ganglia lie in the lumbar region?

The ganglia of the sympathetic chain lie on the anterolateral aspect of the lumbar vertebral bodies. They are separated from the somatic nerves by the psoas fascia and the psoas muscle.

What are the indications for a lumbar sympathectomy?

There are two main indications for this block.

- The diagnosis and treatment of painful lower limb neuropathic conditions associated with dysfunction of the sympathetic nervous system, for example, post-traumatic dystrophy.
- Relief for (mainly elderly) patients with peripheral vascular insufficiency producing severe ischaemic pain, particularly with rest pain and compromised skin nutrition secondary to poor blood flow.

How would you perform this procedure?

- Informed consent must be obtained.
- The block is performed using an image intensifier under full aseptic conditions.
- The patient lies prone with a pillow under the lower abdomen.
- The spinous process of L3 is marked. A point 8–10 cm lateral to the spinous process is then marked.
- The needle is advanced towards the vertebral body of L3. If bony contact is made within 3–4 cm from the skin, this is likely to be the transverse process of L3. Doubling the distance from the skin to the transverse process will find the needle point in the correct position.
- The needle is advanced cranially or caudally to avoid the transverse process and advanced until bony contact is made again.
- The needle is then redirected to slide off the anterolateral aspect of the vertebral body.
- It is sometimes possible to verify the position of the needle with a loss of resistance technique as the needle penetrates the psoas fascia.
- The use of contrast medium allows verification of the correct needle tip position. The contrast should be seen to spread anterior to the L3 vertebral body.

What substances would you inject and at what doses?

This depends on the reason for performing the block:

▪ For the relief of visceral pain 20–30 ml of 0.25% bupivacaine would be reasonable.
▪ To assess whether neurolysis is appropriate, 10 ml of 0.25% bupivicaine mixed with contrast would be appropriate.

Which patients are appropriate for neurolytic lumbar sympathetic blocks?

▪ Vascular patients not suitable for surgery including those with a non-healing ulcer or severe ischaemic rest pain. Lumbar sympathetic neurolysis has been used to provide long-term sympathetic blockade in patients who receive only short-term pain relief with local anaesthetic blocks.
▪ Prior to amputation to demarcate viable from non-viable tissue. It can be performed either by chemical (phenol or absolute alcohol) or by radiofrequency neurolysis.

What are the potential complications of a lumbar sympathectomy?

▪ Hypotension
▪ Intravascular injection
▪ Epidural injection
▪ Intrathecal injection resulting in total spinal block and post-dural puncture headache
▪ Up to 50% of patients may experience transient post-sympathetic neuropathic pain in the anterolateral proximal part of the lower extremity.
▪ Genitofemoral neuralgia (infrequent and usually transient if phenol is used) may occur if the neurolytic agent reaches the genitofemoral nerve. Genitofemoral ethanol neuritis (when alcohol is used as a neurolytic agent) may result in more severe and protracted pain.
▪ Post-sympathectomy allodynia in an L1 distribution may be due to genitofemoral nerve damage from a neurolytic agent, but it may also result from a post-sympathectomy denervation hyperaesthesia.
▪ Ejaculatory failure may occur if bilateral upper level lumbar sympathectomy is performed.
▪ The ureter may be damaged by phenol or alcohol.
▪ Ankle oedema has been reported, particularly in women.

Bibliography

Breivik H, Campbell W, Eccleston C. (2003). *Clinical Pain Management: Practical Applications and Procedures*. London: Arnold.
Wedley J, Gauci C. (1994). *Handbook of Clinical Techniques in the Management of Chronic Pain*. Swizerland: Harwood Academic Publishers.

Lung cyst

A 62-year-old man presents for excision of a right-sided lung cyst

What are the causes of lung cysts?

These may be congenital or acquired.
- **Congenital** Bronchogenic
- **Acquired** Abscess – e.g. tuberculosis, staphylococcal, klebsiella pneumonia, hydatid, septic pulmonary infarction, aspiration
  Tumour – cavitating primary bronchogenic or metastatic
  Bullae secondary to emphysema
  Bronchial obstruction following inhaled foreign body

This man has a right lower lobe abscess that requires resection. He has a history of emphysema. What are the important considerations when assessing this man?

The pre-operative assessment would concentrate on his respiratory function and exercise tolerance. Concomitant medical problems such as ischaemic heart disease are obviously also important. **Poor exercise tolerance, obesity and the presence of cardiovascular disease are strong indicators of a poor prognosis.**
   Routine investigations should include:

- Full blood count
- Electrolytes
- Clotting screen
- ECG
- Chest X-ray
- Pulmonary function tests
- CT/MRI of chest

An echocardiogram may also be indicated.
Post-operative analgesia should be considered and discussed at this stage.

What would you expect the pulmonary function tests to show?

- $\downarrow$ FEV_1
- $\downarrow$ FVC
- $\downarrow$ FEV_1/FVC ratio
- Lung volumes may be normal or increased
- Transfer factor for carbon monoxide is low

What values for FEV_1 and FVC would you consider to be severe?

A predicted post-operative FEV_1 of less than 1L will result in problems with sputum retention and less than 0.8L is a contra-indication to lung resection.

What is maximum breathing capacity?

Maximum breathing capacity (MBC) is the product of maximum respiratory rate and tidal volume. The patient is asked to breathe in and out maximally for 15 seconds. The results are then multiplied by four to give the MBC.

Normal is >60 l/min

Value of 25–50 l/min implies severe respiratory impairment.

What are the options for airway management in this man?

It is important to isolate the infected segment as far as possible by performing endobronchial intubation usually with a double-lumen tube. Re-usable tubes such as the Robertshaw and Carlens (carinal hook) or disposable tubes are suitable. The choice of induction may be influenced by the expected difficulty of intubation or the request by the surgeon to perform rigid bronchoscopy before the tube is inserted. Acceptable techniques include awake fibre-optic intubation, inhalational induction, rapid-sequence induction or even a conventional intravenous induction followed by a non-depolarising relaxant. In the latter technique, strong positive pressure should be avoided until the infected area is isolated. The patient should be positioned semi-sitting, ideally with the abscess-side down for induction.

How do you confirm correct placement of a double-lumen tube?

The procedure for a left-sided tube is as follows:

1. Inflate tracheal cuff (5–10 ml of air) → confirm bilateral breath sounds.
2. Open tracheal lumen to air.
3. Ventilate down bronchial lumen only (proximal clamp on tracheal lumen).
4. Inflate bronchial cuff (1–2 ml) until leak disappears (listen at open tracheal lumen) and breath sounds heard only on left side.
5. Unclamp tracheal lumen.
6. Clamp bronchial lumen → confirm breath sounds heard only on right side.
7. Unclamp both lumens.

NB: The procedure may be altered in the case of a lung abscess where the infected lung needs to be isolated as soon as possible. In this case both cuffs may be inflated before any ventilation to reduce the risk of spillover into the good lung.

The correct position should ideally be confirmed by the use of a fibre-optic bronchoscope. When it is passed down the tracheal lumen of a left-sided tube, the carina should be visible with the bronchial cuff seen within the left main bronchus. The right main bronchus should also be visible and the origin of the right upper lobe bronchus may be seen.

What measures can be used to prevent or treat hypoxaemia during one-lung ventilation?

▓ Administer 100% oxygen.
▓ Check position of DLT with fibre-optic scope.
▓ Oxygen may be insufflated into the collapsed lung via a suction catheter.
▓ PEEP to the dependent lung may expand collapsed alveoli.
▓ This may necessitate the application of CPAP to the collapsed lung to prevent a shift of blood flow secondary to the increase in pulmonary vascular resistance in the dependent lung.
▓ Intermittent two-lung ventilation if surgical access is compromised by the above manoeuvres.
▓ Clamping of the pulmonary artery supplying the collapsed lung may be required.

Note that, in general, ventilator settings used during two-lung ventilation need very little (if any) adjustment when one-lung ventilation is commenced.

What are the options for post-operative analgesia?

▓ Intravenous opioids	Not ideal in patients with limited respiratory reserve Regional techniques are preferable
▓ NSAIDs	
▓ Epidural analgesia	May need supplementing with NSAIDs for shoulder-tip pain.
▓ Paravertebral block	May be less reliable than an epidural but fewer haemodynamic problems.
▓ Interpleural catheter	Placed by the surgeon.
▓ Intercostal blocks	By anaesthetist blind or by surgeon under direct vision.

Bibliography

Coates M. (2001). A practical view of thoracic anaesthesia. *RCA Bulletin 6*, March.
Craft T, Upton P. (1995). *Key Topics in Anaesthesia*, 2nd edition. Bios Scientific Publications.
Gothard JWW. (2005). Principles and practice of thoracic anaesthesia. *Anaesthesia and Intensive Care Medicine*, **6**(12), 428–32.
Kumar P, Clark M. (1994). *Clinical Medicine*, 3rd Edition. Baillière-Tindall.
Morgan GE, Mikhail MS. (1996). *Clinical Anaesthesiology*, 2nd Edition. Appleton and Lange.
Pfitzner J, Peacock MJ, Tsirgiotis E, Walkley IH. (2000). Lobectomy for cavitating lung abscess with haemoptysis: strategy for protecting the contralateral lung and also the non-involved lobe of the ipsilateral lung. *British Journal of Anaesthesia*, **85**(5), 791–4.

Major obstetric haemorrhage

You are asked to assess a 24-year-old woman who is in labour and has had a significant antepartum haemorrhage. What are the causes of major obstetric haemorrhage?

Major haemorrhage occurs in 6.7/1000 deliveries and may be defined as (multiple definitions exist, pick one or two):

- Acute loss of 40% of circulating volume (~2 litres at term).
- Loss of 50% of circulating volume in under 3 hours.
- Loss of one total blood volume in 24 hours.

Antepartum haemorrhage:

- **Placental abruption.** Occurs in 1%–1.5% of pregnancies and is responsible for 20%–25% of antepartum haemorrhages. Blood loss may be concealed and DIC may occur.
- **Placenta previa.** Occurs in 0.5%–1% of pregnancies and is responsible for 15%–20% of antepartum haemorrhages.
- **Uterine rupture.** Blood loss may be concealed and associated with severe abdominal pain.
- Cervical or vaginal lesions.
- Unknown aetiology.

Primary postpartum haemorrhage:

- **Uterine atony.** Most common cause of bleeding (80% of PPH) and more likely with uterine over distension, uterine fatigue (prolonged or augmented labour) or obstruction due to retained products.
- **Trauma to the birth canal**
- **Coagulopathy**
- Uterine inversion
- Uterine rupture
- Placenta accreta.

Secondary postpartum haemorrhage

- Retained products of conception
- Sepsis.

There were 17 maternal deaths due to haemorrhage reported in the 2000–2002 report on the Confidential Enquiry into Maternal Death in the United Kingdom. This represented 16% of all direct deaths.

- Four due to placenta previa.
- Three due to placental abruption.
- Ten due to post-partum haemorrhage.

Anaesthetic care was deemed to be substandard in five of these cases.

How would you manage this lady with a massive antepartum haemorrhage for emergency caesarean section?

The 2000–2002 report into the Confidential Enquiry into Maternal Death in the United Kingdom recommended that a multi-disciplinary massive haemorrhage protocol should be available in all units and regular 'fire drills' should be run.
   Initial resuscitation with ABC and anaesthetic assessment:

- Oxygen via non-rebreathing mask and bag at 15 litres per minute.
- Left lateral position and head down.
- Two large bore (14G) cannulae and rapid infusion to maintain circulating volume (crystalloid or colloid until blood available).
- Blood for FBC, Coagulation screen, 6 unit cross-match.
- Transfuse blood when available (uncrossed O negative blood should be available if needed).
- Call for senior anaesthetic and obstetric help.
- Inform haematology of situation and involve consultant haematologist if coagulopathy present. FFP, cryoprecipitate, platelets and other clotting factors may be required.

Anaesthetic management:

- Consider upgrading monitoring (arterial and central access) when the situation allows.
- Anti-reflux medication may be given if the situation allows.
- Maintain left tilt or uterine displacement.
- Pre-oxygenation.
- Rapid sequence induction and intubation using suxamethonium with cricoid pressure. If shocked, some authors recommend etomidate or ketamine as induction agents instead of thiopentone.
- Endotracheal intubation and ventilation.
- Maintain anaesthesia with volatile agent. If shocked, continue 100% oxygen.
- Continue resuscitation intra-operatively via warming devices. Maintain Hb >8.0 g/dl and maintain circulating volume.
- Correct coagulopathy.
- Cell salvage has been successfully used to reduce homologous blood requirements. Separate suction should be used for amniotic fluid.
- Post-operative stabilisation may be best performed in a critical care setting.

Specific managements:

- Uterine atony:
  - Bimanual massage.
  - Oxytocin. 5iu slow i.v. bolus followed by infusion. May precipitate hypotension.
  - Ergometrine. 250–500 mcg by i.m. injection. Nausea and vomiting are very common.
  - Carboprost (hemabate). 250 mcg by deep intramuscular or intramyometrial injection.
  - Misoprost

■ Coagulopathy:
- Maintain PT <1.5 times normal. 4 units FFP is first line and should be repeated as required.
- Maintain platelets > 75×10^9/l.
- Maintain fibrinogen level >1.0g/l. If not corrected by FFP will require 10 units cryoprecipitate.
- Tranexamic acid – antifibrinolytic.
- Persistent non-surgical bleed may be managed with recombinant activated factor VII (NovoSeven).

■ Surgical management of persistent bleeding:
- Uterine packing
- Uterine artery ligation
- B-lynch sutures
- Hysterectomy

■ Radiological management of persistent bleeding:
- Embolisation of pelvic vessels may prevent the need for hysterectomy.

You mentioned recombinant activated factor VII and carboprost. Tell me about them?

Recombinant activated factor VII (NovoSeven) was initially developed for conditions of factor VII deficiency or inhibition.

The first step in the coagulation cascade is the activation of factor VII by tissue factor. Recombinant activated factor VII was first reported in the management of major traumatic haemorrhage in 1999 (Israeli army) and various case reports of successful use in obstetric haemorrhage have been published.

However, some concern still exists regarding thrombotic complications.

Dosing should follow haematology guidance (40–100 mcg/kg).

Failure of NovoSeven has been associated with profound coagulopathy and acidosis.

Carboprost is a prostaglandin F2 receptor agonist (15-methylprostaglandin F2α). It causes uterine contraction. The major side effects are bronchospasm (contra-indicated in asthma), hypoxia, flushing, nausea and vomiting. Repeated dosing was thought to have contributed to one maternal death between 2000 and 2002.

Bibliography

Banks A, Norris A. (2005). Major obstetric haemorrhage. *BJA CEPD Reviews*, **5**(6), 195–8.
Kenet G. (1999). Treatment of traumatic bleeding with recombinant factor VIIa. *Lancet*, **354**, 1879.
Report on the confidential enquiry into maternal death 1997–1999.
Report on the confidential enquiry into maternal death 2000–2002.
Stein DM. (2005). Determinants on the futility of administration of factor VIIa in trauma. *Trauma*, **59**, 609–15.
Thomas C, Madej T. (2002). Obstetric emergencies and the anaesthetist. *BJA CEPD Reviews*, **2**(6), 174–7.

Malignant hyperthermia

Emergency scenarios you must know include:

- MH
- Cardiac arrest
- Anaphylaxis
- Failed intubation

How does malignant hyperthermia present?

- Rising end-tidal CO_2 is one of the first signs
- Tachycardia
- Arrhythmias
- Sweating
- Muscle rigidity
- Masseter spasm
- Temperature rise   Not necessarily an early sign.
- Rate of rise 2–5 °C/hour

You mentioned a raised $ETCO_2$. How would you differentiate MH from other more common causes of a raised CO_2?

A raised $ETCO_2$ is not uncommon and may be due to:

- **Increased production**   Hypermetabolic states, e.g. severe sepsis
  Thyrotoxic crisis, MH
  Reperfusion, e.g. cross-clamp release
  Bicarbonate administration
- **Decreased excretion**   Decreased minute volume
- **Exogenous administration**   Laparoscopy, rebreathing

It is important to maintain a high index of suspicion of MH, being aware that it has a high mortality if left untreated (70%) – and it is treatable. Therefore, if the $ETCO_2$ was high, one should exclude the more common causes of a raised $ETCO_2$ such as rebreathing or a reduced minute volume. The patient should be observed for sweating, flushing and signs of cardiovascular instability.

Other differential diagnoses are:

- Malignant neuroleptic syndrome
- Ecstasy intoxication
- Inadequate anaesthesia or analgesia.

How do you treat MH?

- **Stop administration** of any likely causative agents (volatiles)
- Change to a **vapour-free machine and circuit.** Use propofol/midazolam/opioids to keep the patient asleep if needed.

- **Inform surgeons** and abandon surgery if possible.
- **Summon help** – both a senior and further skilled anaesthetic assistance.
- Give **100% O$_2$**.
- **Hyperventilate** – increase minute volume by 2–3 times.
- **Dantrolene** give 2–3mg/kg i.v. initially and then 1mg/kg PRN. Average dose needed to reverse MH crisis is 2.5 mg/kg. Assistance will be needed to draw this up, as it is slow to dissolve. Continue for 48 hours at a rate of 1–2 mg/kg every 4–6 hours.
- **Measure core temperature**
- **Cool the patient** with ice/fan/tepid sponging/cold i.v. fluids and cold fluid into the bladder if practical but avoid vasoconstriction. Cardiopulmonary bypass has been used
- Establish **invasive monitoring**: arterial line and CVP/PAFC
- Check K$^+$, CK and blood gases
- Monitor coagulation profile for DIC

What is the molecular basis for the clinical picture?

A genetic trait (mainly autosomal dominant) results in an error in skeletal muscle calcium control. The inborn error leads to a loss of control of calcium flux and an increase in the calcium concentration in the cytosol of skeletal muscle. The proposed site of action is the Ryanodine (a natural plant alkaloid) receptor, which spans the calcium releasing channels on the sarcoplasmic reticulum and T-tubule.

The increase in intracellular free calcium results in the clinical picture of:

- Increased skeletal muscle contraction
- Increased skeletal muscle metabolism
- Glycolysis
- Rhabdomyolysis
- Uncoupling of oxidative phosphorylation

Dantrolene:
Vial containing orange powder
20 mg per vial
3 g of mannitol (to improve solubility)
Sodium hydroxide (to give pH of 9.5)
Reconstitute with 60 ml of water
Protect from light

Testing for MH susceptibility:
Halothane/caffeine/ryanodine
contracture testing – with a strain
gauge
Muscle biopsy from vastus lateralis

Divides into:

MH susceptible – MHS

MH negative – MHN

MH equivocal – MHE

DNA testing is now available

Bibliography
Guidelines for the Management of a Malignant Hyperthermia Crisis. AAGBI, 2007.

Hopkins PM. (2000). Malignant hyperthermia: advances in clinical diagnosis and management. *British Journal of Anaesthesia*, **85**(1), 118–28.

Massive blood transfusion

What is the definition of a massive blood transfusion?

Definitions do vary:

Remember a couple of definitions and stick with them!

■ **Replacement of total blood volume, with stored homologous bank blood, within 24 hours**
■ Acute administration of more than 1.5 times the patient's blood volume
■ A transfusion of half the blood volume per hour
■ A transfusion greater than the total blood volume (10–20 units)
■ 6 units.

What problems are associated with a massive transfusion?

This is a very dry question and the answer is difficult to categorise. It will inevitably consist of a long list of facts.

Clotting abnormalities
Clotting abnormalities occur as a result of:

■ **Blood loss** causing reduced levels of platelets, coagulation factors and inhibitors.
■ **Dilution** of these factors with volume replacement
  ● dilutional thrombocytopaenia
  ● dilutional coagulopathy

Only likely after a blood volume replacement with non-plasma fluid and red cells.

■ **DIC** may occur in 30% of patients who have a massive transfusion.
   Lab results: Increased PT, APTT and FDPs
                  Decreased platelet count
                  Decreased fibrinogen
   DIC is generally due to hypoperfusion, etc. and *not* to transfusion itself.

> **Storage**
> **Platelets** are unstable in stored blood at $4\,^{\circ}C$ and the platelet count falls rapidly in blood stored for more than 24 hours. **Factor V** (50% after 14 days) and **VIII** (50% after 1 day) also lose activity on storage.

Biochemical complications

■ **Hyperkalaemia** K^+ conc. in stored blood = 30 mmol/l after 3 weeks storage

■ **Citrate toxicity**   Metabolised to bicarbonate in the liver resulting in metabolic alkalosis
                         Patients who have liver disease or who are hypothermic are more prone to this
                         >1 unit / 5 min needed to overwhelm citrate metabolism
                         Citrate binds to ionized calcium → hypocalcaemia

■ **Hypocalcaemia**   Causing decreased cardiac output – rare

■ **Acid–base disturbance**   Lactate from red cells
                              Citric acid (the anticoagulant in donor blood)
                              Acid–base balance depends on rate of blood administration, rate of citrate metabolism and the perfusion of the patient

Other problems

■ **Hypothermia**   Left shift of O_2 dissociation curve
                    Platelet and clotting dysfunction

■ **Haemoglobin dysfunction**   Low temperature – left shift of O_2 dissociation curve
                                Acidosis – right shift of O_2 dissociation curve. Decreased levels of 2,3-DPG (especially after 14 days) – left shift of O_2 dissociation curve

■ **Haemolysis**   Due to osmotic fragility

■ **Incompatibility**   Errors occur more easily in extreme clinical situations

■ **Air embolism**   Potential hazard with the use of pressure bags

■ **Anaphylaxis**   3%–5%

Delayed complications

■ Disease transmission   HIV/hepatitis/malaria/bacteria → sepsis
■ **Immunosuppression**   Ca bowel recurrence, infection
■ ARDS
■ Pulmonary oedema

How would you manage a patient requiring a massive transfusion?

> The aim is to restore:
>
> ■ **Circulating volume** – mortality is increased with prolonged shock.
> ■ **Oxygen carrying capacity** – packed cell volume >0.20
> ■ **Haemostasis**
> ■ **Colloid osmotic pressure**
> ■ **Biochemical balance**

Points to mention are:

■ **ABC** approach   High flow O_2
                      Large bore peripheral venous access with fluid warmers
                      Keep the patient warm (warming blankets)
■ **Get help**   Senior assistance
                      Haematologist-**communicate** with the lab!
                      Surgical help -? required to stop bleeding
■ **Monitoring**   Amount of blood loss – suction, weighing swabs
                      Invasive arterial blood pressure
                      CVP/PAWP
                      Blood gases (repeated at intervals)
                      Frequent clotting studies
                      ECG
                      Urinary catheter
                      SaO_2
                      $ETCO_2$
                      Temperature (central and peripheral)
                      A thromboelastograph may prove useful if available.
■ **Equipment**   Rapid infusion device
                      Cell saver
                      Sengstaken–Blakemore tube
                      MAST suit
■ **HDU/ICU**
■ **FFP and platelets** 2 units of FFP and 5 units of platelets have been
                      recommended in the past for every 8–10 units of blood
                      transfused. However, **the need for supplements must be
                      judged by clinical assessment and lab tests**.
                      FFP should be given if the PT is prolonged by more than
                      5 seconds.

Microvascular bleeding due to thrombocytopaenia is more likely to occur if the platelet count is $<50 \times 10^9/l$. Treat with 6–8 units of platelets.

■ **Cryoprecipitate**   Contains more **fibrinogen** and **Factor VIII**

15 packs can be used to help treat **DIC**, which should be suspected if **thrombin time** is doubled.

■ **Drugs**   **Aprotinin** – serine protease inhibitor to inhibit fibrinolysis

Tranexamic acid – antifibrinolytic agent that binds to plasminogen and plasmin and interferes with their ability to split fibrinogen.

Desmopressin/vasopressin – affects circulatory endothelial cells

Calcium chloride

Blood filters – a contentious issue
Designed to remove microaggregates:
■ **Micropore filters:** 2   Depth filters (impaction and adsorption)
   types (20–40 µm)   Screen filters (direct interception principle)
Problems: Impede blood flow, become blocked and activate complement
Haemolysis and platelet depletion (depth filters)

■ **Standard blood filters** (170 µm)

Bibliography

Donaldson MDJ, Seaman MJ, Park GR. (1992). Massive blood transfusion. *British Journal of Anaesthesia*, **69**, 621–30.

Hewitt PE, Machin SJ. (1990). Massive blood transfusion. ABC of transfusion. *British Medical Journal*, **13**, 107–9.

Hoffbrand AV, Pettit JE. (1993). *Essential Haematology.* Oxford, UK: Blackwell Scientific Publications.

McClelland DBL. (2007). *Handbook of Transfusion Medicine*, UK Blood Services. 4th edition. Available online at *www.transfusionguidelines.org.uk.*

Mitral stenosis

A 56-year-old woman is listed for a laparoscopic cholecystectomy. She is known to have mitral stenosis.

What are the symptoms and signs of mitral stenosis?

Symptoms

■ Usually appear when the cross-sectional valve area is less than $2\,cm^2$ (normal $= 5\,cm^2$).

- May be up to 20 years after the initial event, which is almost always rheumatic fever.
- Recurrent bronchitis, dyspnoea, cough with bloodstained, frothy sputum (pulmonary oedema) and palpitations (secondary to atrial fibrillation). Eventually, there is fatigue and peripheral oedema with the onset of right heart failure. There may also be symptoms related to systemic emboli and, rarely, a hoarse voice secondary to compression of the left recurrent laryngeal nerve by the enlarged left atrium.

Signs
- Malar flush
- Irregularly irregular pulse
- Tapping, undisplaced apex beat ($\equiv$ palpable first heart sound)
- Left parasternal heave
- On auscultation there is an opening snap (mitral valve) followed by a mid-diastolic, rumbling murmur localized to the apex.
- There may also be signs of left and right heart failure and tricuspid regurgitation secondary to the back pressure from the left side.

ECG
- If in sinus rhythm, there will be biphasic P waves and signs of right heart strain.
- Atrial fibrillation

Would you like any special investigations?

An **echocardiogram** would give an indication of the severity of the mitral stenosis in terms of the valve area and the pressure gradient across it.

Mitral stenosis is described as severe when the cross-sectional area is less than 1 cm².

What are the principles involved in anaesthetising this lady?

The problems associated with mitral stenosis will be complicated by the added effects of laparoscopy. This is a complex case, as the haemodynamic changes associated with laparoscopy in a patient with mitral stenosis may make it very hazardous. The benefits of laparoscopic surgery would have to be weighed up against the risks of haemodynamic instability. An open cholecystectomy should be considered.

The principles involved in anaesthetising a patient with mitral stenosis are as follows:

- Establish **intra-arterial blood pressure monitoring.** Consider pulmonary artery catheter placement prior to induction, although a pulmonary artery catheter has certain limitations in this situation. It may precipitate atrial fibrillation (if the patient is in sinus rhythm) with disastrous consequences and it may not reflect the true left ventricular end-diastolic pressure.
- **Avoid tachycardia** (which would reduce LV filling).

- **Maintain pre-load** without overdoing it. Hypovolaemia may lead to a marked reduction in cardiac output and overfilling could easily result in pulmonary oedema.
- **Avoid falls in SVR** – fixed cardiac output.
- **Avoid increases in PVR:** hypoxia, hypercarbia, N_2O.
- **Avoid vasodilators:** care with volatile agents.
- **Maintain sinus rhythm** – be prepared to shock if patient goes into AF Volatiles may lead to junctional rhythm with loss of atrial kick.
- **Antibiotic prophylaxis** against endocarditis – BNF, probably amoxycillin and gentamicin in this case.
- Post-operatively either HDU or ICU care would be appropriate.

Bibliography

Deakin CD. (1998). *Clinical Notes for the FRCA*. Edinburgh, UK: Churchill Livingstone.
Looney Y, Quinton P. (2005). Mitral valve surgery. *Continuing Education in Anaesthesia, Critical Care and Pain*, **5**(6), 199–202.
Morgan GE, Mikhail MS. (1996). *Clinical Anaesthesiology*, 2nd edition. Appleton and Lange.

Mitral valve disease (chest X-ray)

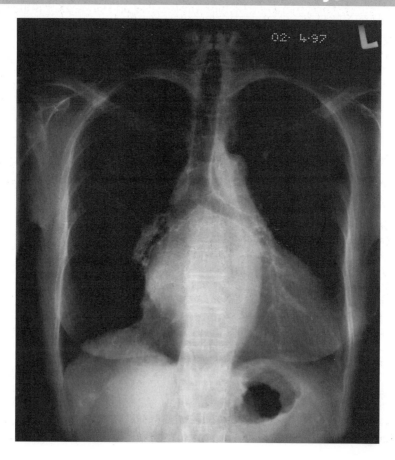

Have a look at this chest X-ray. What does it show?

This is a PA chest X-ray of a female patient.

The film is not rotated and is adequately penetrated.

There is a **double heart border** on the right and straightening of the upper left heart border suggesting an enlarged left atrium. The **carina is splayed greater than 60°** and there is **upper lobe blood diversion**.

These features suggest mitral stenosis. In addition, there is cardiomegaly (CT ratio>0.5) which only occurs in the presence of co-existing mitral regurgitation.

The diagnosis is therefore **mixed mitral valve disease**.

What are the additional X-ray features that suggest severe, late disease?

These are the features of pulmonary hypertension and pulmonary oedema. In addition, the mitral valve annulus may be a calcified.

X-ray features of pulmonary hypertension and oedema

- Pulmonary arteries prominent in perihilar regions but 'pruned' peripherally.
- Upper lobe blood diversion (mild venous hypertension).
- Interstitial oedema (moderate) – fluid in fissures, pleural effusions and Kerley B lines.
- Alveolar oedema (severe) – pleural effusions, areas of consolidation and mottling of the lung fields.

Myasthenia gravis

What is myasthenia gravis?

This is a rare condition characterised by **fatiguable weakness** classically affecting the **ocular, bulbar and proximal limb muscles**. There is **destruction of the acetylcholine receptor** protein at the (largely post-junctional) neuromuscular junction, resulting in the failure of neuromuscular transmission. Serum **acetylcholine receptor antibodies** (polyclonal IgG) are present in 90% of generalised cases. It is twice as common in females, is associated with **thymoma in 10%–15%** of cases and may be associated with other autoimmune conditions, e.g. thyrotoxicosis, rheumatoid arthritis, pernicious anaemia and SLE.

What is myasthenic syndrome?

This is a **paraneoplastic syndrome** also known as **Eaton–Lambert syndrome** (ELS) characterised by proximal muscle weakness that typically affects the

lower extremities. It is most commonly associated with **small-cell carcinoma** of the lung.

Can you compare and contrast the two conditions?

The two conditions differ in several ways.

- **At a molecular level**, Eaton–Lambert syndrome results from a pre-junctional defect in the quantal release of acetylcholine, which may be due to antibodies directed against calcium channels. Myasthenia gravis is due to a post-junctional defect as already described.
- **Clinically**, Eaton–Lambert syndrome more commonly affects the lower limbs. It can also produce autonomic effects (hypotension, gastroparesis or urinary retention).
- **Exercise** causes improvement in the weakness with Eaton–Lambert syndrome ('second wind phenomenon'), but worsening with myasthenia gravis. This can be easily demonstrated electrophysiologically (incrementing response as opposed to decrementing).
- **Anticholinesterases** do not cause an improvement with Eaton–Lambert syndrome. Instead, guanidine hydrochloride and 4-aminopyridine often help by enhancing Ach release by acting on calcium and potassium channels.
- **Response to neuromuscular blockers**. ELS patients are sensitive to both depolarizing and non-depolarizing muscle relaxants. Myasthenia gravis patients are resistant to depolarizing muscle relaxants.

What problems does a patient with myasthenia gravis pose for the anaesthetist?

Some form of categorizing this question is worth learning.
The problems of anaesthetizing a myasthenic patient breakdown into:
The problems of. . .. 1. Altered response to drugs, esp. muscle relaxants.
2. The type of surgery being performed.
3. Severity of disease.
4. Co-existent medical (auto-immune) disease.
5. Intercurrent medication – steroids, etc.
6. Exacerbation of disease.
7. Post-op respiratory failure.

- **Altered response to drugs**, especially muscle relaxants. The response to suxamethonium is unpredictable. Relative resistance (ED_{95} reported as 2.6 times normal), prolongation or a phase II block may be seen. Opioids or barbiturates may produce profound respiratory depression. Patients are often extremely sensitive to non-depolarising relaxants. Either avoid (patients can often be intubated with volatile alone) or use at about 1/10 of the usual dose. However, atracurium has been used without problems because of its rapid metabolism. A nerve stimulator must be used.

- **The type of surgery** being performed. With a thymectomy there is a risk of damage to the SVC and a risk of pneumothorax. Venous access in the lower limbs may be prudent. After trans-sternal thymectomy 50% of patients require post-operative ventilation.

- **Severity of disease:** Respiratory or bulbar muscle involvement? Increased risk of aspiration Arterial blood gases/CXR/PFTs will be needed to assess respiratory embarrassment.

- **Co-existent auto-immune disease**
- **Current treatment** may include steroids, azathioprine, cyclophosphamide, cyclosporin and anticholinesterases (typically pyridostigmine which lasts about 3–4 hours). Medical treatment should be optimised. This may include plasmapheresis. There is debate about whether to reduce or stop anticholinergics before surgery. Patients are better off being slightly myasthenic rather than cholinergic.

Anticholinesterases may cause:

  Increased vagal reflexes (? pre-medicate with atropine) The possibility of disrupting bowel anastomosis. Prolonged action of ester-type local anaesthetics and suxamethonium (inhibition of plasma cholinesterase).

- **Exacerbation of the disease** may be caused by surgery, stress, infection, aminoglycosides, hypokalaemia and pregnancy.
- **Post-operative respiratory failure**.

Increased risk with: Disease duration >6 years Co-existing pulmonary disease Vital capacity <40 ml/kg Pyridostigmine dose >750 mg/day Poor bulbar function.

Apart from needing surgery, how else may you be asked to help with the management of a myasthenic patient?

- **Intensive care management**
- Performance of an **edrophonium ('Tensilon') test** -distinguishing a myasthenic crisis from a cholinergic crisis. There is a risk of bradycardia and bronchoconstriction.

What is the difference between a myasthenic crisis and a cholinergic crisis?

- **A cholinergic crisis** is due to excessive administration of anticholinesterases and causes increased weakness with pronounced muscarinic effects:
  Bradycardia
  Salivation
  Sweating

Small pupils

Lacrimation

Abdominal pain

Diarrhoea

Edrophonium will exacerbate the weakness.
- **A myasthenic crisis** is due to under-treatment with anticholinesterases. Weakness will improve after administration of edrophonium.

Bibliography

Baraka A. (1992). Anaesthesia and myasthenia gravis. *Canadian Journal of Anaesthesia*, **39**(5), 476–86.

Craft TM, Upton PM. (1995). *Key Topics in Anaesthesia*, 2nd Edition. Bios Scientific Publishers Limited.

Hirsch NP. (2007). Neuromuscular junction in health and disease. *British Journal of Anaesthesia*, **99**(1), 132–8.

Schady W. (1997). Myasthenia. *Current Anaesthesia and Critical Care*, **8**, 279–84.

Myotonic dystrophy

A 35-year-old male patient with mild myotonic dystrophy presents for wisdom teeth extraction.

What is the underlying metabolic problem with this disorder?

It is an intrinsic muscle disorder. There is **delayed muscle relaxation due to abnormal closure of sodium/chloride channels** following depolarisation. This causes repetitive discharge and contraction.

What are the clinical features associated with myotonic dystrophy?

- **General** Frontal balding

  'Lateral' smile

  Muscle wasting – especially sternocleidomastoids, shoulders and quadriceps

  Gonadal atrophy → infertility

  Ptosis

  Cataracts

  Low serum IgG

- **Neurological** Bulbar problems Slurred speech

  Dysphagia

  Can lead to **aspiration**, a frequent cause of death

  Decreased tone and reflexes with muscle wasting

  Foot drop

  Decreased IQ in 40%

- **Cardiac** — Conduction defects (primary heart block, bundle-branch block and widened QRS) – may need pacing
  Increased QTc and increased PR interval
  Cardiomyopathy → cardiac failure
  Mitral valve prolapse
- **Respiratory** — Respiratory muscle fatigue → poor cough → LRTI
  Restrictive lung defect
  Centrally mediated decreased ventilatory response to CO_2
  Obstructive sleep apnoea
  Chronic hypoxaemia → Cor pulmonale
- **Gastrointestinal** — Constipation
  Delayed gastric emptying
- **Endocrine** — Diabetes
  Hypothyroidism

What are the problems when anaesthetizing these patients?

- **Undue sensitivity to anaesthetic drugs** (opioids, barbiturates and volatiles)
- **Precipitation of myotonia** by: — Anaesthetic and surgical interventions
  Diathermy
  Cold (monitor temperature)
  Pregnancy (atonic uterus and PPH also reported)
  Shivering (avoid high volatile concs.)
  Suxamethonium
  Non-depolarising muscle relaxants
  Anticholinesterase drugs
  K^+ containing solutions
  Exercise

- **Cardiovascular and respiratory problems** – especially the risk of aspiration.
- **Control of blood sugar** as many of these patients have diabetes.
- **Drug interactions** with concomitant drug treatment: phenytoin, quinine, procainamide.
- **Presentation** may be late on in the disease (second–fourth decade) and the disease may therefore present undiagnosed to the anaesthetist.

(NB. No proven link with malignant hyperthermia.)

What anaesthetic techniques can be used?

- **Pre-operatively** these patients should have:
  An ECG (24-hour if appropriate)
  Full blood count, urea, electrolytes (NB. K^+) and a blood sugar
  Pulmonary function tests
  Arterial blood gases
  Chest X-ray.
- **Pre-medication** – respiratory depressants should be avoided.
- Antacids are advisable.

- **Invasive monitoring** would be appropriate (arterial line/CVP/PAFC) if there is a history of arrhythmias or cardiomyopathy.
- **Temperature** must be monitored and maintained. Warming mattresses and warmed i.v. fluids should be used.
- **Induction and maintenance**. Propofol has been shown to be safe. Extreme caution with dosing. Intubation is necessary to protect against aspiration. High concentrations of volatiles should be avoided as they can cause shivering and hence myotonia.
- **Regional techniques** will avoid the use of general anaesthetic drugs that can precipitate myotonia. Nerve blockade will not, however, prevent the myotonic reflex. Local anaesthetic infiltration into the *muscle* can prevent this reflex.
- If a **muscle relaxant** must be used, then the agent of choice would be atracurium. Neuromuscular block monitoring is essential.
- **Post-operatively**, HDU or ICU care should be considered. Early feeding should be avoided due to the possibility of aspiration.

Bibliography

Driessen, Jacques J. (2008). Neuromuscular and mitochondrial disorders: what is relevant to the anaesthesiologist? *Current Opinion in Anaesthesiology*, **21**(3), 350–5.

Goldstone JC, Pollard BJ. (1996). *Handbook of Clinical Anaesthesia*. Edinburgh, UK: Churchill Livingstone.

Morgan GE, Mikhail MS. (1996). *Clinical Anaesthesiology*, 2nd edition. Appleton and Lange.

Russell SH, Hirsch NP. (1994). Anaesthesia and myotonia. *British Journal of Anaesthesia*, **72**, 210–16.

Obesity

A 40-year-old female (weight = 120 kg, height = 155 cm,) is on your list for an abdominoplasty.

How can you classify obesity?

There are numerous classification systems for categorising the relationship between height and weight. The two commonest are:

- The **body mass index** (BMI) is a useful method and is calculated by
    BMI = weight (kg)/height squared (m²)
    22–25 is normal.
    25–30 is considered overweight.
    >30 is obesity.
    >40 or >35 with obesity-related comorbidity is morbid obesity. (from AAGBI)
- The **Broca Index** is another method and has a different formula for males and females.
    Normal weight (kg) for males = height (cm) – 100
    Normal weight (kg) for females = height (cm) – 105

This lady's BMI is 49, which would define her as morbidly obese.

What are the problems that her obesity may pose for anaesthesia?

> There are two approaches to this question. The one you choose will be a combination of personal choice and the way in which the question is asked.
>
> 1. A **body systems** approach – describing the pathophysiology of each system.
>   The danger with this method is that it is easy to omit practical problems, e.g. cannulation, positioning and monitoring.
> 2. A more practical, **chronological approach** listing the problems encountered from the pre-operative, through to the post-operative period.

Cardiovascular
- **Increased blood volume and cardiac output** leading to cardiomegaly, left ventricular hypertrophy (therefore reduced compliance and diastolic function) and a potential for left ventricular failure.
- **Hypertension** and **ischaemic heart disease** are common.
- **Venous access** can sometimes be difficult.
- **Thromboembolism** risk is increased.

Respiratory
- **Increased work of breathing**.
- **Reduced compliance** (both chest wall and lung) and **reduced FRC** will pre-dispose to atelectasis, increased shunt and hypoxia. These patients must be pre-oxygenated as they desaturate much quicker than non-obese (3–5 times).
- Pulmonary vasoconstriction, **pulmonary hypertension** and right ventricular hypertrophy.
- Oxygen consumption and carbon dioxide production are increased.
- **Obstructive sleep apnoea** is relatively common and 5% have **Pickwickian syndrome** in which there is a loss of the sensitivity to hypercarbia resulting in a combination of **hypoxia, cor pulmonale and polycythaemia**.
- There is a higher incidence of **difficult laryngoscopy**.

This presents the anaesthetist with a patient who may be difficult to bag-mask ventilate, difficult to intubate and will desaturate quickly.

Gastrointestinal
- **Increased acidity and volume** of gastric contents.
- **Hiatus hernia** and **gallstones** are common associations.
- **Increased intra-abdominal pressure**.
- There is a higher risk of **regurgitation and aspiration** requiring rapid sequence induction if a difficult airway is not anticipated.
- Tracheal extubation should be undertaken with the patient awake.

Endocrine
- There is an association with **glucose intolerance**.

Morphological
- **Positioning**
- **Transferring**
- **Monitoring** (arterial line may be needed if NIBP is problematic)

How would you assess this lady's airway?

History	Symptoms of obstructive sleep apnoea including snoring and daytime hypersomnolence. The patient's partner may give a useful description of apnoeic episodes.
	Previous anaesthetic charts should be reviewed to determine if there were problems with airway maintenance in the past.
Examination	Assessment of head and neck movement
	Mouth opening
	Mandibular movement
	Thyromental distance
	Nostril patency
Investigations	Indirect laryngoscopy may be useful.
	Radiology

The incidence of difficult intubation in morbid obesity is around 13%

Altered anatomy:	Increase in soft tissue
	Reduced head and neck mobility
	Large tongue
	Short neck
	Large breasts
	Anterior larynx
	Restricted mouth opening

Tell me how you would anaesthetise this lady.

There is no one right answer to this question. Whichever method is chosen should be systematic and start with history, examination and investigations. Conduct of anaesthesia, including pre-medication and post-operative management, should then be discussed. The examiner may stop you and jump to an issue they wish to explore.

Having taken a history, examined the patient and performed appropriate investigations, consideration should be given to pre-medication. Anti-emetics and sodium citrate may be prescribed and an anticholinergic agent should be given if fibre-optic intubation is to be performed.

If a difficult intubation is not anticipated, then the patient should be pre-oxygenated (in the head up position if possible) for at least 3 minutes and a rapid sequence induction performed with cricoid pressure. All difficult airway adjuncts should be immediately available. Once the airway is secured with an endotracheal tube, the patient should be ventilated. Compared with non-obese patients a higher FiO_2 and the addition of PEEP may be required to help prevent basal atelectasis. However, the addition of PEEP may adversely affect venous return and cardiac output.

A combination of general and regional anaesthesia has many advantages but:

- Regional blocks can be technically difficult as anatomical landmarks may be obscured. Longer needles may be necessary.
- Epidural local anaesthetic dose requirements are reduced as the volume of the epidural space is reduced.

Analgesia with intravenous paracetamol, an NSAID such as parecoxib and morphine would be reasonable. Anti-emetics should not be forgotten and post-operative analgesia could be provided with a combination of regular paracetamol and brufen with PCA morphine.

Important post-operative considerations include:

- Extubate awake, sitting up.
- HDU care, may need CPAP.
- Oxygen and oximetry.
- Obstructive sleep apnoea is most common *some days after* surgery.

- Adequate analgesia to allow deep breathing/coughing.
- Physiotherapy
- DVT prophylaxis

Bibliography

Adams JP, Murphy PG. (2000). Obesity in anaesthesia and intensive care. *British Journal of Anaesthesia*, **85**(1), 91–108.
Brodsky JB. (1998). Morbid obesity. *Current Anaesthesia and Critical Care*, **9**, 249–54.
The Association of Anaesthetists of Great Britain and Ireland. (2007). Perioperative Management of the Morbidly Obese Patient.

Obstructive sleep apnoea

A 45-year-old man is referred to your pre-operative anaesthetic clinic. During your routine assessment, he reveals that he is troubled by day-time somnolence and his partner says that his snoring could wake the dead. His weight is 135 kg and he is 175 cm tall.

What concerns you about his history?

He has symptoms suggestive of obstructive sleep apnoea (OSA) almost certainly related to his weight.

Can you define and classify this condition

- Apnoea is defined as cessation of airflow for more than 10 seconds.
- Sleep disordered breathing encompasses obstructive and central sleep apnoea.
- Obstructive sleep apnoeas are present when there is persistent effort without airflow.
- Obstructive sleep apnoea syndrome is defined as OSA accompanied by day-time symptoms such as hypersomnolence.
- The Respiratory Disturbance Index (Apnoea/Hypopnoea Index – the number of apnoeas/hypopnoeas per hour of sleep) is used to classify the severity of OSA syndrome together with the degree of associated symptoms and hypoxaemia.
  - 5–15 mild
  - 15–30 moderate
  - >30 severe

What are the predisposing factors for OSA syndrome?

- Obesity
- Increasing age
- Male gender

- Alcohol, sedatives, analgesics, anaesthetics
- Smoking
- Nasal obstruction
- Pharyngeal/laryngeal obstruction
- Endocrine /metabolic
- Neuromuscular disorders
- Chronic renal failure

What other symptoms may you elicit from the history?

Patients may commonly report restless or unrefreshing sleep, whilst their partners may have witnessed apnoeic episodes. Less commonly, patients report nocturnal sweating, morning headaches, nocturia and reduced libido.

What are the potential complications of OSA?

Cardiovascular	Hypertension
	Right heart failure
	Ischaemic heart disease
	Cerebrovascular disease
Respiratory	Pulmonary hypertension
	Hypoxaemia and hypercapnia
Endocrine	Reduced growth hormone/testosterone levels
	Diabetic instability
CNS	Impaired cognition
	Accident risk
	Anxiety/depression
	Chronic headache
GIT	Gastro-oesophageal reflux

What pathophysiological changes occur during an episode of hypopnoea/apnoea?

During sleep, the narrow floppy airway in patients with OSA collapses as a result of the decrease in dilator muscle activity and the sub-atmospheric pressure generated during inspiration. Depending on whether the collapse is partial or complete, snoring or apnoea will result. Arousal is caused by a decreasing PaO_2, increasing $PaCO_2$ and increased respiratory efforts. The arousal response is accompanied by an abrupt increase in BP and heart rate.

How is the diagnosis of OSA syndrome made?

Overnight polysomnography (PSG) is regarded as the gold standard investigation. EEG and submental EMG are recorded for the purpose of staging sleep, ECG, pulse oximetry, respiration and body position are monitored. The PSG data is divided into epochs of 30s.

What treatment modalities are available?

Mild cases

- Weight loss
- Smoking cessation
- Alcohol and sedative intake reduction
- Mandibular repositioning devices

Moderate

- Measures mentioned above
- Nasal CPAP – pneumatically splints the airway

Severe

- Initially bi-level non-invasive ventilatory support followed by CPAP once control of respiratory failure has been achieved.

What is the role of surgery for OSA syndrome?

There is very little evidence that tongue base reduction or uvulopalatopharyngoplasty confers any significant long lasting benefit. Where OSA is due to tonsillar or adenoid hypertrophy or tumours of the larynx or pharynx, the surgical treatment is clear. Life threatening OSA may require a tracheostomy.

How would you manage this patient peri-operatively?

Pre-operative assessment must establish:

- Severity and complications of the apnoea
- Causes of OSA
- Mode of treatment and compliance.

Anaesthetic management depends on:

- Impact of the surgery on the OSA
- Requirements for post-operative analgesia.

Pre-operatively, patients who use CPAP should take the equipment with them to theatre and the staff should be instructed in its use.

Intra-operatively a regional technique will circumvent issues of airway maintenance and suppression of arousal responses. Where a general anaesthetic is considered, a difficult intubation should be anticipated. Opioids should be used with care.

Post-operative care should involve nursing in an appropriate environment with the application of CPAP if required.

Bibliography

Davies R, Stradling J. (1993). Acute effects of obstructive sleep apnoea. *British Journal of Anaesthesia*, **71**, 725–9.

Loadsman JA, Hillman DR. (2001). Anaesthesia and sleep apnoea. *British Journal of Anaesthesia*, **86**, 254–66.

Pacemakers

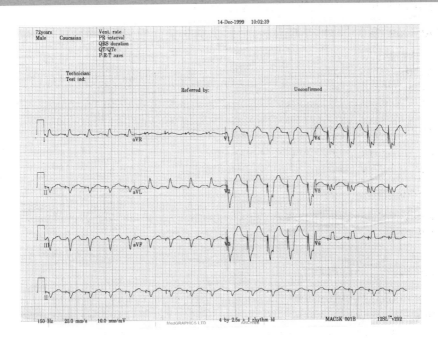

14-Dec-1999   10:02:39

| 72years Male   Caucasian | Vent. rate PR interval QRS duration QT/QTc P-R-T axes |
| Technician: Test ind: |

Referred by: Unconfirmed

150 Hz   25.0 mm/s   10.0 mm/mV   MedGRAPHICS LTD   4 by 2.5s + 1 rhythm ld   MAC5K 001B   12SL™ v252

Have a look at this ECG

The ECG shows paced rhythm from a ventricular pacemaker with a rate of approximately 100 bpm. The QRS complexes are broad and bizarre looking in keeping with the abnormal pathway through slower conducting ventricular tissue.

How are pacemakers classified?

There is a **five-letter code** that describes the characteristics of each permanent pacemaker. The first three letters are the most important. The North American Society of Pacing and Electrophysiology (NASPE) and the British Pacing and Electrophysiology Group (BPEG) produced a pacemaker code (NBG) in 1987. This was revised in September 2001.

Letter

I	Chamber paced	O = No action
		A = Atrium
		V = Ventricle
		D = Dual
II	Chamber sensed	O = No action
		A = Atrium
		V = Ventricle
		D = Dual
III	Response to sensed information	O = No action
		T = Pacemaker triggered
		I = Pacemaker inhibited

$$D = \text{Dual (ventricular sensed events lead to inhibition but atrial sensed events trigger ventricular output)}$$

IV Programmability, rate modulation	The ability of the pacemaker to alter the pacing rate in response to physiological variables such as increased activity, respiration or blood temperature. Generally, the sensors respond to increased movement or increased minute ventilation.
	O = No action
	R = Rate modulation
V Multisite Pacing	O = No action
	A = Atrium
	V = Ventricle
	D = Dual

The commonest pacemaker modes are: VVI (16.9%), VVIR (24.8%), DDD (27.3%) and DDDR (25.4%)

CRT (Cardiac resynchronisation therapy), or **biventricular pacing**, is used to improve cardiac performance in patients with heart failure.

ICDs (Implantable cardioverter defibrillators) can be complex and tailored to individual patients. They, too, have NASPE/BPEG codes to describe their function.

BPEG defibrillator codes

Chamber shocked (I)	Anti-tachycardia pacing chamber (II)	Anti-tachycardia detection (III)	Pacing chamber (IV)
O = No action	O = No action	E = Electrogram	O = No action
A = Atrium	A = Atrium	H = Haemodynamic	A = Atrium
V = Ventricle	V = Ventricle	V = Ventricle	D = Dual
D = Dual	D = Dual		

What is the anaesthetic management of a patient who is fitted with a pacemaker and requires surgery?

The main peri-operative problems in a patient with a permanent pacemaker are due to the effects of anaesthetic agents, altered physiology and surgical diathermy.

Pre-operative assessment

Usual anaesthetic assessment plus:

■ In 2005 the **ASA** made some recommendations regarding peri-operative management. The MHRA (Medicine and Healthcare products Regulatory Agency) and Heart Rhythm UK (HRUK) have also produced some guidance in 2006.

- **Establish the original indication** for inserting the pacemaker, what type it is, when it was last checked and information about any programmed functions it may have. If it's an ICD, has it shocked them?
- Look for symptoms that may suggest problems with pacing, e.g. syncope or palpitations
- Pacemakers with rate-responsive or anti-tachycardia modes should probably have them deactivated pre-operatively
- **Check pacemaker function:**   ECG
  If the intrinsic rate is higher than that set on the pacemaker, then a Valsalva manoeuvre may be employed to check function. CXR will identify number and integrity of leads
- **Check electrolytes** – especially K^+ Hypokalaemia → loss of capture.
  Hyperkalaemia
  → ventricular irritability
- Acid–base disturbances, some anti-arrhythmic drugs, digoxin toxicity and hypothermia may influence capture. These should be addressed and corrected if necessary.
- If in doubt, get a cardiology opinion – may require temporary pacing.

Intra-operative management

- Appropriate monitoring based on pre-op assessment.
- An alternative means of pacing must be immediately available: external, transvenous or oesophageal.
- Care at induction – may result in stimulation or inhibition of the pacemaker due to alterations in myocardial conduction or sensed muscular contractions (e.g. etomidate or suxamethonium) depending on the pacemaker programme.
- Volatile agents do not significantly alter the pacing threshold
- Etomidate and ketamine may be best avoided due to the possibility of myoclonic movements.
- Avoid hypoxaemia and hypercarbia – ectopics and arrhythmias.
- Rate-responsive pacemakers may induce a tachycardia in response to a high respiratory rate set on the ventilator (trans-thoracic impedance).
- **Diathermy** The use of diathermy may reprogramme the pacemaker, cause microshock or induce VF. Bipolar should be used if possible or, if unipolar is essential, the plate should be placed as far away from the heart as possible. Short bursts followed by long pauses should be used.
- **Magnets** In general should not be used. If placed over a programmable pacemaker in the presence of electromagnetic interference (e.g. diathermy), there may be unpredictable reprogramming. The magnet may also initiate a 'threshold test' whereby the output current gradually decreases until failure of capture occurs! Although the 'magnet rate' is usually written on the packaging for each pacemaker, most anaesthetic references now recommend that magnets are not used.
- Peripheral nerve stimulators may interfere with pacing.

- If DC cardioversion is required, the paddles should be placed perpendicular to the direction of the pacing wire (i.e. in anterior and posterior positions). The box is designed to protect itself by diverting current away from the internal circuitry, which may then pass down a damaged lead resulting in burns.
- Isoprenaline may be required as a holding measure, while emergency pacing is achieved in the event of pacemaker failure.

Post-operatively

- Pacemaker function should be checked at the pacemaker clinic.

Bibliography

Allen M. (2006). Pacemakers and implantable cardioverter defibrillators. *Anaesthesia*, **61**(9), 883–9.

Bennett DH. (1994). *Cardiac Arrythmias*, 4th edition. BH Publishing.

Bourke M. (1996). The patient with a pacemaker or related device. *Canadian Journal of Anaesthesia*, **43**(5), R24–32.

Deakin CD. (1998). *Clinical Notes for the FRCA*. Edinburgh, UK: Churchill Livingstone.

Morgan GE, Mikhail MS. (1996). *Clinical Anaesthesiology*. Appleton and Lange.

Rastogi S, Goal S, Tempe DK, Vivani S. (2005). Anaesthetic management of patients with cardiac pacemakers and defibrillators for noncardiac surgery. *Annals of Cardiac Anaesthesia*, **8**, 21–32.

Paediatric day-case surgery

You are asked to anaesthetise a fit 3-year-old child for circumcision as a day case. Is this an appropriate patient for day case anaesthesia?

Yes, provided the child has a suitable social set-up and no potential issues with general anaesthesia.

Suitability for day case may be assessed on four areas.

Patient factors

- Either fit and well or well-controlled systemic diseases such as asthma.
- Age > 50–60 weeks post-conceptual age if pre-term due to apnoea risk.
- Absence of active viral or bacterial infections particularly respiratory tract infections (excluding isolated runny noses, as this is usually benign seasonal rhinitis and is very common). **The presence of respiratory tract infections should result in deferral of surgery for 2–4 weeks** to reduce the risk of intra-operative laryngospasm, bronchospasm and post-operative hypoxia.
- Absence of undiagnosed murmurs (should be investigated pre-operatively) or significant congenital heart disease.
- Absence of diabetes mellitus.

Surgical factors

- Duration <1 hour
- Surface or laparoscopic procedures
- Minimal anticipated blood loss
- Anticipated post-operative pain controllable with simple analgesics.

Anaesthetic factors
■ Absence of known anaesthetic problems such as difficult airway or family history of MH.

Social factors
■ Adequate parental support, cooperation and understanding of instructions
■ Telephone in home or nearby
■ Access to transport and proximity to hospital (<1 hour away)

The child with a cold

> ■ It is very common to have a child with a runny nose.
> ■ Probably OK to continue if the child is at the end of a cold, is constitutionally well and has a normal temperature and no chest signs, otherwise postpone.
> ■ Increased risk of laryngospasm, bronchospasm, airway secretions and airway obstruction.
> ■ Postpone for 2 weeks for an URTI and 4 weeks if lower respiratory tract signs are present.

What would be your lower age cut-off for day case anaesthesia?

Pre-term infants with post-conceptual ages less than 50–60 weeks are unsuitable for day case because of increased apnoea risk in the post-operative period. Some centres will not accept term infants below this age while others will consider well, term infants for minor procedures.

What pre-medication would you consider using in paediatric day case?

■ Cutaneous local anaesthesia with EMLA (eutectic 2.5% lidocaine and 2.5% prilocaine) or Ametop (4% tetracaine gel – Tetracaine was previously known as Amethocaine in the UK, hence the name Ametop).
EMLA should be applied > 1 h before cannulation and is unlicensed below 1 year. Ametop has a more rapid onset and may be applied >45 min before cannulation. It is not recommended below 1 month of age.
■ Profoundly anxious children or those with behavioural or learning difficulties may require sedative pre-medication.
Midazolam 0.5 mg/kg orally or nasally will usually result in adequate sedation if given 30–45 min prior to induction. While post-operative sedation is seldom a problem, it may occur. Other traditional sedatives result in too much post-operative sedation to be used in day case.
■ Simple analgesia may be given pre-emptively as a pre-med.

What anaesthetic agents would you use in paediatric day case?

■ **Induction** with either intravenous Propofol (2.5–4 mg/kg) or inhalation with Sevoflurane are acceptable techniques. Thiopentone may result in delayed recovery.

■ **Maintenance** with a volatile agent in oxygen/air or oxygen/nitrous oxide may be used and facilitate spontaneous breathing. The use of nitrous oxide in day case has not been shown to increase the incidence of PONV in children. Sevoflurane offers rapid emergence and is well tolerated, though in short procedures there is not likely to be a benefit in terms of discharge time compared with isoflurane that justifies the extra cost. Desflurane has been advocated due to rapid wake up but may cause airway irritation and coughing in spontaneously breathing patients. TIVA with Propofol may be of use if PONV is anticipated.

What analgesics would you use in paediatric day case and how would you administer them?

■ **Paracetamol** may be given orally as pre-med (single loading dose of 20 mg/kg if aged over 3/12 or 15 mg/kg below), rectally (single dose of 40 mg/kg) or intravenously (15 mg/kg).

■ **NSAIDs** are suitable agents for day case and Ibuprofen 5 mg/kg orally pre-operatively or Diclofenac 1mg/kg orally or rectally are the most commonly used. The majority of children with asthma do not have NSAID sensitivity, the exception being those with nasal polyps.

■ **Opioids** may produce significant sedation and PONV. Ideally, only short-acting agents such as fentanyl (1–2 ug/kg i.v.) or weak opioids such as codeine (1 mg/kg orally) should be considered.

■ **Local anaesthetic blocks** may reduce or obviate the need for opioids.

How would you anaesthetise this child?

■ **Pre-operative:** Full anaesthetic history from the parents including fasting status and examination of the child including weight measurement. Explanation and consent for penile block under general anaesthesia and consent for rectal analgesia. Cutaneous anaesthesia with EMLA or Ametop on the ward and calculation of drug doses. Preparation of emergency drugs, atropine 20 ug/kg and suxamethonium 1.5–2 mg/kg.

■ **Induction:** Full anaesthetic monitoring. i.v. induction with Propofol or inhalation with Sevoflurane if cannulation is difficult. Insertion of LMA (probably size 2).

■ **Analgesia:** Penile block after induction. IV Paracetamol and Diclofenac.

■ **Maintenance:** Spontaneously breathing on Sevoflurane in oxygen/air mix (or oxygen/nitrous oxide). Intravenous fluid if prolonged starvation (either 10 ml/kg bolus or calculation of deficit and replacement). Some anaesthetists advocate prophylactic anti-emetics, particularly in high risk patients. Suitable agents are Ondansetron 0.15 mg/kg and Dexamethasone 0.15 mg/kg.

- **Emergence:** 100% oxygen in left lateral position.
- **Discharge criteria post-operatively:**
  - Stable vital signs.
  - Pain and nausea controlled.
  - Able to pass urine and drink fluids.

What other blocks may you consider?

An alternative to a penile block would be a caudal block. The potential problems with a caudal in an ambulatory child would be temporary leg weakness and the risk of urinary retention, which may delay discharge.

Explain how you would perform a penile and caudal block.

Penile block:
- Take consent from the parents.
- Full preparation with trained assistant and resuscitation equipment available.
- Calculate toxic dose of local anaesthetic to prevent over-dose. (Bupivacaine or levobupivacaine 2 mg/kg). Adrenaline containing local anaesthetics must be avoided.
- After induction of anaesthesia leave the patient in the supine position.
- Full asepsis with skin preparation.
- **Palpate the distal symphysis pubis**.
- Pass a 21G block needle just distal to the palpating finger.
- When the needle contacts the distal edge of the symphysis pubis, it should have passed through **Buck's fascia** and be in proximity to the dorsal nerves of the penis.
- After careful aspiration, inject local anaesthetic (Bupivacaine 0.5% 1ml + 0.1 ml/kg). Some advocate performing injections either side of the midline because of a possible midline septum.
- The block is completed by subcutaneous injection across the base of the penis (Bupivacaine 0.5% 2 ml).

Caudal block:
- Take consent from the parents.
- Full preparation with trained assistant and resuscitation equipment available.
- Calculate local anaesthetic dose to be delivered. According to the regimen of Armitage this would be 0.5 ml/kg of Bupivacaine 0.25% for a lumbosacral block.
- After induction of anaesthesia, place the child in the left lateral position (if a right-handed approach).
- Full asepsis with skin preparation.
- Locate the sacral hiatus (defect due to failure of the fusion of the fifth and sometimes fourth sacral laminae). The sacral hiatus may be located by:

(a) The sacral hiatus forms the apex of an equilateral triangle with the posterior superior iliac spines.
(b) Place your index finger along the curve of the sacrum in the midline with the tip on the tip of the coccyx. Withdraw the finger cephalad until a depression is felt.

In both techniques the sacral cornua can be palpated just cephalad to the sacral hiatus.

■ Insert a 22G cannula at 45 degrees aiming cephalad until a 'click' is felt. Bring the cannula to a more shallow angle (approximating the long axis of the spinal column) and advance the plastic cannula forward a short distance (the dural sack may terminate at S2 or lower).
■ Careful aspiration for blood or CSF should be performed before injection of local anaesthetic.
■ If resistance is encountered or swelling occurs, injection should be terminated and the cannula should be repositioned.

Regimen of Armitage for caudal blocks

■ 0.25% Bupivacaine
■ Volume based on weight and the level to be blocked
■ Lumbosacral block up to L1 – 0.5 ml/kg
■ Block up to T10 – 1 ml/kg
■ Block up to T6 – 1.25 ml/kg
■ It can be seen that the higher blocks use more than the suggested maximum dose of Bupivacaine of 2 mg/kg. However, this is a well-recognised and widely used formula.

Bibliography

Brennan LJ, Prabhu AJ. (2003). Paediatric day-case anaesthesia. *British Journal of Anaesthesia CEPD Reviews*, **8**(5), 134–8.
Morton NS. (2004). Local and regional anaesthesia in infants. *British Journal of Anaesthesia CEPD Reviews*, **4**(5), 148–51.
Payne K, Moore EW, Elliott RA, Moore JK, McHugh GA. (2003). Anaesthesia for day case surgery: a survey of paediatric clinical practice in the UK. *European Journal of Anaesthesiology*, **20**(4), 325–30.
Pinnock CA, Fischer HB, Jones RP. (1998). *Peripheral Nerve Blockade*. Churchill Livingstone.
Sasada M, Smith S. (1997). *Drugs in Anaesthesia and Intensive Care*. Oxford, UK: Oxford Medical Publications.

Paediatric fluid management

You are asked to anaesthetise a 6-year-old child who has acute appendicitis and has been unwell for the past 2 days. There are no significant findings in your medical or anaesthetic assessment. What problems do you need to address in the peri-operative period?

The main issues are:

- Physiological effects of acute illness (dehydration and SIRS) – does the child need resuscitation prior to theatre?
- Emergency anaesthetic in a child.
- Risk of aspiration.
- Post-operative analgesia.

How would you assess the degree of dehydration clinically?

- Calculation of **water deficit** due to dehydration using clinical signs is usually inaccurate and only gives an approximation of the true deficit
- A history of vomiting, diarrhoea, poor urine output (wet/dry nappies in babies) and poor oral intake should be sought

---

Clinical assessment of dehydration – (Classifications vary)
Mild/no dehydration (<5%)
- No clinical signs

Severe dehydration (>10%)

Moderate dehydration (5%–10%)
- Cool pale peripheries
- Prolonged capillary return time
- Dry mouth
- Decreased skin turgor
- Sunken fontanelle (infant)
- Sunken eyes
- Deep (acidotic) breathing
- Tachycardia may be present
- Increased thirst

- Cold, sweaty, grey, cyanosed
- Irritability/lethargy
- Dry mouth and mucus membranes
- Markedly decreased skin turgor
- Sunken eyes
- Markedly sunken fontanelle (infant)
- Deep and rapid respiration
- Tachycardia present/feeble pulse
- Reduced blood pressure
- Reduced urine output

If the child was 10% dehydrated clinically and weighed 20 kg, how would you calculate the fluid deficit?

The formula is: **Wt (kg) × % Dehydration × 10**

- For this child: 20 × 10 × 10 = 2000 ml.
- Fluid deficits should be replaced over 24 hours and added to maintenance fluids.

What fluid would you use?

- **Resuscitation** – bolus doses of 10–20 ml/kg of 0.9% (isotonic) sodium chloride.
- **Deficits** – infusion over 24 hours of 0.9% sodium chloride with glucose 5% (isotonic solution) or normal saline alone.

■ **Maintenance** – 0.45% sodium chloride with glucose (5% or 2.5%) or Hartmann's solution.

Wouldn't you use 0.18% (one-fifth) normal saline with glucose 4%.

■ This is a markedly hypotonic solution and risks **hyponatraemia.**
■ Hyponatraemia is particularly problematic in the peri-operative period, but also with the dehydrated, septic, head injured or a chronically unwell child.
■ The risks of iatrogenic hyponatraemia have recently been highlighted by the **National Patient Safety Agency.**
■ One-fifth normal saline should be reserved for specialist units such as cardiac or renal wards.

What other considerations are there when it comes to fluid therapy?

■ **U&Es** should be monitored at baseline and every 24 hours.
■ **Ongoing losses** should be assessed every 4 hours.
■ **Glucose**-containing solutions should be administered to prevent hypoglycaemia in the fasting child.
■ **Potassium** should be added at up to 40 mmol/l guided by U&E results.
■ **Enteral fluid** administration should be considered regularly and instituted as soon as tolerated.

General points for fluid replacement

■ Ongoing losses should be replaced with 'like-for-like' fluids that reflect the electrolyte composition of the fluid being lost.
■ Losses can usually be replaced with isotonic solutions with or without the addition of potassium.
■ There is currently not enough evidence to recommend one glucose containing solution over another.
■ 2.5% glucose (with 0.45% saline or Hartmann's) is probably enough to prevent hypoglycaemia in the fasting child.
■ Higher concentrations of glucose combinations are hyperosmolar and may require multiple cannulations or even central access for prolonged intravenous fluid therapy.

How would you provide post-operative analgesia for this child?

■ **Multi-modal analgesia**
■ **Paracetamol**
  - 15 mg/kg i.v. or
  - 40 mg/kg (p.r.) loading
  - 15 mg/kg maintenance 4–6 hourly
  - Max 90 mg/kg per day
■ **NSAID** such as Diclofenac – 1 mg/kg 8 hourly

- **Opioids** such as morphine
  - 0.15 mg/kg i.v.
  - 0.3 mg/kg p.o. 2–3 hourly
- **Wound infiltration** with local anaesthetic
  - Bupivicaine 0.25% (up to 2 mg/kg)
- **Anti-emetics**: combination therapy would be reasonable in this case.
  - Ondansetron 0.15 mg/kg
  - Dexamethasone 0.15 mg/kg

Fluid requirements

- Fluid requirements in infants are greater than in adults or older children because of their higher metabolic rate and their greater surface area to weight ratio.
- This results in higher insensible water loss.
- The reduced renal concentrating capacity also results in increased obligatory water loss.
- Formula for daily maintenance fluid requirements
  - First 10 kg   4 ml/kg per hour   (100 ml/kg per 24 hours)
  - Second 10 kg   2 ml/kg per hour   (50 ml/kg per 24 hours)
  - Subsequent kgs   1 ml/kg per hour   (20 ml/kg per 24 hours)

Solution	Osmolarity (mOsmol/l)	Sodium content (mequiv/l)	Osmolality (compared to plasma)	Tonicity
0.9% sodium chloride	308	154	Isosmolar	Isotonic
0.45% sodium chloride with 5% glucose	432	75	Hyperosmolar	Hypotonic
5% glucose	278	–	Isosmolar	Hypotonic
0.9% sodium chloride with 5% glucose	586	150	Hyperosmolar	Isotonic
0.18% sodium chloride with 4% glucose	284	31	Isosmolar	Hypotonic
Hartmann's solution	278	131	Isosmolar	Isotonic

Bibliography

National Patient Safety Agency. (2007). Patient Safety Alert 22. *Reducing the risk of hyponatraemia when administering intravenous infusions to children.* March.

Stewart P. (2007). New maintenance fluid guidelines for children : is 0.9% sodium chloride with 5% glucose a good choice? *Anaesthesia*, **62**, 319–24.

Penetrating eye injury

You are asked to anaesthetise a 15-year-old girl who sustained a penetrating eye injury 1 hour ago. She is fit and well but had fish and chips just prior to her injury.

What are the issues here?

There are two major and conflicting priorities in this case.

1. The need to minimize the risk of aspiration in a patient requiring emergency anaesthesia with a full stomach.
2. The need to avoid a rise in intra-ocular pressure (IOP).

What are the determinants of intra-ocular pressure?

- Normal IOP is 12–20 mmHg.
- The eye can be thought of in a similar way to the skull. If any of the contents of this 'rigid' sphere (such as blood or aqueous humour) increase, then the IOP will increase.
- Raised IOP may be caused by direct pressure on the eye, raised CVP, hypertension, hypercarbia, hypoxia, coughing, straining or alterations in production/drainage of aqueous humour.
- When the globe is open, the IOP is equal to atmospheric pressure, therefore anything that would normally lead to raised IOP will lead to extrusion of intra-ocular contents.

How do induction agents alter IOP?

Most reduce IOP with the exception of ketamine, which may cause an increase via hypertension. (Ketamine may also cause nystagmus and blepharospasm.)

How do volatile anaesthetics alter IOP?

All modern inhalational agents reduce IOP in proportion to the depth of anaesthesia. The fall in BP with increasing depth of anaesthesia reduces choroidal blood volume and relaxes the extra-ocular muscles. The pupillary constriction aids aqueous drainage. There may also be a direct action on central control mechanisms.

How do muscle relaxants alter IOP?

Non-depolarising agents have minimal effect on IOP.
Suxamethonium increases IOP by around 5–10 mmHg for 5–10 minutes.

Why does suxamethonium have this effect?

The extra-ocular muscles have a more prolonged contraction compared with other skeletal muscles due to their innervation by multiple neuromuscular junctions ('en-grappe' – bunch of grapes) on each muscle fibre.

How will you manage this case?

Local anaesthesia is not suitable, as IOP will be raised by injecting around the globe. Discuss the degree of urgency with the surgeon. It may be possible to delay surgery until an adequate starvation time has elapsed though eye injury may result in gastric stasis and the surgery is likely to be urgent.

The surgeon feels that the surgery is urgent and must be performed straight away.

What will you do?

- Reduce the risk of aspiration and its consequences as much as possible.
- Rapid sequence induction
- Obtund response to suxamethonium/laryngoscopy/intubation

This is **not a life-threatening emergency.** However, the surgery is urgent. Giving metoclopramide will encourage gastric emptying, ranitidine will raise the pH of any remaining contents and 0.3M sodium citrate will neutralise remaining gastric acid.

The patient will require a **rapid sequence induction** with cricoid pressure. The main issue is the use of suxamethonium. If airway assessment suggests that intubation will be straightforward, then rocuronium could be considered, but if there is any doubt then protection of the airway should come first. If rocuronium is used, then it is important to give it adequate time to work (at least 60 seconds). Coughing at this stage may be disastrous. In a study of RSI using suxamethonium in 228 patients with penetrating eye injury, there was no loss of vitreous through the eye wound (Libonati et al., 1985).

Fentanyl (3–5 mcg/kg), **alfentanil** (20 mcg/kg) or **lignocaine** (1.5 mg/kg) could be used to obtund the hypertensive response to laryngoscopy. Pre-treatment with a non-depolarising muscle relaxant will also reduce the IOP rise associated with suxamethonium.

Remifentanil (1 mcg/kg immediately prior to induction) has also been shown to effectively obtund the IOP response to suxamethonium and intubation.

Attention should be given to general measures to prevent a rise in IOP. These are similar to those used in the management of raised intracranial pressure. Anti-emetics should be given to try to prevent vomiting in the post-operative period.

Coughing on the tube at emergence is a risk. However, if the patient is deemed to be at risk of aspiration, then protection of the airway takes priority and the patient should be extubated awake. If the risk is low, then consider changing the tube for an LMA whilst still paralysed or under deep anaesthesia.

If IOP increases intra-operatively what would you do?

- Look for a cause and treat.
- Other therapeutic measures

Ensure adequate depth of anaesthesia and analgesia. Hypercarbia and hypoxia should be addressed as should any obstruction to venous flow. Mannitol (0.5 g/kg) or acetazolamide (500 mg) could be considered.

What is the oculo-cardiac reflex and how is it managed?

It may occur following pressure on the eyeball, traction on the extra-ocular muscles, pain or raised IOP. There may be bradycardia, nodal rhythm, ectopic beats, sinus arrest or even ventricular fibrillation.

The afferent passes via the ophthalmic division of the trigeminal nerve to the sensory nucleus in the fourth ventricle. The efferent is supplied via the vagus.

Management involves asking the surgeon to stop operating for the time being, ensuring adequate depth of anaesthesia and analgesia and administering atropine or glycopyrrolate if it persists.

> The management of penetrating eye injury is not black and white. There are many different techniques described in the literature. An informed presentation of the issues surrounding its management and a safe approach should hopefully win the day!

Bibliography

Craft TM, Upton PM. (1995). *Key Topics in Anaesthesia* 2nd edition. Bios Scientific Publishers Limited.

Deakin CD. (1998). *Clinical Notes for the FRCA*. Churchill Livingstone.

Libonati MM, Leahy JJ, Ellison N. (1985). The use of succinylcholine in open eye surgery. *Anaesthesiology*, **62**, 637–40.

Mergatroyd H, Bembridge J. (2008). Intraocular pressure. *Continuing Education in Anaesthesia, Critical Care and Pain*, **8**(3), 100–3.

Morgan GE, Mikhail MS. (1996). *Clinical Anaesthesiology*, 2nd edition. Appleton and Lange.

Ng H-P, Chen F-G, Yeong S-M, Wong E, Chew P. (2000). Effect of remifentanil compared with fentanyl on intraocular pressure after succinylcholine and tracheal intubation. *British Journal of Anaesthesia*, **85**(5), 785–7.

Phaeochromocytoma – peri-operative management

You are asked to anaesthetise a patient for resection of a phaeochromocytoma. What is a phaeochromocytoma?

A phaeochromocytoma is a functionally active, catecholamine-secreting tumour of the neuroendocrine **chromaffin** cells found in the sympathetic nervous system. They account for about 0.1% of cases of hypertension. They are usually benign and localised to an adrenal gland. These tumours are important to the anaesthetist because they can present unexpectedly peri-operatively and the mortality is high.

- They may secrete any combination of
  - Noradrenaline
  - Adrenaline
  - Dopamine
  - Occasionally vasoactive intestinal peptide (VIP) or ACTH.

How does it present?

- The commonest presentation is **sustained hypertension.**
- The classic presentation is of **paroxysms of sympathetic crises** (in 35% of cases).
  - Severe hypertension
  - Flushing
  - Sweating
  - Palpitations
  - Headache
  - Anxiety
  - Weakness
  - Lethargy
- Paroxysms may be precipitated by multiple factors:
  - Simple activities such as exercise
  - Manoeuvres that increase intra-abdominal pressure such as sneezing, voiding and defaecating.
  - Histamine releasing drugs and succinylcholine
  - Anaesthetic procedures (particularly intubation)
- If undiagnosed, it may present with end-organ damage:
  - Heart failure
  - Pulmonary oedema
  - Myocardial ischaemia
  - Cerebro-vascular events
- Presentation may be determined by the dominant catecholamine secreted:
  - Mainly noradrenaline   Hypertension, headaches, Slow, thudding palpitations

- Mainly adrenaline   Tachycardias
                      Anxiety attacks
- Mainly dopamine   Nausea and vomiting

Effects of adrenoreceptors

- α_1 Vasoconstriction
  Sweating
  ↓ insulin and glucagon release
- α_2 Inhibition of noradrenaline release
- β_1 Chronotropy
  Inotropy
  Renin secretion
- β_2 Smooth muscle relaxation   -bronchi
                                          -vascular wall
                                          -uterus

  ↑ insulin and glucagon release

How is the diagnosis confirmed?

- Clinical suspicion on the basis of history or hypertension.
- Traditionally by measuring **urinary catecholamines** or their metabolites (vanillylmandelic acid [VMA] and metanephrine).
- **Clonidine Suppression Test** – lack of suppression suggests phaeochromocytoma (prevents noradrenaline reuptake).
- Genetic testing may identify familial cases.
- **CT** can localise adrenal tumours with 93%–100% sensitivity.
- **MRI** scan of the abdomen has a slightly higher sensitivity for extra-adrenal tumours.
- An **isotope scan** may help to localise an extra-adrenal tumour. A radio-labelled iodine isotope, ^{123}I-metaiodobenzylguanidine (**MIBG**), is taken up by the chromaffin cells.
- Selective vena caval sampling.

What is the 10% rule?

- 10% are extra-adrenal and can be anywhere along the sympathetic chain from skull base to pelvis.
- 10% are bilateral.
- 10% are malignant.
- 10% occur in children.

Are there any associations with other conditions?

- **Multiple endocrine neoplasia** (MEN) Syndrome Type 2
  - Type 2A – medullary thyroid carcinomas and parathyroid adenomas
  - Type 2B – medullary thyroid carcinomas and Marfanoid features.

- **Von Hippel–Lindau disease** (Phaeochromocytomas, cerebellar haemangioblastomas, and renal cell carcinoma).
- **Neurofibromatosis Type I** (von Recklinghausen disease) – 1% incidence of phaeochromocytoma.
- **Familial carotid body tumours.**

If you saw this person 10 weeks pre-operatively, what investigations and treatment would you institute?

- The aim of pre-operative management is to:
  - Determine the site of the tumour and what it secretes.
  - Normalize the blood pressure.
  - Allow the resolution of catecholamine cardiomyopathy.
  - Correct hypovolaemia (contracted intravascular volume).
- An echocardiogram is useful to assess left ventricular function and to exclude cardiomyopathy.
- ECG
- α and β-adrenoceptor blockade
  - Controls the symptoms and hypertensive swings
  - Reduces the hypertensive surges associated with tumour handling.
- **α-adrenoceptor blockade should be instituted prior to β-blockade.**

> **Regarding β-blockers**
>
> - Theoretically unopposed β-blockade should be avoided. This can block compensatory β_2 vasodilatation and precipitate a hypertensive crisis. Cardiac failure may also occur due to the reduced contractility in the presence of a high afterload.
> - Selective β_1-blockade is used in adrenaline secreting tumours.
>
> NB It is not uncommon for patients to have been commenced on a β-blocker for treatment of their hypertension, usually without adverse effects.

Does it matter which alpha blocker you use?

- **Phenoxybenzamine** is a non-selective α_1 and α_2 blocking drug
  - It binds covalently and irreversibly to the receptors.
  - It has a long duration of action and may contribute to post-operative hypotension.
  - α_2 blocking can inhibit pre-synaptic noradrenaline re-uptake
  - Usually necessitates the use of β-blockade to treat secondary tachycardia
- **Prazosin** and **doxasosin** are shorter acting competitive α_1 selective blocking drugs
  - Less tachycardia
  - May not require adjuvant β-blockade unless the tumour is secreting adrenaline.

Do you need a cardioselective β-blocker?

In theory, avoiding β_2 blockade will allow β_2-mediated vasodilatation to continue but in practice a selective β_1-blocker is not necessary. β-blockers are usually added to control tachycardia secondary to α-blockade. Selective β_1-blockers may be used for adrenaline secreting tumours or to treat the tachycardia associated with the use of phenoxybenzamine.

Assuming that this patient has been adequately treated pre-operatively, how would you anaesthetise them for laparoscopic tumour removal?

- Sedative pre-medication
- Invasive arterial and central venous monitoring is essential.
- Large bore i.v. access
  - The patient may be intravascularly depleted after prolonged sympathetic over-stimulation.
  - Large fluid shifts are possible.
- Cardiac output monitoring is useful in those with cardiomyopathy
- Induction with remifentanil and propofol. Remifentanil may be useful in this instance as it has short-acting sympatholytic properties.
- Vecuronium to paralyse the patient to avoid the potential histamine (and therefore catecholamine) release associated with other agents.
- Intubate the patient and maintain anaesthesia with a mixture of oxygen, air, sevoflurane and remifentanil.
- Opioid-based analgesia is reasonable for a laparoscopic technique.
- Thoracic epidural for an open procedure.

What drugs would you have drawn up or immediately available?

Blood pressure swings can be dramatic but transient and so the available drugs must be potent and short-acting.

- **Phentolamine** (a non-selective α-antagonist) may be given as an infusion or a bolus (1–2 mg increments). It acts within one circulation time.
- The heart rate should be kept below 100 bpm. Short-acting β-blockers such as **Esmolol** or **Metoprolol** may be useful for this.
- **Magnesium** blocks catecholamine release and the adrenoceptor response to noradrenaline. It also has anti-arrhythmic activity.
- **Labetalol** is a combined α and β blocker ($\sim$1:10 α: β activity). Onset in 5 minutes but effect may last hours.
- There can be hypotension during these procedures too, particularly once the tumour has been removed.
- There may be profound hypovolaemia necessitating several litres of fluid.
- Vasopressors such as **epinephrine and metaraminol** should also be immediately available.

> **Surgical technique**
>
> ■ Open lateral retroperitoneal approach
>   ● Quicker
>   ● Fewer catecholamine surges
>   ● More painful
> ■ Laparoscopic approach
>   ● Long operation
>   ● Shorter recovery time
>   ● Greater surgical manipulation – more instability.

How would you treat post-operative hypotension?

Post-operative hypotension is a common problem as the source of catecholamines has been removed but the adrenergic blockade remains.

■ Assessment of pre-load/volume status, cardiac function, inotropy and the peripheral vascular resistance should guide treatment.
■ Catecholamine infusions in 'normal' doses may be ineffective, therefore **fluid** and **posture** may need to be the mainstays of treatment.
■ Early extubation helps by negating the need for sedation.
■ Adrenaline can be useful if there is evidence of left ventricular failure.
■ Noradrenaline or Vasopressin may be useful in refractory vasodilatation.
■ When both adrenals have been removed, **hydrocortisone** is required immediately.

What other specific problems may occur post-op?

■ **Hypoglycaemia:** Hyperglycaemia is often associated with the catecholamine surges and following tumour removal the patients may become hypoglycaemic.
■ The symptoms of this may be masked by β-blockade so the glucose should be measured regularly.
■ **Glucocorticoid and mineralocorticoid deficiency** requiring supplementation with hydrocortisone and fludrocortisone.
■ **Electrolyte and fluid imbalance**

Bibliography
Allman K, Wilson I. (2002). *Oxford Handbook of Anaesthesia* (Oxford Handbooks) 2nd edition. Oxford, UK: Oxford University Press. ISBN: 0192632736.

McIndoe AK. (2002). Recognition and management of phaeochromocytoma. *Anaesthesia and Intensive Care Medicine*, 3(9), 319–24.

Prys-Roberts C. (2000). Phaeochromocytoma – recent progress in its management. *British Journal of Anaesthesia*, **85**, 44–57.

Pneumonectomy

A 67-year-old man is listed for a right pneumonectomy for carcinoma of the lung.

What histological types of bronchial carcinoma are there?

- Squamous   35%
- Small (oat) cell   25%
- Adenocarcinoma   20%
- Large cell   20%

What are the symptoms and signs of bronchial carcinoma?

The commonest **symptoms** are cough, haemoptysis and dyspnoea, followed by chest pain, wheeze and weight loss.

Signs include clubbing, wheeze, stridor and supraclavicular lymph nodes.

The signs of the *complications* of bronchial carcinoma are varied and can be categorised into:

- **Intra-thoracic** Pleural effusion
  SVC obstruction
  Recurrent laryngeal nerve palsy
  Phrenic nerve palsy
  Horner's syndrome
  Pericarditis, cardiac arrhythmias (especially AF)
  Rib erosion
- **Non-metastatic** Ectopic hormone secretion, e.g. ADH/ACTH from oat cell tumours
  Neuromuscular, e.g. mixed sensorimotor peripheral neuropathy, encephalopathy, proximal myopathy, Eaton–Lambert (myasthenic) syndrome and polymyositis
  Haematological, e.g. anaemia, polycythaemia, bleeding disorders
  Weight loss
  Hypertrophic pulmonary osteoarthropathy
  Thrombophlebitis migrans
- **Metastatic** Brain, bone, liver, adrenals, skin, kidney

What are the risk factors for developing a bronchial carcinoma?

The biggest risk factor is **cigarette smoking** but others include:

- Increasing age
- Male > female
- Asbestos exposure
- Radiation

What are the important considerations in your pre-operative assessment?

There are now guidelines to aid the selection of patients with lung cancer for surgery. These assess a patient's fitness for surgery, based heavily on age, pulmonary function and cardiovascular fitness. Risk is stratified into minor, intermediate and major.

Age

Peri-operative morbidity for lung cancer surgery increases with age. Mortality rates for pneumonectomy average 14% in the elderly (higher than in younger patients), and therefore age should be a factor in assessing suitability for pneumonectomy.

Pulmonary function

1. If $FEV_1 > 2.0$ l then no further respiratory function tests are required.
2. If $FEV_1 < 2.0$ l then *post-operative* FEV_1 and T_{LCO} need to be estimated and compared to predicted values for normal patients.

> Estimated post-operative $FEV_1 > 40\%$ predicted
> Estimated post-operative $T_{LCO} > 40\%$ predicted } average risk
> Saturation $> 90\%$ on air
>
> Estimated post-operative $FEV_1 < 40\%$ predicted
> Estimated post-operative $T_{LCO} < 40\%$ predicted } high risk
>
> All others – exercise testing

High-risk patients need formal multi-disciplinary discussion and consideration of alternative treatment.

Cardiovascular fitness

There is little specific information relating to the cardiac risks of patients who are undergoing pneumonectomy and most data surrounds the 'non-cardiac surgery' group. Clinical predictors of increased peri-operative cardiovascular risk include:

■ **Major**	Recent MI
	Grade 3 or 4 angina (Canadian Cardiovascular Society)
	Decompensated CCF
	Significant arrhythmias
	Severe valvular disease
■ **Intermediate**	Grade 1 or 2 angina (CCS)
	Prior MI
	Compensated CCF
	Diabetes mellitus
■ **Minor**	Advanced age
	Abnormal ECG
	Rhythm other than sinus
	Low functional capacity
	History of stroke

Other considerations pre-operatively are weight loss, nutritional status and other medical co-morbidities.

Bibliography
British Thoracic Society. (2001). Guidelines on the selection of patients with lung cancer for surgery. *Thorax*, **56**, 89–108.
Kumar PJ, Clark ML. (1990). *Clinical Medicine*, 2nd edition. Baillière-Tindall.

Post-operative confusion

You are asked to see a 65-year-old lady, in recovery, post-total abdominal hysterectomy. She is confused and aggressive.

What are the causes of post-operative confusion?

Another very broad question . . .

■ Questions where the answer is an enormous list of causes, are never as easy as they appear.

■ You **must** categorise your answer. Not only does this demonstrate organised thinking in the stress of the exam, but it demonstrates that, in the 'real' world, you have a clear, logical approach to clinical problems.

■ ABC – exclude emergency causes, e.g. airway obstruction/respiratory distress
■ The common causes are:

Physiological effects of anaesthesia and surgery
- Hypoxaemia
- Hypotension
- Hypercapnia/Hypocapnia
- Metabolic
  - Hypoglycaemia
  - Hyponatraemia
  - Hypercalcaemia
- Pain or discomfort (including bladder distension)
- Sepsis
- Hypothermia/Hyperthermia

Pharmacological effects
- Drugs
  - Anticholinergics
  - Opioids
  - Ketamine/propofol
  - Benzodiazepines
  - Volatiles
- Withdrawal
  - Delirium tremens
  - Benzodiazepines

Specific patient events

- Pre-existing cognitive dysfunction
- CVA (emboli – especially with by-pass)
- Hepatic failure
- Renal failure

Post-operative cognitive dysfunction (POCD)

- Post-operative confusion may be multi-factorial.
- Many studies are conflicting over causation.
- There are changes in **neurotransmitter levels** (catecholamines and the cholinergic system).
- Increased **cortisol** levels post-operatively may play a role in post-operative delirium in the elderly.
- The incidence reported varies considerably between studies.
- ~25% of patients over 60 years of age will have evidence of cognitive dysfunction at 1 week.
- **Emergency surgery** and increased **blood loss** are implicated.

What are the causes of hypoxia in the post-operative period?

- Hypoventilation is the most common cause and can itself result from a number of peri-operative situations:
  - Residual effects of anaesthetics, benzodiazepines and/or opioids
  - Incomplete reversal of neuromuscular blockade
  - Airway obstruction (laryngospasm, laryngeal oedema, reduced conscious level, retained airway packs, etc.)
  - Pain, particularly from thoraco-abdominal procedures can also lead to hypoventilation.
- Atelectasis and lobar collapse
- Pulmonary oedema
- Pneumonia (and aspiration pneumonitis)
- Bronchospasm (and anaphylaxis)
- Pneumothorax
- Pulmonary embolism
- Shock
- Pre-existing lung disease.
- It is important to note that there is a significant alteration in normal respiratory physiology with advancing age, e.g. closing capacity encroaches on FRC, reduced elastic recoil, increased V/Q mismatch, all of which result in much less respiratory reserve and faster onset hypoxia.

How would you manage this lady?

- After giving supplementary oxygen, perform an examination of the patient following an ABC approach.
- Review the patient's medical and operative history.
- Pay particular attention to what drugs had been given and intra-operative haemodynamic and respiratory stability.

■ Urinary retention should be remembered as a frequently encountered and easily remedied cause of confusion.
■ Arterial blood gases, FBC, U & Es, chest X-ray, and ECG may form part of the assessment.
■ Lateralising neurological deficits will require further investigation with CT scan if persistent.

Correction of causative factors for post-operative confusion forms the mainstay of treatment and this should be done following the ABC hierarchy. **Pharmacological management** should be reserved for patients with profound delirium and for those with withdrawal.

■ Haloperidol 0.5–5 mg i.v. (low dose in elderly patients)
■ Benzodiazepines may be necessary but current evidence suggests that these drugs are more of a cause of the problem than a solution
■ Chlordiazepoxide 10–20 mg p.o. for alcohol withdrawal. Thiamine may be added if there are concerns regarding Korsakoff's psychosis.

Delirium on ICU

■ Recognition is the key to treatment
■ 3 Motoric subtypes -Hyperactive
　　　　　　　　　　　 -Hypoactive
　　　　　　　　　　　 -Mixed
■ Confusion Assessment Method for ICU (CAM ICU) – popular delirium assessment scale
■ Age/Severity of illness/Lorazepam – three biggest risk factors
■ 8 out of 10 ventilated patients suffer with delirium
■ Treatment　　　　　-Non-pharmacological (environment etc.)
　　　　　　　　　　　 -SCCM based guideline – haloperidol preferred

Bibliography

Chung FF. Postoperative delirium in the elderly. *ASA website.*
Dodds C, Allison J. (1998). Postoperative cognitive deficit in the elderly surgical patient. *British Journal of Anaesthesia*, **81**, 449–62. www.icudelirium.org.
Fines DP, Severn AM. (2006). Anaesthesia and cognitive dysfunction in the elderly. *BJA Continuing Education in Anaesthesia, Critical Care, and Pain*, **6**(1), 37–40.

Post-operative hypotension

You are asked to see a 40-year-old lady in recovery after an elective right hemicolectomy. The nurse is concerned because her blood pressure is 80/40. What are the causes of hypotension in recovery?

Questions like this can be difficult because, although they appear simple, their scope is large. Start simply and categorise your answers, mentioning common things first.

Mean arterial pressure is determined by the formula MAP = CO × SVR. Cardiac output is determined by heart rate and stroke volume (which is dependent on pre-load, after-load, and contractility). Therefore, hypotension may be caused by:

- **Reduced SVR:**
  - Residual anaesthetic agents.
  - Sympathetic blockade from spinal or epidural anaesthesia.
  - Opioids.
  - Systemic inflammatory response or sepsis.
  - Hypothermia or pyrexia.
  - Anaphylaxis or anaphylactoid reactions.
  - Actions of patient's normal medication especially ACEIs and Angiotensin 2 blockers.
  - Hypercapnia (though sympathetic stimulation usually produces hypertension).
- **Low heart rate:**
  - High epidural or spinal block with cardiac sympathetic block.
  - Myocardial ischaemia or infarction (particularly inferior).
  - Pre-operative beta-blockade or digoxin (particularly if hypokalaemic).
  - Opioids.
  - Hyperkalaemia.
  - Hypothermia.
  - Profound hypoxia.
- **Reduced pre-load:**
  - Absolute hypovolaemia due to bleeding or other intra-operative losses.
  - Relative hypovolaemia due to vasodilatation. Similar to causes of reduced SVR.
  - Obstruction to venous return such as tension pneumothorax or right to left obstruction due to pulmonary embolism.
- **Reduced contractility:**
  - Myocardial ischaemia or infarction
  - Hypoxia
  - Hypocalcaemia
  - Hyperkalaemia
  - Hypothermia
  - Beta-blockade
  - Cardiac insufficiency in TUR syndrome.

The commonest causes of Low MAP peri-operatively are:

- Volume related (relative or absolute) as volume is the biggest determinant of cardiac output.
- A low SVR – as many anaesthetic drugs affect SVR.

How would you approach this problem?

I would familiarise myself with the patient's history and peri-operative records to identify relevant factors such as cardiac history, pre-operative medication, pre-operative and intra-operative blood pressure, anaesthetic agents and techniques used, and intra-operative fluid loss and fluid management.

I would also perform an Airway, Breathing and Circulation assessment of the patient and rectify problems as I identified them.

Tell me what you would be looking for in each part of your examination and what you would do?

Airway   **Look for obstruction leading to respiratory failure. I would give supplementary oxygen to all patients:**
- Mechanical obstruction due to low conscious level or residual neuromuscular blockade. Use airway opening manoeuvres and airway adjuncts. Naloxone or neostigmine may be indicated.
- Laryngospasm. PEEP should be applied via a bag and mask. Propofol may be useful to loosen the spasm, but suxamethonium should be available if re-intubation becomes necessary.
- Physical obstruction due to retained airway packs or vomitus.
- Airway oedema. May warrant re-intubation and dexamethasone.

Breathing   **Look, listen and feel noting respiratory rate, pattern, breath sounds, and oxygen saturation:**
- Hypo-ventilation due to residual anaesthesic agents, opioids or neuromuscular blockade. Naloxone or neostigmine may be indicated.
- Pulmonary oedema. Diuretics, nitrates and facial CPAP can be used but may compromise blood pressure. Severe cases will require re-intubation.
- Aspiration.
- Pneumothorax. If tension pneumothorax is suspected, needle thoracocentesis in the second intercostal space followed by formal intercostal drainage is indicated.
- Atelectasis.
- Hypo-ventilation due to high spinal. May require re-intubation and sedation until block descends.
- Pulmonary embolism.

Circulation   **Look, listen and feel noting heart rate, rhythm, blood pressure, capillary refill, urine output, drains output, fluid management, and evidence of occult bleeding:**
- Hypovolaemia due to haemorrhage or other flood loss. Treat with fluid resuscitation and blood products as needed. May require surgical input if bleeding.

- Vaso-dilatation. First line treatment should be fluid resuscitation but vasopressors may be required. Adrenaline may be required if anaphylaxis is suspected.
- Cardiac insufficiency. Signs of ischaemia or infarction should be sought and an ECG performed. Correction of hypoxia, hypovolaemia, hypothermia, and electrolyte imbalance may improve cardiac output. Inotropes may be required.

Bibliography

ATLS Manual. (2004). American College of Surgeons.

Comfere T. (2005). Angiotensin system inhibitors in a general surgical population. *Anesthesia and Analgesia*, **100**(3), 636–44.

Kumar P, Clark M. (1994). *Clinical Medicine*. Baillière Tindall.

Power I, Kam P. (2001). *Principles of Physiology for the Anaesthetist*. London: Arnold.

Rassam SS, Counsell DJ. (2005). Perioperative fluid therapy. *BJA CEPD Reviews*, **5**(5), 161–5.

Post-herpetic neuralgia

What do you understand by the term neuralgia?

This is simply a mononeuropathy of a named nerve.

Can you tell me something about the pathogenesis of post-herpetic neuralgia?

Following chicken-pox, the varicella-zoster virus lies dormant in the dorsal horn of the spinal cord. Shingles develops after reactivation of the dormant varicella zoster virus causing infection of a nerve. The infection causes nerve fibre damage by inflammation and ischaemia in both sensory and motor (usually subclinical) nerves. These lesions are at the dorsal root, dorsal root ganglion and dorsal horn. Post-herpetic neuralgia is a persistent nerve pain after the rash of shingles has disappeared.

What are the clinical features?

The initial herpes zoster is painful and has a variable time course. There is no set definition of post-herpetic neuralgia, but some authors use the presence of pain persisting at 1 month as diagnostic.

The syndrome occurs predominantly in patients over the age of 50 and is normally isolated to a single dermatomal segment, frequently unilateral. Thoracic dermatomes and the ophthalmic division of the trigeminal nerve are common sites.

The pain itself is severe with constant aching, burning or itching. There may be superimposed bouts of stabbing pain. Pigmentation and scarring may also occur.

What are the treatment options available?

- **Simple analgesics**
- **Tricyclic anti-depressants**
  These currently appear to be the most effective drugs used. Amitriptyline is commonly used as first line and changed or added to if not wholly effective. Tricyclics usually begin to ease the pain within a few days, but they may take several weeks to gain maximum benefit. They should ideally be continued for a month after the pain has gone. The doses needed are lower than those for depression.
- **Capsaicin cream**
  Acts by depleting the neurotransmitter substance P in small afferent fibres. The 0.075% cream is applied 3–4 times per day for 6 weeks. Capsaicin cream should not be used on broken or inflamed skin. Even on healthy skin, it may cause an intense burning feeling when it is applied.
- **Anti-convulsants**
  Phenytoin and carbamezepine have both been used successfully. More recently, gabapentin has been used with some success.
- **Opioids**
- **TENS**

Bibliography

Charlton E. (2001). *Post-herpetic Neuralgia*. Nuffield Department of Anaesthesia.
Grady KM, Severn AM. (1997). *Key Topics in Chronic Pain*. Bios Scientific Publishers.

Pre-eclampsia

What is the definition of pre-eclampsia?

Pre-eclampsia is a multi-system disorder occurring during pregnancy and characterised by:

- Sustained hypertension beginning after 20 weeks' gestation (systolic >140 or diastolic >90)
- Proteinuria – significant if 2^+ on dipstick testing or >300 mg/24 h

It is associated with significant potential morbidity and mortality to mother and baby.

What is the underlying pathophysiology?

In normal pregnancy, there is invasion of the spiral arteries by trophoblast. They dilate and thus their resistance decreases. In pre-eclampsia, this does not occur. Instead, the **spiral arteries maintain their muscular layer and contractile**

ability. This may be due to alterations in cytokine physiology. There is **placental ischaemia** and **membrane dysfunction in other organs**. The release of a tissue factor from the ischaemic placenta may be responsible for the widespread effects on maternal endothelial cells resulting in occlusive arteriolar spasm.

What are the main problems associated with pre-eclampsia?

- Hypertension
- Oliguria with difficulty in assessing fluid balance and risk of pulmonary oedema
- Impaired coagulation
- Abnormal liver function (HELLP) and risk of hepatic rupture
- Intra-uterine growth retardation
- Seizures

What are the principles of management?

- Control of hypertension
- Seizure prophylaxis
- Fluid balance
- Establish epidural analgesia early if possible.
- Timing and mode of delivery of the baby
- Anaesthetic techniques for delivery
- Post-delivery care

- **Control of hypertension**
  Drug therapy may include **labetolol** (either orally or intravenously) if it is not contraindicated, nifedipine (orally not sublingual) or intravenous **hydralazine**, **Epidural analgesia** may also be considered as an adjunct in the management of hypertension if the platelet count and coagulation screen are OK. This is very much a risk versus benefit decision. Haemodynamic measurements tend to divide the patients into two groups. The larger, low-risk, group consists of patients with hyperdynamic left ventricular function and a moderately raised SVR. The high-risk group patients have a failing heart in association with a very high SVR. Hence, a pulmonary artery catheter (or other method of measuring CO and SVR) may be required in very severe cases to establish the haemodynamics and guide management.
- **Seizure prophylaxis and recurrent seizures**
  Magnesium is the drug of choice. The management of seizures may be divided up into seizure prophylaxis, treatment of the first seizure and prevention of recurrent seizures.
  Seizure prophylaxis
  This is prevention of the first seizure. The MAGPIE study has shown that magnesium is effective in reducing the risk of seizures. It should be continued for 24 hours after delivery or 24 hours after the last seizure (whichever is later).

Treatment of acute seizures
Remember ABC. Magnesium is the drug of choice. It is recommended at a dose of 4 g over 5–10 minutes followed by an infusion of 1 g/hr. (2 g bolus if already on a magnesium infusion.) Diazepam, phenytoin and thiopentone may be used, but are not first-line therapies.

Prevention of recurrent seizures
The **Collaborative Eclampsia Trial** showed magnesium to be clearly superior to phenytoin and diazepam.

Magnesium therapy:

- **Dose = 4 g bolus** over 10 minutes followed by an **infusion of 1–2 g/h.**
- **Therapeutic level = 2–3.5 mmol/l**
- **Continue for 24 hours after last seizure.**
- **Magnesium 1 g $\equiv$ 4 mmol**

Symptoms and signs of hypermagnesaemia:

- Nausea and flushing
- Somnolence
- Double vision
- Slurred speech
- ↓ **patellar reflexes – first sign**   > 5 mmol/l
- Respiratory depression   > 6 mmol/l
- Respiratory arrest   6.3–7.1 mmol/l
- Cardiac arrest at   12.5–14.6 mmol/l

Magnesium may work by prevention of cerebral vasospasm through the block of Ca^{2+} influx via NMDA glutamate channels.

- **Fluid balance**
  Assessment of fluid balance is very difficult. There is a **contracted intra-vascular space but a tendency towards capillary leakage** and reduced colloid osmotic pressure. It is easy to give too much fluid to treat the oliguria and **pulmonary oedema is common particularly post-delivery** when interstitial fluid is mobilized. It has been shown that mothers are far more likely to die as a result of the effects of fluid overload than from renal failure secondary to hypovolaemia. Central venous pressure monitoring is only useful when the value is low to help diagnose hypovolaemia but, when greater than 6 mmHg, is not a reliable indicator of left ventricular filling pressure. It is important to **monitor input and output closely and avoid giving excessive volumes of fluid.** There is no difference in outcome if colloids are used instead of crystalloids.

- **Establish epidural analgesia**
  If timing and the clinical state of the patient permit, then siting an epidural under controlled conditions is ideal. It will suppress the hypertensive response to pain and may improve placental blood flow. If a caesarean section is required later and the **epidural** has already been sited then it can be topped-up for theatre. Coagulation tests and platelet count need to be checked prior to the procedure.

- **Timing and mode of delivery**
  This needs to be decided by the obstetrician and anaesthetist in collaboration and will be determined by the clinical situation. If there is

time, then optimisation of hypertension, anti-convulsant therapy and fluid balance is indicated prior to delivery.

Anaesthetic techniques for delivery

If an urgent caesarean section is required, and there is no time to establish an epidural, then the choice is limited to spinal or general anaesthesia. **Spinal** anaesthesia theoretically may result in hypotension and uteroplacental insufficiency although several publications in the recent literature describe its successful use and safety. If a regional block is contra-indicated, for example, because of coagulopathy, or there is no time because of severe fetal distress, then **general anaesthesia** will have to be undertaken. Factors making GA in pre-eclampsia particularly hazardous include a higher chance of difficult intubation and a marked pressor response at laryngoscopy and intubation. There is a significant risk of intracerebral haemorrhage secondary to severe hypertension. Invasive monitoring should be established pre-induction if there is time.

Post-delivery care

Convulsions can occur up to 23 days after delivery. In the UK, up to 44% of fits occur in the puerperium. Fluid balance can remain difficult in the post-operative period. The most common time for pulmonary oedema to occur is in the first 48–72 hours post-delivery. This is probably as a result of large volumes of fluid given peri-operatively (in the face of oliguria and capillary-leak syndrome) mobilising from the extravascular space as the patient improves. Platelet count is lowest in the 24–48 hours post-delivery and HELLP presents after delivery in 30% of cases. This demonstrates that, although delivery of the baby is the 'cure', it may not be the end of the problem. The decision to send a patient to **intensive care** is made on the basis of her clinical condition (a patient may also be considered for intensive care pre-operatively).

Bibliography

Brodie H, Malinow AM. (1999). Anaesthetic management of pre-eclampsia/eclampsia. *Review article, International Journal of Obstetric Anaesthesia*, April.

Engelhardt T, Maclennan FM. (1999). Fluid management in pre-eclampsia. *Review article, International Journal of Obstetric Anaesthesia*. October.

Mortl MG, Schneider MC. (2000). Key issues in assessing, managing and treating patients presenting with severe pre-eclampsia. *Review article, International Journal of Obstetric Anaesthesia*. January.

Royal College of Obstetricians and Gynaecologists. (2006). The management of severe pre-eclampsia. March.

Pre-medication

What are the indications for pre-medication in modern anaesthetic practice?

This question can be answered in a list fashion in the knowledge that the examiner will want you to elaborate on a number of your answers. The main indications are as follows:

> **Think of the seven As**
>
> ■ Anxiolysis
> ■ Amnesia
> ■ Anti-emesis
> ■ Analgesia – systemic and topical (for venepuncture)
> ■ Antacids
> ■ Antisialogogues
> ■ Additional – oxygen, nebulisers, steroids, heparin, etc.

Tell me what you would use for: 'anxiolysis/amnesia'

It is worth mentioning that the **pre-operative visit** is possibly the most important component of anxiolysis by establishing a rapport with the patient, discussing the anaesthetic technique and answering any questions they may have. Parental anxiety in paediatric practice can also be addressed at this stage.

■ **Benzodiazepines** are probably the most commonly prescribed pre-medicants. They act by enhancing GABA, an inhibitory neurotransmitter that causes an influx of chloride ions thereby hyperpolarising the neurone. They produce anxiolysis, amnesia and sedation and can be given orally, intramuscularly or intranasally. Typical doses are:

Temazepam	10–30 mg orally in adults
	0.5–1 mg/kg orally in children upto 20 mg
Midazolam	0.2–0.75 mg/kg orally in children (max 20 mg)
	5–10 mg i.m.
	0.2–0.3 mg/kg intranasally
Lorazepam	2–4 mg orally
Diazepam	5–10 mg orally in adults
	0.2–0.4 mg/kg orally in children

■ **Trimeprazine** (2 mg/kg), a phenothiazine with anticholinergic, antihistamine, antidopaminergic and α-blocking properties is used less commonly
■ The α_2-**agonists** clonidine and dexmedetomidine reduce sympathetic outflow and have been used as pre-medicants with sedative, anxiolytic and analgesic properties.

'Anti-emesis'

Most anaesthetists would target specific groups of patients at high risk of post-operative nausea and vomiting for pre-operative anti-emetics:

■ Previous history of PONV / motion sickness (three incidences of PONV)
■ Those having 'high risk' surgery, e.g. gynaecological, upper abdominal, middle ear and squint surgery.
■ Females (2–4 that of males)

- Obese patients
- Other risk factors – use of opioids, nitrous oxide, volatile versus TIVA.

The choice of anti-emetics is then from 5-HT$_3$, dopamine, histamine or muscarinic antagonists.

Dopamine antagonists:	This group includes the phenothiazines (commonly prochlorperazine), butyrophenones (droperidol) and metoclopramide. The evidence for the efficacy of these drugs is often variable and they can produce extra-pyramidal side effects, e.g. dyskinesia, tremor, dystonia and oculogyric crisis.
Histamine antagonists:	These act directly on the vomiting centre, e.g. cyclizine
Muscarinic antagonists:	This group, which includes hyoscine and atropine, is probably used less commonly than in times when reducing excessive secretions was an important component of pre-medication. Side effects include dry mouth, blurred vision, sedation and disorientation in elderly patients.
5HT$_3$ antagonists:	The advantage of these drugs, e.g. ondansetron is their efficacy and side effect profile compared to the more traditional agents. They are, however, more expensive.

Other modalities include:

Dexamethasone	The mechanism of action of dexamethasone is poorly understood.

- Acupuncture and acupressure
- NK$_1$ antagonists
- Cannabinoids

It should be noted that the use of anti-emetics as part of a pre-med does not reduce PONV any more than giving them at the end of surgery.

'Analgesia'

Routine opioid pre-medication for elective surgery is used less frequently than in years gone by and the concept of pre-emptive analgesia (modulating spinal cord nociceptive transmission) has yet to be translated into a proven clinical entity. Treating acute preoperative pain should be guided by the clinical situation.

In paediatric practice, EMLA™ cream is commonly used as a topical anaesthetic before venepuncture. This is the eutectic mixture of local anaesthetics and is a mixture of the unionised forms of lignocaine and prilocaine. It should be applied for at least 1 hour with an occlusive dressing covering it.

'Antacids'

The overall incidence of aspiration related to anaesthesia has been quoted as 1:3216, with a higher incidence for emergency surgery (1:895). Of these, 64% do not develop any further symptoms and 20% require mechanical ventilation. It is interesting to note that Warner *et al.* (1993) found no difference in the aspiration rate if pharmacoprophylaxis was used or not.

There are many risk factors that have been associated with peri-operative aspiration, e.g. emergency surgery, obstetrics, obesity and hiatus hernia. Historically, a significant residual volume of gastric juice (>0.4 ml/kg) and low pH (below 2.5) were thought to be important factors. This has since been questioned.

The main drugs used to alter gastric secretions are:

■ H_2-antagonists – these agents, e.g. ranitidine alter both the production and pH of gastric contents.
■ Sodium citrate is used to neutralize the pH of gastric contents, particularly in the obstetric setting
■ Prokinetic agents such as metoclopramide

Bibliography

Ahmed AB, Hobbs GJ, Curran JP. (2000). Randomised, placebo-controlled trial of combination antiemetic prophylaxis for day-case gynaecological laparoscopic surgery. *British Journal of Anaesthesia*, **85**(5), 678–82.
Warner MA, Warner ME, Weber JG. (1993). Clinical significance of pulmonary aspiration during the perioperative period. *Anaesthesiology*, **78**, 56–62.

Previous anaphylaxis

A patient with a history of anaphylaxis during general anaesthesia 3 months ago now presents for an evacuation of retained products of conception.

Discuss the anaesthetic management of this patient

The details of the episode must be established from the notes and the patient. The reaction may have been:

■ True anaphylaxis (Type I IgE mediated or Type III immune complex, IgG mediated)
■ Anaphylactoid (histamine release directly or by complement)
■ An alternative diagnosis that was misinterpreted either by the anaesthetist or the patient, such as:
  ● Asthma
  ● MH
  ● Angio-oedema
  ● Vaso-vagal episode.

All drugs given during the previous episode should be avoided if possible. Volatile anaesthetics have not been reported to cause anaphylaxis, so an inhalational technique would be safe if the patient was not thought to be at risk of regurgitation. A spinal anaesthetic may also be considered, although local anaesthetic allergy is possible.

There is insufficient time to establish the cause of the anaphylaxis and the surgery is urgent. The safest method of proceeding may be with a gas induction and maintenance of anaesthesia with avoidance of colloids and latex exposure.

- Avoid any drugs given in the initial anaesthetic if these can be identified, unless a specific drug has been implemented.
- There is significant cross over in related drugs, especially non-depolarising muscle relaxants (NDMRs)
- Do not give cephalosporins or imipenem to those with suspected or confirmed penicillin anaphylaxis.
- There may be a history of non-pharmacological reaction. The quaternary ammonium group of NDMRs are shared by some foods, cosmetics and hair-care products.
- There have been no reports of anaphylaxis to volatile anaesthetic agents, so an inhalational technique is possible.

What investigations for anaphylaxis would this patient have undergone post-operatively?

- **Serum tryptase**:
  - Released by degranulating mast cells in an IgE reaction.
  - It should be measured ideally at 0, 1, 6 and 24 hours (in reality the zero time means as soon as possible after resuscitation).
  - The half-life of tryptase is 2.5 hours.
  - Peak concentration at 1 hour (may be earlier in cases with associated hypotension).
  - The peak may be missed if the early samples are not taken.
- **Radioallergosorbent test (RAST)**
  - Involves laboratory exposure of antigen to patient serum to identify IgE reactions. Coated allergen particle (CAP) is a newer test.
  - Only really useful for suxamethonium, latex and penicillin, although many other RASTs exist (with lower specificity).
- **Skin prick testing**
  - Gold standard
  - Remember all the possible allergens such as latex, chlorhexidine, antibiotics, colloids and lidocaine.
  - If skin prick testing is negative and there remains a strong clinical suspicion, then intradermal testing can be considered.

When should you perform skin testing?

- Skin prick testing should be performed 4–6 weeks after the event to allow IgE stores to regenerate.

■ It needs to be done at a centre experienced in the performance and interpretation of such tests.
■ Resuscitation equipment should be available.

What is the evidence for pre-medicating this patient with an antihistamine in these circumstances?

Some would advocate pre-medication with an antihistamine and hydrocortisone, but there is no convincing evidence that this reduces the incidence of anaphylaxis.

Which induction agent is least likely to cause anaphylaxis?

■ There is not enough data to state which induction agent is more or less likely to cause a reaction but thiopentone has the longest safety history of all currently used agents.
■ Reactions to anaesthetic drugs are rare and the incidence in the UK is unknown.
■ The RCA estimates the risk of life-threatening anaphylaxis to be between 1 in 10 000 and 1 in 20 000 anaesthetics.

> ### Further information regarding anaphylaxis
>
> ■ In France, the incidence of anaphylaxis to neuromuscular blocking agents (NMBs) is 1 in 6500 anaesthetics.
> ■ In one study of 477 confirmed reactions, NMBs accounted for 62%, latex 17%, antibiotics 8%, hypnotics 5% and colloids, opioids and others approximately 3% each.
> ■ 17% of allergies to NMBs had not had a previous anaesthetic.
> ■ With allergy to NMBs, previous exposure was found in less than 50% of patients.
> ■ **Previous exposure to the allergic agent is not necessary.**

How would you recognise anaphylaxis if the patient was anaesthetised?

■ 88% present with signs of cardiovascular collapse related to distributive shock. There may be:
  ● Tachycardia
  ● Hypotension
  ● Low cardiac output state (seen as a reduced ET CO_2).
■ Cardiovascular collapse is the only feature in 10% of cases.
■ 36% present with bronchospasm due to histamine release.
■ Angio-oedema is present in 24% of cases.

■ Isolated cutaneous erythema is often seen due to local histamine release, commonly after atracurium, morphine or thiopentone injections. This is usually trivial but may represent the first sign of impending anaphylaxis.

If this patient presented for a peripheral limb operation, how would you anaesthetise her?

A regional technique such as spinal, supraclavicular or interscalene block could be performed, but care must be taken as the causative agent may have been latex, chlorhexidine, local anaesthetic agent or colloid.

Bibliography

Axon AD, Hunter JM. (2001). Anaphylaxis and anaesthesia – all clear now? *British Journal of Anaesthesia*, **93**, 501–4.

Fisher M, Doig G. (2004). Prevention of anaphylactic reactions to anaesthetic drugs. *Drug Safety*, **27**(6), 393–410.

Laxenaire M, Mertes P. (2001). Anaphylaxis during anaesthesia. Results of a two-year survey in France. *British Journal of Anaesthesia*, **87**(4), 549–58.

Problems of the premature baby

A 10-week-old female infant weighing 3.5 kg is scheduled for inguinal hernia repair. She was delivered prematurely at 34 weeks. What would you enquire about specifically in your pre-operative assessment?

■ A detailed history from the parents and the notes is required, particularly if the child spent any time on the neonatal ICU.
■ Details of any previous operations.
■ Time spent on a ventilator.
■ Any medical conditions or congenital problems diagnosed.
■ General health since leaving hospital – putting on weight, feeding (associated breathlessness?).
■ Special precautions or procedures required eg NG feeding, handling.
■ Any medications, including oxygen therapy.

Premature babies are defined as those born before 37 weeks' gestation and account for about 13% of UK births. They are susceptible to the following:

■ Increased risk of congenital abnormalities (especially 'small for dates' babies).
■ Hyaline membrane disease
■ Bronchopulmonary dysplasia
■ Patent ductus arteriosus

■ Intra-ventricular (brain) haemorrhage
■ Retinopathy of prematurity
■ Hypoglycaemia
■ Anaemia
■ Increased susceptibility to infection
■ Lack of thermoregulation.

What potential problems are there in anaesthetising her?

■ A **difficult airway** should be suspected if there has been prolonged intubation.
  ● This may be subglottic or be part of a congenital abnormality.
■ Previously ventilated neonates can have **poorly compliant lungs.**
  ● Adjust ventilation to minimise high airway pressures.
  ● Avoid high FiO_2.
■ Fluctuations in blood pressure should be avoided to minimise the risks of hypoperfusion (and resultant ischaemia) and haemorrhagic cerebral injury.
■ **Venous access** may be difficult after prolonged i.v. access in NICU.
■ **Drug metabolism** may be impaired due to immature liver and enzyme systems.
■ **Drug elimination** is impaired due to immature renal function.
■ **Hypoglycaemia** should be avoided by:
  ● Minimising the starvation time.
  ● Administering glucose containing i.v. fluids.
  ● Regular monitoring of the serum glucose concentration.
■ Meticulous attention should be paid to **maintaining normothermia.**
■ The general problems of anaesthetising a baby also apply (see box).

What precautions would you take post-operatively?

■ Post-operative **apnoea** is a common problem.
■ Apnoea is significant if >15 seconds or if associated with cyanosis or bradycardia.
■ An apnoea alarm is mandatory in the post-operative period.
■ **Caffeine** 10 mg/kg on induction reduces the incidence by 70%.
■ **CPAP** may be helpful by distending the chest wall and triggering stretch receptors.

How would you provide post-operative analgesia?

■ The principles of **multimodal analgesia** should be used.
    However:
  ● Avoid opioids if possible due to apnoea risk.
  ● NSAIDs should be used with caution as they reduce renal function by up to 20% and may affect ductus arteriosus closure in the very young neonate.
  ● Paracetamol dosing intervals are extended due to reduced metabolism.
  ● Paracetamol is given at a dose of 15 mg/kg 8 hourly.

- Use local anaesthetic infiltration where possible, e.g. Bupivicaine 2 mg/kg.

General considerations when anaesthetising a baby airway

- The airway is prone to obstruction because the head is relatively large with a prominent occiput and the tongue is large.
- Infants and neonates breathe mainly through their nose.
- The epiglottis is large, floppy and U-shaped.
- The trachea is short (endobronchial intubation).
- The glottis is more anterior and the narrowest part of the airway is at the cricoid ring.

Respiratory

- Ventilation is diaphragmatic and rate dependent.
- Horizontal ribs reduce mechanical advantage.
- Closing capacity encroaches into FRC during tidal breathing.
- Increased airway resistance (50% nasal).

Cardiovascular

- Rate-dependent cardiac output.
- Poor ventricular compliance.
- Low SVR.
- High vagal tone.

Gastrointestinal

- Immature enzyme systems until 12 weeks alter drug handling.
- Prone to hypoglycaemia.

Renal

- Functionally immature.
- Altered sodium and drug excretion.

Poor thermoregulation

- High surface area : volume ratio.
- Minimal fat.

Some other definitions . . .

Neonate	First 44 weeks post-conceptual age
Premature infant	Less than or equal to 37 weeks' gestation
Neonates	First month of life
Infants	1–12 months
Low birth wt	Less than or equal to 2.5 kg

Bibliography

Berg S. (2005). Special considerations in the premature and ex-premature infant. *Anaesthesia and Intensive Care Medicine*, **6**(3), 81–3.

Raised intracranial pressure

When treating a patient with a severe head injury on the intensive care unit, we talk about using cerebral protection. What does this mean?

Cerebral protection means controlling the physiological and biochemical milieu of the brain to **decrease the likelihood of secondary brain injury**.

Several factors have been shown to be associated with poor outcome after severe head injury. These are:

- Increasing age
- Low admission GCS
- Pupillary signs
- Systolic blood pressure <90 mmHg
- Low arterial O_2 tension
- High arterial CO_2 tension
- ICP >20 mmHg
- High blood glucose

Attention must therefore be paid to controlling these factors. An adequate cerebral perfusion pressure (some suggest >70 mmHg or until pressure waves disappear from the ICP waveform) must be maintained and hypoxia should be avoided at all costs. A 'low-normal' $PaCO_2$ (35–40 mmHg) is current best practice. Any patient with a severe head injury should have their ICP monitored and should preferably be cared for in a neurosurgical intensive care unit.

What are the causes of primary cerebral injury?

This is the damage that occurs at the time of the initial insult and may be the result of:

- Trauma
- Haemorrhage
- Tumour.

What is secondary brain injury?

This is additional ischaemic neurological damage that occurs after the initial injury as a result of:

- Hypoxaemia
- Hypercapnia
- Hypotension
- Raised ICP
- Cerebral arterial spasm
- Hyperglycaemia.

Possible mechanisms:
Glutamate and aspartate act on NMDA receptors causing increased intracellular calcium, activation of phospholipases, breakdown of arachidonic acid and generation of free radicals.

What CO_2 do we aim for and why?

At a $PaCO_2$ between 3.0 kPa (23 mmHg) and 7.0 kPa (53 mmHg) cerebral blood flow is directly proportional to the $PaCO_2$. In the past, hyperventilation has been used to decrease CBF and CBV, but it has been shown that **hyperventilation (CO_2 less than 35 mmHg) is associated with a poorer outcome** because it may produce ischaemia secondary to a severe reduction in CBF. A **'low-normal' CO_2 of just over 4.0 kPa (35 mmHg)** is now the accepted target.

How can we treat raised ICP?

Treatment of raised ICP should be initiated if >20–25 mmHg and is aimed at reducing the volume of the three components making up the intracranial contents: namely brain, blood and CSF. Firstly, **maintenance of an adequate cerebral perfusion pressure** should be ensured. Arterial blood gases should be corrected. The patient should be sedated to a satisfactory level. Attention can then be paid to the following:

Decreasing the brain volume

- Mannitol (0.25–1.0 g/kg) is frequently used to reduce cerebral oedema.
- Loop diuretics, e.g. frusemide (0.5 mg/kg) given within 10–15 min of mannitol produce a synergistic effect. They encourage a more hypotonic diuresis that prolongs the duration of intravascular osmotic load produced by mannitol.
- Cerebral oedema may be worsened with inattention to the serum osmolarity, which should be kept between 300 and 310 mosmol. Hypotonic solutions should be avoided. Treat diabetes insipidus with DDAVP.
- Surgical removal of brain tissue.
- Hypertonic saline administration in patients with head injury or brain tumour have demonstrated a reduction in ICP, however the overall results of studies are inconclusive and require further trials to define its role.

Decreasing cerebral blood volume (CBV)

- Surgical removal of blood (i.e. clot).
- Avoid impeding venous drainage by tight tube ties, high ventilation pressures or excessive neck rotation.
- Venous drainage can be aided by a 30° head-up position.
- Hyperventilation can be effective in the short term but should not be used in the long term because of the potential for causing ischaemia (can be monitored by jugular bulb venous oxygen saturation and cerebral oximetry).

■ Reducing cerebral metabolic requirements with thiopentone will decrease cerebral blood volume by decreasing cerebral blood flow, but has the disadvantage of prolonged sedation.

■ Hyperglycaemia has deleterious effects on metabolism and cerebral perfusion. Blood glucose should be maintained between 4.5 and 8 mmol/l.

■ Control of fitting (fitting increases $CMRO_2$ and therefore cerebral blood flow).

■ Avoidance of pyrexia will help to prevent increases in the $CMRO_2$ and associated increases in CBF and ICP. Induced hypothermia has been used in an attempt to improve outcome. However, a recent multicentre study does not support its routine use.

Head injury and hypothermia

A study published in the *New England Journal of Medicine* (Feb 2001) looked at the effect of induced hypothermia (to 33 °C) on outcome at 6 months after closed head injury. The trial was stopped after 392 patients (500 planned) because there was no improvement in outcome and, in fact, patients in the over-45 years group did worse. The authors recommended not deliberately cooling patients who were normothermic on admission. However, if they were hypothermic on admission, then they should not be aggressively warmed. Studies of head-injured patients with severe intracranial hypertension have demonstrated a beneficial effect in mild hypothermia.

Decreasing the CSF volume

■ CSF can be drained via an external ventricular drain (EVD).
■ Production is reduced by mannitol and frusemide.

Mannitol

■ Osmotic diuretic
■ Rheological effects ↓ red cell rigidity (rbc membrane) ↓ haematocrit (haemodilution)
■ Free-radical scavenger
■ Dose is usually 0.5 g/kg rapid infusion
■ Giving frusemide 0.5 mg/kg 10–15 minutes after mannitol prolongs its effect (see above)
■ Efficacy depends on intact BBB.

Bibliography

Clifton GL, Miller ER, Choi SC. (2001). Lack of effect of induction of hypothermia after acute brain injury. *New England Journal of Medicine*, **344**(8), 556–63.

Galley HF. *Critical Care Focus 3: Neurological Injury*. BMJ Books.

Kaufmann L, Ginsburg R. (1997). *Anaesthesia Review 13*. Churchill Livingstone.

Mishra LD, Rajkumar N, Hancock SM. (2006). Current controversies in neuroanaesthesia, head injury management and neuro critical care *CEACCP*, **6**, 79–82.

Stone DJ, Sperry RJ, Johnson JO, Spiekermann BF, Yemen TA. (1996). *The Neuroanaesthesia Handbook*. Mosby.

The management of raised intracranial pressure. CME Core Topic. *BJA Bulletin*. May 2000.

Rheumatoid arthritis

What are the clinical features of rheumatoid arthritis?

This is a chronic multisystem autoimmune disease of unknown cause. It principally affects the joints causing a **symmetrical inflammatory polyarthritis**. This presents as **pain and stiffness**. Most patients have several joints involved, especially the hands, wrists, elbows, shoulders, cervical spine, knees, ankles, and feet.

Other findings are **Sjögren's syndrome** (dry eyes and dry mouth), **Felty's syndrome** (splenomegaly and neutropaenia), **anaemia** and **thrombocytopaenia**.

Other systems involved include:

■ **Respiratory system**	Pleural effusions
	Diffuse fibrosing alveolitis
	Nodules
	Caplan's syndrome
	Small airways disease
■ **Cardiovascular system**	-up to 35% of patients
	Pericarditis
	Nodules causing conduction defects
	Tamponade – rarely
	Endocarditis (usually mitral)
■ **Haemopoietic system**	Anaemia (see later)
	Effects of drug treatment
■ **Kidneys**	40% have impaired renal function
	Amyloidosis
	Drug toxicity
■ **Skin**	Leg ulcers
	Vasculitic lesions
■ **CNS**	Polyneuropathy
	Carpal tunnel syndrome
	Atlanto-axial subluxation

What airway problems can rheumatoid arthritis present?

■ **Cervical instability** caused by weakening of the transverse ligament of the atlas resulting in potential cord compression. Assess with flexion and extension X-rays looking for a 3 mm gap between odontoid peg and posterior border of anterior arch of atlas

- **Limited cervical spine movement**
- **Fixed flexion deformity** is not uncommon.
- **Cricoarytenoid involvement** can result in upper airway obstruction (hoarseness and stridor).
- **Temporomandibular joint** involvement may limit mouth opening.

A **difficult intubation** is therefore likely, and consideration should be given to spinal / epidural anaesthesia or a LMA technique. Otherwise an awake fibreoptic intubation may be necessary.

What are the other *problems associated with anaesthesia in these patients?*

These are:

- **Respiratory problems**
  A restrictive lung defect may be present and will warrant investigation with pre-op pulmonary function tests, a chest X-ray and blood gases.
- **Anaemia**
  Anaemia of chronic disease (normochromic, normocytic)
  Iron deficiency – GI bleeding from use of NSAIDs.
  Bone marrow suppression from gold and penicillamine.
  Haemolytic anaemia
  Felty's syndrome causing hypersplenism.
- **Other systemic complications** of the disease, e.g. CVS / renal problems.
- **Positioning**
  Care is required due to fixed deformities, tendon and muscle contractures and fragile skin (long-term steroid therapy). Access for local anaesthetic techniques may be difficult.
- **Monitoring**
  Inserting invasive monitoring lines can be very difficult for the same reasons.
- **Altered response to drugs**
  Renal dysfunction
  Decreased serum albumin
  Increased α1-acid glycoprotein
- **Concomitant drug therapy**
- **Post-operatively**
  May be unable to use a PCA.

What are the complications of drug therapy?

Commonly prescribed medication includes:

NSAIDs	Renal impairment, gastric erosions→bleeding
	Fluid retention
Steroids	Hypertension, electrolyte imbalance, diabetes
	Easy bruising, osteoporosis, obesity, myopathy, mania
	Peptic ulcer disease, etc.

Penicillamine	Bone marrow suppression (thrombocytopaenia, neutropaenia, agranulocytosis)
	Haemolytic anaemia
	Nephrotic syndrome
	SLE-like syndrome
	Myasthenia-like syndrome
Chloroquine	Retinopathy
	Cardiomyopathy
Gold	Fatal blood disorders
	Pulmonary fibrosis
	Hepatotoxicity
	Nephrotic syndrome
Azathioprine	Bone marrow suppression
	Abnormal LFTs
Methotrexate	Pulmonary toxicity (esp. in rheumatoid patients)
	Cirrhosis
	Blood dyscrasias
Sulphasalazine	GI side effects
	Haematological toxicity
Cyclosporin	Nephrotoxicity

Bibliography

Nicholson G, Burrin JM, Hall GM. (1998). Peri-operative steroid supplementation. *Anaesthesia*, **53**, 1091–104.
Skues MA, Welchew EA. (1993). Anaesthesia and rheumatoid arthritis *Anaesthesia*, **48**, 989–97.

Secondary brain injury

You are called to A&E to see a 40-year-old man with a GCS of 6, who was brought in with a history of spontaneous headache and then a grand mal fit.

What do you think the differential diagnosis could be?

This is a fairly classic history for a spontaneous sub-arachnoid haemorrhage, although a history of trauma should be sought, backed up by careful clinical examination.

- The other major differential diagnosis is an infective CNS cause such as bacterial or viral meningitis or encephalitis.
- Other causes of a fit include
  - Primary epilepsy
  - Secondary epilepsy from a space occupying lesion or intra-cerebral haemorrhage or infarct
  - Electrolyte disturbances
  - Hypoglycaemia

Assuming someone is dealing with his airway, breathing and circulation, what tests do you want to do immediately?

- Blood sugar
- Arterial blood gas
  - Hypoxia
  - Hypercapnia
  - Profound acidosis
- Ideally, the ABG would rapidly show relevant electrolytes such as sodium and calcium.

Assuming his GCS remains the same, what would you do?

He needs intubating and ventilating in order to

- Secure his airway
- Prevent aspiration
- Control his pO_2 and CO_2.

Does he need an anaesthetic?

- Yes! Even though he is unconscious, reducing the $CMRO_2$ and minimising ICP and MAP surges associated with intubation require adequate doses of anaesthetic agents.
- The quickest and safest way to secure his airway would be to use suxamethonium.

Does suxamethonium have an effect on ICP?

- Probably. Animal data have demonstrated a rise in ICP and this has been both confirmed and rejected by small human studies.
- This has to be weighed against securing the airway safely and effectively.
- The technique could be modified with the use of an opioid or pre-treatment with a small dose (10% ususal dose) of a non-depolarising muscle relaxant to minimise the rise in ICP.
- This may lead onto the next question!

Doesn't using an opioid alter the basis of the rapid sequence induction?

- This is again something that has to be balanced carefully.
- If the airway assessment does not reveal any cause for concern, then the use of an opioid in such situations would minimise the risk of ICP changes.
- If there is any doubt about safely securing the airway, then this has to be the priority and a simple RSI may be the safest option.

Would you use Remifentanil?

- There have been case reports of remifentanil (and other opioids) causing asystole when delivered by bolus injection.
- Combination with the vagotonic effects of suxamethonium or a raised ICP has also led to profound bradycardias and asystole being reported.
- Current advice is to avoid remifentanil and suxamethonium together unless you can justify the benefits (profound, short-acting, blunting of the pressor response to laryngoscopy).
- Pre-treatment with a vagolytic such as glycopyrrolate would also be an option.

What do you understand by the term secondary brain injury?

This is any ischaemic neurological damage that occurs after the primary injury. Significantly worse outcome has been demonstrated in traumatic severely brain injured patients with:

- Hypotension defined as systolic blood pressure <90 mm Hg
- Hypoxia with PaO_2 <9 kPa
- (or apnoea, cyanosis or an oxygen saturation <90%).

These factors must be monitored and avoided if possible and, at the very least, corrected immediately.

- The mean arterial blood pressure should be maintained above 90 mm Hg.
- Infusion of fluids to attempt to maintain cerebral perfusion pressure (CPP) greater than 60 mm Hg.
- Hypotonic solutions should be avoided as they can contribute to cerebral oedema.

What are your targets with regard to ventilation?

- PaO_2 greater than 13 kPa.
- Low normocapnia with $PaCO_2$ around 4.0 – 4.5 kPa.
- Aggressive hyperventilation to sub-normal $PaCO_2$ has been shown to worsen outcome even in the face of raised ICP due to compromise of the cerebral blood flow.

What other options do you have to lower an acutely raised ICP?

- Mannitol is effective for control of raised ICP after severe head injury.
- Effective doses range from 0.25 g/kg body weight to 1 g/kg body weight.
- The indications for the use of mannitol prior to ICP monitoring are
  - Signs of transtentorial herniation
  - Progressive neurological deterioration not attributable to extra-cranial causes.
- Serum osmolarity should be kept below 320 mOsm/l.
- Euvolemia should be maintained by adequate fluid replacement.
- A urinary catheter is essential in these patients.
- Central venous pressure monitoring is usually required.
- Intermittent boluses of mannitol may be more effective than continuous infusion.

Other points of note in managing head injuries:

- Simple ICU nursing care can be of great benefit in reducing ICP.
- Ensure good venous drainage of the head – by ensuring that the neck veins are not occluded or kinked.
- Sit the patient 15 degrees head up.
- Avoid coughing by paralysis and minimal tracheal suctioning.
- Paralysing a patient can result in fits going undetected so deep sedation is usually preferred if paralysis is not essential.
- Adequate sedation for procedures can also minimise ICP rises.

Guidelines were published in 2003 (and updated in 2007) from the National Institute for Clinical Excellence regarding the immediate management of head injury. They broadly follow the ATLS scheme for immediate attention to the airway with cervical spine control, breathing, and circulation. In traumatic cases, there should be a concurrent assessment of other injuries and stabilisation if appropriate. There is further evidence to guide imaging, referral to a tertiary centre, and when to measure and control ICP.

Intubation and ventilation of the head injured may be required for several reasons.

- To facilitate CT scanning in the obtunded or intoxicated patient.
- To facilitate transfer in certain circumstances (long distances, likely deterioration).
- GCS <8 or loss of laryngeal reflexes.
- Ventilatory insufficiency as judged by blood gas estimation.
  - $PaO_2 < 9kPa$ on air (or 13 kPa on oxygen)
  - $PaCO_2 > 6$
  - $PaCO_2 < 3.5$ due to spontaneous hyperventilation.
- If the patient needs transferring and there are facial injuries or a dropping GCS which may need intervention en-route.

Would you use an anti-convulsant in this patient?

- Anti-convulsants may be used to prevent early post-traumatic seizures in patients at high risk for seizures following head injury.
- Phenytoin and carbamazepine have been demonstrated to be effective in preventing early post-traumatic seizures.
- However, the available evidence does not indicate that prevention of early post-traumatic seizures improves outcome following head injury.

Would you tape the patient's eyes shut for a transfer?

- This is a balance of the risks of sustaining a corneal injury, or missing the signs of a raised ICP or intra-cerebral problem causing a III cranial nerve palsy.
- I would lightly tape the eyes and ensure that I regularly inspected the pupils.

Bibliography

American College of Surgeons Committee on Trauma. (1997). *Advanced Trauma Life Support Manual*. Chicago: American College of Surgeons.

Brain Trauma Foundation, Inc, American Association of Neurological Surgeons, Congress of Neurological Surgeons, Joint Section on Neurotrauma and Critical Care. Guidelines for the management of severe traumatic brain injury: cerebral perfusion pressure. New York (NY): Brain Trauma Foundation, Inc. March 2003, p14–22.

Clancy M, Halford S, Walls R, Murphy M. (2001). In patients with head injuries who undergo rapid sequence intubation using succinylcholine, does pretreatment with a competitive neuromuscular blocking agent improve outcome? A literature review. *Emergency Medicine Journal*, **18**, 373–5.

EAST. (1998). Practice management guidelines for identifying cervical spine injuries following trauma. http://www.east.org.

Helm M. (2002). A prospective study of the quality of pre-hospital emergency ventilation in patients with severe head injury. *British Journal of Anaesthesia*, **88**(3), 345–9.

Joo HS, Salasidis GC, Kataoka MT. et al. (2004). Comparison of bolus remifentanil versus bolus fentanyl for induction of anesthesia and tracheal intubation in patients with cardiac disease. *Journal of Cardiothoracic and Vascular Anesthesia*, **18**(3), 263–8.

National Institute for Clinical Excellence (NICE). (2003). *Clinical Guideline number 4. Head injury. triage, assessment, investigation and early management of head injuries in infants, children and adults*. June 2003.

National Institute for Clinical Excellence (NICE). (2007). NICE clinical guideline 56. Head injury: triage, assessment, investigation and early management of head injury in infants, children and adults. September.

Reed M J. (2005). Can we abolish skull X-rays for head injury? *Archives of Disease in Childhood*, **90**, 859–64.

Young KD, Okapa PJ, Sokolove PE. *et al.* (2004). A randomized, double-blinded, placebo-controlled trial of phenytoin for the prevention of early post-traumatic seizures in children with moderate to severe blunt head injury. *Annals of Emergency Medicine*, **43**(4), 435–46.

Sickle cell

An unbooked Afro-Caribbean primagravida arrives on the ward in advanced labour. Fetal distress is diagnosed and the obstetricians wish to do an emergency caesarean section. Her full blood count shows an Hb of 8.3 g/dl with a microcytic picture (normal platelets). Time will not permit electrophoresis.

What may explain the blood picture?

A haemoglobin concentration of less than 10.5 g/dl is due to something other than the dilutional anaemia of pregnancy. Some causes of a microcytic anaemia with normal platelets are:

- Iron deficiency
- Hb SS (Sickle cell disease) – the patient would know this diagnosis
- **Hb AS** (Sickle cell trait)
- **Hb SC**
- α-Thalassaemia
- β-Thalassaemia (less common in Africans)
- Some anaemias of chronic disease.

The blood film should be examined and electrophoresis should be organised because it may influence future management.

Sickle cell trait (AS)
- Usually no clinical abnormality unless exposed to extreme hypoxia (sickling if $PaO_2 < 15$ mmHg).
- Increased risk of pyelonephritis during pregnancy.

Sickle cell haemoglobin C (SC) disease
- Less severe clinical course than SCD but can suffer the same complications.
- Prevalent in West Africans.
- May not develop symptoms until late pregnancy (splenic sequestration and marrow necrosis).
- Can develop proliferative retinopathy.

How would you manage anaesthesia for the Caesarean section?

Pregnancy exacerbates the complications of sickle cell anaemia. Maternal mortality of 1% is due to pulmonary infection and infarction.
Blood transfusions are indicated for:

- Severe anaemia
- Hypoxaemia
- Pre-eclampsia
- Septicaemia
- Renal failure
- Acute chest pain syndrome
- Anticipated surgery.

A haemoglobin concentration of 10 g/dl is commonly aimed for in patients having a caesarean section.
   Either regional or general anaesthesia is acceptable. Principles of management are:

- Oxygen
- Crystalloids for intravascular volume
- Transfusion to maintain oxygen carrying capacity
- Venous stasis prophylaxis
- Normothermia.

Anaesthetic problems with Sickle cell disease

- Avoidance of precipitants of sickle crises
- Difficult i.v. access
- Pain/opioid tolerance
- Anaemia and high output failure
- Infection (salmonella)
- Psychiatric problems
- Intra-operative crisis/thrombo-embolic phenomena
- Acute chest syndrome
- Renal impairment
- Pulmonary hypertension.

Precipitants of a Sickle crisis

- Dehydration
- Hypoxia
- Cold
- Alcohol
- Stress
- Infection
- Menstruation

■ Vascular stasis
■ Acidosis.

Surgery proceeds uneventfully, but post-operatively she develops acute pleuritic chest pain. What may be causing this?

Possible causes
■ Pulmonary embolus
■ Acute chest syndrome
■ Pneumothorax
■ Pneumonia.

If this were a Sickle crisis, how would you manage the case?

The mainstays of management of a Sickle crisis are:

■ Analgesia
■ Fluid replacement
■ Avoidance of hypoxia.

Types of Sickle crisis:

■ **Aplastic**   Depression of erythropoiesis secondary to infection (esp. parvovirus) or folate deficiency in pregnancy.
■ **Sequestration** This can result from massive pooling in the spleen (esp. with SC disease).
■ **Infarctive**   These are vaso-occlusive events, often in the abdomen, back or long bones.

■ **Pain**   Can be very severe (and often underestimated).
                                        Treat with: High dose opioids (PCA may be used)
                                        NSAIDs
                                        Epidural
                                        Paracetamol
                                        Fentanyl patches
                                        Tricyclic antidepressants
                                        Benzodiazepines for spasms and anxiolysis.
■ **Dehydration**   Causes increased haematocrit and increased sickling.
■ If **fever** is present: Search for focus of infection (**cultures** of blood, sputum and urine).
                                        It may be due to the **crisis itself**.
                                        Broad-spectrum antibiotics, which must cover strep. Pneumonii (hyposplenism).
■ If refractory: **Exchange transfusion**
                                        Steroids have been used (Methylprednisolone).

Acute chest syndrome

Cause	Unknown exactly ? Hypoventilation due to pain from rib infarcts ? infarcted marrow embolism ? PE
Signs	Acute chest pain Fever Cough Basal X-ray changes $\downarrow SaO_2$
Treatment	O_2/CPAP/IPPV Exchange transfusion with HbS < 30% causes a response within 1–2 days.

Sickling mechanism

The HbS tetramer undergoes a conformational change in the **deoxygenated** state and leaves **hydrophobic residues** (valine instead of glutamic acid) exposed. These react with other globin chains forming an **insoluble polymer.** Hb S begins to aggregate at a PO_2 of less than 50 mmHg. The process is also time dependent.

When exposed to **oxidant stress**, HbS produces **free radicals** that damage the erythrocyte membrane proteins. **Abnormal adhesion to endothelium** then occurs.

Infection or minor sickling events cause leucocytes to produce **IL-6, IL-1 and TNF** that **up-regulate cell adhesion molecules** (CAMs) on the vascular endothelium. These cause **activation of the haemostatic mechanism.** Platelets and sickle reticulocytes bind easily to CAMs causing **clot formation and vascular occlusion** → **hypoxia** → more sickling.

Bibliography

Chestnut DH. (1994). *Obstetric Anesthesia: Principles and Practice.* Mosby.

Esseltine DW, Baxter MRN, Bevan JC. (1988). Sickle cell states and the anaesthetist. *Canadian Journal of Anaesthesia,* **35**(4), 385–403.

Hatton C, Mackie PH. (1996). Haemoglobinopathies and other congenital haemolytic anaemias. *Medicine,* **24**(1), 14–19.

Hoffbrand AV, Pettit JE (1993). *Essential Haematology,* 3rd edition. Oxford, UK: Blackwell Scientific Publications.

Vijay V, Cavenagh JD, Yate P. (1998). The anaesthetist's role in acute sickle cell crisis. *British Journal of Anaesthesia,* **80**, 820–8.

Spontaneous pneumothorax

A young man presents to the accident and emergency department with an acute onset of dyspnoea. You are asked to see him.

What course of action would you take?

Assess the patient with an ABC approach.

- Airway patency
- Breathing (resp rate, auscultation, expansion, SaO_2, **give oxygen** 15 l/min via mask with reservoir bag).
- Circulation (HR, BP, peripheral perfusion).

If possible, take a history from the patient or relative. This may give a clue to the diagnosis, especially:

- Speed of onset (i.e. gradual or sudden) and duration of symptoms
- Similar previous episodes
- Current medication including inhalers
- General health.

What are the likely causes of this presentation?

- Respiratory causes include
  - Asthma
  - Pneumothorax
  - Infection
  - Pleural effusion
  - Systemic allergic reaction.
- Cardiovascular causes include
  - Pulmonary embolism
  - Pulmonary hypertension
  - Pulmonary oedema.
- Physiological responses to underlying metabolic disorders should be considered, e.g. acute abdomen, DKA, etc.

What are the causes of a pneumothorax?

Trauma	Penetrating chest injury
	Fractured rib
Spontaneous	Usually young thin males
	Associated with Marfan's syndrome
	Ascent in aeroplanes
	Wind instrument players!
2° to underlying chest disease	Pneumonia/TB/lung abscess
	Diffuse lung disease
	Emphysematous bulla
	Carcinoma
	Asthma
Iatrogenic	Central line insertion
	IPPV

How would you differentiate between a flail chest and a pneumothorax?

Flail chest

- Occurs when there are two or more fractures in a rib or one fracture and costo-chondral dislocation.
- Clinically, the flail segment shows **paradoxical movement**, i.e. on inspiration it is drawn inwards and on expiration it is pushed outwards.
- There is pain and respiratory distress.

Pneumothorax

- Symptoms include pleuritic pain and shortness of breath.
- Signs include
  - Reduced movement or expansion on the affected side
  - Hyper-resonant percussion note
  - Reduced breath sounds
  - Tracheal deviation away from the affected side with a large pneumothorax.

NB Pneumothorax and flail segment may both be present at the same time.

> **Tension pneumothorax**
> The above features plus . . .
>
> - Contralateral mediastinal shift
> - Cardiovascular collapse.

How do you treat a patient with a pneumothorax?

- Pneumothoraces are designated 'small' or 'large', depending on the visible rim of air between lung and chest wall seen on a PA CXR.
- The cut off is 2 cm.
- 50% of lung volume may be lost in the presence of a 2 cm rim.

> **Management of pneumothorax**
>
> - Small pneumothorax, patient not breathless – observe.
> - Small pneumothorax and patient breathless – reassess, but if symptoms remain then aspirate.
> - Large, primary pneumothorax – aspirate.
> - Large secondary pneumothorax – unlikely to treat definitively with aspiration:
>
>   especially if age > 50 years but may be attempted.
>   Likely to need intercostal drain.
>
> - Aspiration should improve symptoms and drain at least 2.5 litres of air.
> - Otherwise, consider repeat aspiration or intercostal tube drainage.

Describe how a chest drain is inserted.

- The patient should be adequately prepared and consented.
- Establish i.v. access.
- Infiltrate the area with local anaesthetic (10–20 ml of 1% lignocaine).
- Insertion should be in the 'safe triangle' bordered by the anterior border of the latissimus dorsi, the lateral border of the pectoralis major muscle, a line superior to the horizontal level of the nipple, and an apex below the axilla.
- **Traditional blunt dissection.**
  - A small incision (parallel to and just superior to the rib).
  - Dissection as close to the top of the rib as possible to avoid the neuro-vascular bundle.

- Puncture the pleura with blunt forceps.
- Finger sweep into the pleural cavity to ensure that the lung is not adherent to the insertion site.
- Clamp the proximal end of the tube and insert without the trocar.
- Direct the tube towards the apex (towards the base for fluids – not essential).
- Connect the tube to an underwater drainage system.
- Suture in place and apply dressing.
- Obtain a chest X-ray.

- **Seldinger technique**
  - A guide-wire is passed through a needle into the pleural cavity
  - Followed by dilators and then the drain.
- Seldinger drains are smaller, generally cause less of a scar and the technique is familiar to most anaesthetists.
- The complication rates for both techniques are similar.

> **Ventilated Patients**
>
> If the patient is on a ventilator, then the BTS advice is to disconnect the ventilator prior to entering the pleural cavity and inserting the drain. This will help avoid lung lacerations.

What can you connect the drain to?

All chest tubes should be connected to a single flow closed drainage system.

- An underwater seal (UWS) bottle or
- A flutter (Heimlich) valve

Tell me about underwater seals?

The intercostal tube is placed with the tip lying 2–3 cm under the surface of the water. This provides a one-way valve system for the drainage of air. Fluid will drain with gravity. The underwater seal system needs to be kept below the level of the patient so that fluid does not drain back into the chest under hydrostatic pressure.

Spontaneous breathing
On inspiration, a negative intrapleural pressure is created (around −8 cm of water in tidal breathing). The fluid level in the tube will therefore rise. If the underwater seal was not present, air would be sucked into the pleural cavity. On expiration, intrapleural pressure will become positive if chest wall pressure exceeds alveolar pressure. If this occurs, then air will be expelled via the drain.

IPPV
On inspiration, a positive intrapleural pressure is created, which results in the drainage of air. On expiration, the intrapleural pressure will still be positive if there is PEEP applied to the lungs and therefore air will still drain.
A potential problem may arise when using traditional chest drain bottles to drain fluid and air simultaneously. As the fluid level in the bottle (and thus the submerged end of the tube) rises, a higher positive intrapleural pressure will be required to drain air. Hence, the lung may not fully re-expand and in the case of a persistent leak a tension pneumothorax could develop (or may just drain at a higher pressure). Modern chest drain bottles are now designed to maintain the submerged end of the intercostal drain at less than 2–3 cm below the level of the fluid.

How far beneath the water must the tube be placed?

■ In a closed UWS bottle the tube is placed under water at a depth of approximately 3 cm with a side vent which allows the escape of air.
■ The UWS allows you to see:
  ● Air bubble out as the lung re-expands in the case of pneumothorax.
  ● Fluid evacuation rate in empyemas, pleural effusions, or haemothorax.
■ Continuous bubbling suggests a visceral pleural air leak (bronchopleural fistula).
■ The respiratory swing in the fluid in the chest tube is useful for assessing tube patency and confirms the position of the tube in the pleural cavity.

What is the significance of the depth of the underwater seal?

■ The effective drainage of air, blood or fluids from the pleural space requires an airtight system to maintain subatmospheric intrapleural pressure.
■ With a collection chamber of approximately 20 cm diameter and a 3 cm depth of water, this ensures minimum resistance to drainage of air and maintains the underwater seal even in the face of a large inspiratory effort.
■ The chamber should be 100 cm below the chest as subatmospheric pressures up to −80 cmH_2O may be produced during obstructed inspiration.
■ Lifting the drainage system above the patient's chest will cause siphoning of the contents back into the pleural cavity.

Tell me about suction applied to intercostal drains?

Suction can be used to increase the drainage from the pleural space. Only high volume, low pressure pumps should be used. A pressure of 10–20 cmH_2O is adequate for a pneumothorax. Low volume, high pressure pumps are *dangerous and should not be used. The low volume displacement may not be able to cope with large air leaks, resulting in tension. High pressure may result in damage to the visceral surface of the lung.*

When would you clamp an intercostal drain?

This is controversial. Some authorities state that there are no indications to clamp a drain. Some points to note are:

- Never clamp a bubbling chest drain.
- Drains should not be clamped during transfer.
- Drains should be clamped after a pneumonectomy. If they are not, then catastrophic mediastinal shift can occur. Every hour the drain should be unclamped briefly to look for significant post-operative bleeding.

Large effusions can drain rapidly resulting in re-expansion pulmonary oedema (may be unilateral). This can cause chest discomfort and tightness and has resulted in death. Clamping the drain for a period of time (4 hours has been suggested.

Chest drains – additional information

The underwater seal

UWS first used in 1875, but used in its modern form since 1916 when Kenyon described a 'siphon method of draining traumatic haemothorax'. It has potential hazards apart from insertion in that the UWS system must be kept upright and the draining tube must always be under the water. A bubbling chest tube should never be clamped, as this risks creating a tension pneumothorax if there is persistent air leak.

Does size matter?

There is no evidence that large tubes (20–24 F) are any better than small tubes (10–14 F) in the management of pneumothorax. The initial use of large (20–24 F) intercostal tubes is not recommended, although it may become necessary to replace a small chest tube with a larger one if there is a persistent air leak. Larger tubes are used when one wishes to drain blood or viscous fluids.

Pre-drainage risk assessment

- Risk of haemorrhage
  - Where possible, any coagulopathy or platelet defect should be corrected prior to chest drain insertion.
  - Routine measurement of the platelet count and prothrombin time are only recommended in patients with known risk factors.
- Differential diagnosis between a pneumothorax and bullous disease requires careful radiological assessment.

- Similarly, it is important to differentiate between the presence of collapse and a pleural effusion when the chest radiograph shows a unilateral 'whiteout'.
- Lung densely adherent to the chest wall throughout the hemithorax is an absolute contraindication to chest drain insertion.
- Drainage of a post-pneumonectomy space should only be carried out by or after consultation with a cardiothoracic surgeon.

Tension pneumothorax

If tension pneumothorax is present, a cannula of adequate length should be promptly inserted into the second intercostal space in the mid clavicular line and left in place until a functioning intercostal tube can be positioned.

Bibliography

Anaesthesia UK. 24/4/2006. Underwater chest drain. www.anaesthesiauk.com/article.aspx? articleid=245.

Argall J, Desmond J. (2003). Seldinger technique chest drains and complication rate. *Emergency Medicine Journal*, **20**, 169–70.

ATLS Course for Physicians. (1993). American College of Surgeons.

Hall M, Jones A. (1997). Reducing morbidity from insertion of chest drains. (Letter) *British Medical Journal*, **315**, 313.

Harriss DR, Graham TR. (1991). Management of intercostal drains. *British Journal of Hospital Medicine*, **45**, 383–6.

Henry M, Arnold T, Harvey J (on behalf of the BTS Pleural Disease Group). (2003). BTS guidelines for the management of spontaneous Pneumothorax. *Thorax*, **58**(Suppl II), ii39–ii52.

Hyde J, Sykes T, Graham T. (1997). Reducing morbidity from chest drains. *British Medical Journal*, **314**, 914–15.

Kumar P, Clark M. (1994). *Clinical Medicine*, 3rd edition, Baillière Tindall.

Laws D, Neville E, Duffy J. (2003). BTS guidelines for the insertion of a chest drain. *Thorax*, **58**, 53–9.

Oh TE. (1997). *Intensive Care Manual*, 4th edition, BH publishing.

Skinner D, Driscoll P, Earlam R. (1991). *ABC of Major Trauma*. BMJ Publishing.

Squint surgery

A 4-year-old boy is on your theatre list for squint surgery. You visit the ward pre-operatively and find the mother by the bed and the child playing in the playroom.

How do you approach your assessment?

It is important to establish a rapport with both the child and the mother. The mother, in particular, is likely to be extremely anxious. It is an opportunity to assess the child for anaesthesia, answer questions and address any anxieties. The options for induction of anaesthesia and post-operative analgesia should also be discussed.

Do you go and see the child or leave him playing?

Most of the information can be obtained from the mother, but a useful assessment of the child can be gained from a distance, observing how he interacts and whether his behaviour and physical skills are appropriate for his stage of development. It is important to directly interact with the child at some point and to perform a physical examination. If the child is happier in the playroom, then take the mother to the playroom. The child is not disturbed, but still gets some contact with you. Getting down to the child's level is also important.

What associations are there with squint?

- Cerebral palsy
- Noonan's syndrome (key points: cardiac defects, difficult intubation, platelet and coagulation defects, renal dysfunction).
- Down's syndrome
- Hydrocephalus
- Malignant hyperpyrexia.

What information do you want from mum?

The usual medical and anaesthetic history, including details of

- Gestational age
- Birth and neonatal problems
- Milestones
- Recent vaccinations
- Any recent coughs or colds
- Try to get an idea of whether a sedative pre-med will be needed.
- Obtain consent for and explain rectal analgesia.

What information do you give her?

- Brief explanation of 'the journey' through the theatre complex.
- Include an explanation of what will happen if
  - The child gets upset
  - Failed cannulation.
- Who will escort the parent from the anaesthetic room.
- Details of post-operative analgesia (including suppositories) are important to allay anxiety.

What other methods are there of explaining anaesthesia?

- Optimum choice depends on the intellectual ability of the child.
- Leaflets
- Videos
- Pre-op visits and clinics.

Tell me about fasting times for children prior to surgery?

■ Solids – 6 hours
■ Formula milk – 6 hours
■ Breast milk – 4 hours
■ Clear fluids – 2 hours

Breast milk is more easily absorbed (4 hours fasting time).

Formula milk should be considered as a solid, as should sweets and chewing gum (6 hours fasting time).

> **Children and fasting**
>
> ■ Children are positively encouraged to have clear fluids right up to 2 hours before surgery.
> ■ Rapid fluid turnover and high metabolic rate makes dehydration and hypoglycaemia more likely in the fasting child than potential aspiration.
> ■ Children who have had unrestricted clear fluids until 2 hours prior to surgery have residual gastric volumes equal to or less than those fasted overnight.
> ■ Good hydration may reduce post-operative nausea and vomiting.

How would you anaesthetise him?

Unless the history pointed towards one particular technique, describe your chosen method. For example:

■ Establish routine monitoring.
■ i.v. access following prior use of EMLA cream.
■ Induction with i.v. fentanyl 1 mcg/kg and propofol 3 mg/kg.
■ Maintain an airway with an appropriate LMA.
■ Maintenance: spontaneously breathing in oxygen, air and sevoflurane.

Can your anaesthetic influence the surgery?

■ Suxamethonium increases the ocular tone for up to 20 minutes. This can make surgical correction difficult.
■ Controlling CO_2 helps control the intra-ocular pressure. Reducing the ET CO_2 reduces the incidence and severity of the oculocardiac reflex.
■ Ensure sufficient depth of anaesthesia to achieve neutral gaze.

What potential complications are associated with the surgery?

■ Bradycardia via the oculocardiac reflex (Aschner phenomenon). Not helped by high vagal tone in children.
■ High incidence of post-operative nausea and vomiting (PONV).

Describe the oculocardiac reflex

> **The oculocardiac reflex**
>
> ■ Traction on the extra-ocular muscles or pressure on the eyeball results in arrhythmias, in particular bradycardia but VEs, sinus arrest or VF may also occur.
> ■ Afferents via ophthalmic division of trigeminal nerve (V) to reticular formation and visceral motor nucleus of vagus nerve (X).
> ■ Efferents via the vagus nerve (X) to sino atrial node.

Do anticholinergics given prophylactically prevent the oculocardiac reflex?

■ Atropine and glycopyrrolate both obtend the oculocardiac reflex if given prophylactically.

How would you avoid PONV?

■ General measures
  ● Haemodynamic stability
  ● Control of oxygenation
  ● Adequate hydration.
■ Technique
  ● Avoidance of paralysis and neostigmine
  ● Avoidance of nitrous oxide (controversial)
  ● Avoid intubation
  ● Avoid opioids.
■ Prophylaxis
  ● Combination therapy with agents such as ondansetron 0.1 mg/kg and dexamethasone 0.1 mg/kg.
■ It has been suggested that the oculocardiac reflex predisposes to PONV and preventing its occurrence reduces the incidence of PONV.

How would you treat post-operative pain?

■ This is usually mild and treated with a combination of local anaesthetic drops and simple analgesics.
■ Paracetamol 40 mg/kg rectally or 20 mg/kg orally to load
■ Brufen or voltarol
■ Opioids can usually be avoided
■ Regular paracetamol and NSAID post-operatively.
■ Topical NSAID drops may also be used.

Bibliography
Aitkenhead AR, Rowbotham DJ, Smith G. (2001). *Textbook of Anaesthesia*, 4th Edition. Churchill Livingstone ISBN: 0443063818
Allman K, Wilson I. (2002). *Oxford Handbook of Anaesthesia* (Oxford Handbooks) 2nd edition. Oxford, UK: Oxford University Press. ISBN: 0192632736.
Association of Anaesthetists Guidelines and Information for patients. www.youranaesthetic.info.
Perioperative fasting in adults and children, Nov 2005. www.rcn.org.uk/publications.

Statistics – errors in the interpretation of data from clinical trials

What do we mean by evidence-based medicine?

Decisions regarding the care of patients must be made through the diligent, unambiguous and thoughtful use of current best evidence. Evidence-based medicine is an exhortation to integrate individual clinical proficiency with the best available evidence from systematic research.

What is the null hypothesis?

A hypothesis is a statement of belief about how something occurs. The hypothesis is generated from the research question, can only be disproved and cannot be proved with certainty, e.g. there is no difference between drug X and placebo.

What are alpha and beta errors?

Type I or alpha: A difference is found statistically where none exists. The null hypothesis is wrongly rejected (false-positive). There is no difference between drug X and placebo, but a statistical difference is found.
Maximum p value is usually taken to be 0.05. Whatever the value of p, however, there will always be a random chance of making a Type I error (although the lower the p-value is, the less likely this becomes). Confidence level is (1-alpha).

Type II or beta: The null hypothesis is false in reality but the p-value obtained is ≥ 0.05. We have incorrectly concluded that the sample groups are similar – we have missed a real difference. This is a Type II statistical error. The main cause of Type II errors is inadequate sample size. This is a false-negative, e.g. drug X is found not to be superior to placebo when it is. Power (1-beta) is a measure of the trial detecting a difference if one exists. Most editors of scientific journals require the power of a study to be at least 80% and sometimes 90%.

How do we judge the usefulness of a clinical test?

- To be truly useful, a clinical test must positively identify those who have a disease as well as positively exclude those who do not.
- The methods of quantifying these measures are called the **sensitivity** and **specificity**.
- The **sensitivity** is a measure of how good the test is at correctly identifying those patients afflicted with the disease. It is defined as the number of patients who test positive as a fraction of those who really have the abnormality, i.e. the proportion of positives that are correctly identified by the test.
- The **specificity** is a measure of how good the test is at excluding those patients who do not have the condition. It is defined as the number of patients who test negative as a fraction of those who do not have the abnormality, i.e. the proportion of negatives that are correctly identified by the test.

$$\text{Sensitivity} = \frac{\text{True positives}}{\text{True positives} + \text{False-negatives}}$$

$$\text{Specificity} = \frac{\text{True negatives}}{\text{True negatives} + \text{False-positives}}$$

What are the positive and negative predictive values of a test?

- The **positive predictive value** quantifies how an abnormal result of a test predicts a true abnormality.

  It is defined as the number of patients who both test positive and who really are positive as a fraction of the total with a positive test, i.e. the proportion of those with a positive test who are correctly diagnosed.
- The **negative predictive value** quantifies how a normal result of a test excludes an abnormality.

  It is defined as the number of patients who both test negative and who really are negative as a fraction of the total with a negative test, i.e. the proportion of those with a negative test who are correctly diagnosed.

What is the difference between a systematic review and a meta-analysis?

- A **systematic review** is the formal process of identification, appraisal and evaluation of primary studies and other relevant research to draw conclusions about a specific issue.
- A **meta-analysis** is the **statistical discipline** of assimilating data from similar smaller studies to measure an overall effect size with improved precision. Commonly, it is invoked as part of a *systematic review* of the available literature.

Problems with meta-analysis
Bias

- **Significance** Greater propensity for studies with positive or statistically significant results to be published by scientific journals.
- **Replication** Occurs when the same data are published in multiple articles.
- **Language** Occurs due to failure to search for articles other than in English.
- **Selection** Occurs when citations are specifically derived from articles such as narrative reviews or expert opinion.

Statistical heterogeneity
For studies to be combinable, they should demonstrate homogeneity or similarity particularly with respect to the subjects, pre-test variables and methodology. Combining heterogeneous studies may lead to irrelevant and erroneous conclusions.

Sensitivity analysis
This involves checking to see whether alterations of the analyses by the omission of trials originally included in the meta-analysis materially affect the overall result.

Bibliography
Columb M, Lalkhen A. (2005). Systematic reviews and meta-analyses. *Current Anaesthesia and Critical Care*, **16**(6), 391–4.
Sacket DL, Rosenberg WMC, Gray JAM, Haynes RB, Richardson WS. (1996). Evidence based medicine: what it is and what it isn't. *British Medical Journal*, **312**, 71–2.

Stridor post-thyroidectomy

You are called to recovery urgently to see a patient with stridor 1 hour following a total thyroidectomy.

What are the common causes of stridor in this situation?

- **Wound haematoma** Bleeding is probably the most common cause of early stridor and can lead to life-threatening respiratory obstruction. Removal of clips or sutures may help, or at least buy time, but tracheal intubation will be required for serious cases.
- **Bilateral RLN palsy** Unilateral damage will cause hoarseness, but bilateral damage will lead to adduction of both vocal cords and stridor.

- **Tracheal oedema**   This would be an unusual cause of stridor at such an early stage.
- **Tracheal collapse**   Tracheomalacia may occur intra- or post-operatively. It tends to occur more commonly in large or malignant goitres. A clue to its presence may be observed at the end of the operation with the absence of a leak around the cuff of the E.T. tube when it is deflated.

How would you manage this situation?

This is a life-threatening scenario:

- The patient should be given 100% oxygen.
- A consultant anaesthetist and ENT surgeon should be summoned immediately.
- If there is evidence of an expanding haematoma, the skin clips should be removed, although it may be necessary to open deeper layers.
- Nebulised adrenaline (5 mls of 1/1000, i.e. 5 mg) if there is a suspicion of oedema.
- Heliox (if immediately available) could be considered. NB Heliox is only 21% oxygen.
- The remaining causes would necessitate urgent tracheal intubation or tracheostomy.

The patient deteriorates further without evidence of haematoma and requires intubation. How would you undertake this?

The anaesthetic management of this situation is contentious.
  The options are:

- Gas induction
- i.v. induction followed by neuromuscular blockade.
- Surgical airway

Several factors may help when deciding on the most appropriate management:

- Time. The choice of technique will be limited by the speed of deterioration of the patient and the availability of equipment.
- Ability to achieve any ventilation. If ventilation is not possible and the patient is becoming severely hypoxic, then gas induction is clearly not going to be an option.
- The most likely diagnosis. The surgeon who performed the operation would know if tracheomalacia was likely – the operation note could help. Tracheomalacia may be expected to be an easier intubation than airway oedema.
- The difficulty of the original intubation

■ Availability of a skilled ENT surgeon. If the wound is open, there is no haematoma and if the surgeon is present, then a surgical airway could be considered.

If the patient is partially obstructed and therefore still self-ventilating, a gas induction could be performed. The patient should be immediately transferred to theatre, where facilities for difficult intubation are more readily available. The patient is pre-oxygenated and gas induction of anaesthesia performed with sevoflurane or halothane in 100% oxygen. The trachea can then be intubated under deep inhalational anaesthesia without a muscle relaxant. The ENT surgeon should be scrubbed and ready to perform an emergency tracheostomy if oral intubation is impossible. Rigid bronchoscopy (by an experienced ENT surgeon) or transtracheal jet ventilation may be used as holding measures.

Bibliography
Malhotra S, Sodhi V. (2007). Anaesthesia for thyroid and parathyroid surgery. *CEACCP*, **7**, 55–8.
Marshall P. (2002). *Oxford Handbook of Anaesthesia*. Oxford, UK: Oxford University Press.

Tension pneumothorax

A 35-year-old man has sustained a fall from a ladder and presents to the accident department with increasing shortness of breath.

What does his CXR show?

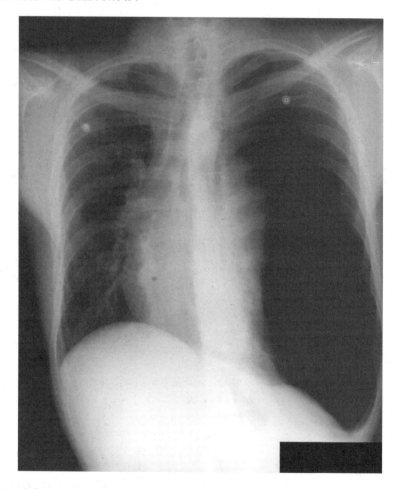

This is a **left tension pneumothorax**. There is gross mediastinal shift to the right. This needs immediate treatment.

How would you treat this?

- Administer high-flow oxygen.
- Identify the second intercostal space in the midclavicular line on the side of the pneumothorax.
- Surgically prepare the chest and locally anaesthetise the area if time permits.
- Insert a cannula (14 or 16 gauge) into the space passing just superior to the rib and puncturing the parietal pleura to enter the pleural cavity.

- Remove the needle and listen for a rush of air to confirm placement and diagnosis.
- Insert a definitive chest drain and remove the original cannula.
- Obtain a chest X-ray.

What are the complications of this procedure?

- Pneumothorax
- Local bleeding (intercostal vessel damage)
- Local cellulitis
- Pleural infection.

Bibliography

American College of Surgeons. (2004). *Advanced Trauma Life Support Course for Physicians*, 7th edition. American College of Surgeons.
Saayman AG, Findlay GP. (2003). The management of blunt thoracic trauma. *British Journal of Anaesthesia CEPD Reviews*, **3**(6), 171–4.

Tetanus

A 47-year-old farmer presents with dysphagia, malaise and muscle pains, following a minor accident at work 6 days earlier.

Tell me some causes of dysphagia.

It is useful to have some form of sieve for an answer like this that you may not have directly thought about before. You will know most of the causes, but delivering them in a structured format will impress.

Mechanical	Benign internal stricture, e.g. oesophageal web
	Malignant internal stricture, e.g. oesophageal/gastric cancer
	Extrinsic pressure, e.g. lung cancer, retrosternal goitre
	Pharyngeal pouch
Motility problems	Bulbar palsy
	Pseudobulbar palsy
	Achalasia
	Systemic sclerosis
	Myasthenia gravis
	Rare infective causes, e.g. tetanus, Chagas' disease
Others	Oesophagitis

What is the likely diagnosis in this farmer?

The most likely diagnosis from the history is tetanus.

What is the causative organism?

The disease is caused by **exotoxins produced by *Clostridium tetani*,** an obligate anaerobic, spore-bearing, Gram-positive bacillus. The spores exist in the soil and in the gastrointestinal tract of humans and animals. The organism is non-invasive, but the spores can gain entry through wounds, ulcers etc. where they can proliferate and produce the toxins **tetanospasmin** (an extremely potent protein) and tetanolysin. In 20% no entry site is identified. Tetanospasmin is taken up and transmitted by motor neurones to the central nervous system where it **preferentially binds to GABA** inhibitory interneurones. Tetanospasmin cleaves synaptobrevin preventing neurotransmitter release thereby blocking these pathways and allowing uninhibited afferent stimuli.

   C. tetani is difficult to culture and only identified in about one-third of cases.

What is the natural course of the disease?

The incubation period is between 3 and 21 days (average 7 days). There is a prodrome of non-specific stiffness, fever, malaise, headache and dysphagia. This is followed by the classical symptoms of:

- Trismus   'Lockjaw' due to masseter spasm
- Risus sardonicus   Rigidity and spasm in the facial muscles
- Opisthotonus   Arched body secondary to paravertebral muscle spasm
- Painful spasms may eventually compromise respiration
- Sympathetic overactivity   Tachycardia, arrhythmias, paroxysmal hypertension, sweating, pyrexia and gastrointestinal stasis.

The spasms can be precipitated by noise, handling or even light. Several grading systems of severity of the disease are in use but the most widely used is that proposed by Ablett (Grades I–IV represent mild to very severe).

How would you treat this man?

- In the first instance an ABC approach is adopted and further management guided by clinical findings.
- The wound should be cleaned and debrided.
- Give metronidazole for 7–10 days to eradicate the causative organism. Penicillin use results in significantly worse mortality rates.
- To neutralise the free toxin, human tetanus immunoglobulin is given i.m.
- General nursing care is very important. These patients should be nursed in a quiet, isolated, darkened room.
- Diazepam or chlorpromazine should be given initially to try and control the spasms.
- Dantrolene and intrathecal baclofen have been used in the treatment of tetanic spasms.

- Magnesium may also be used to control spasms.
- Intensive care may be indicated with paralysis and ventilation.
- Ventilation is likely to be prolonged if required and early tracheostomy should be considered.
- Autonomic dysfunction often occurs after the onset of respiratory symptoms. Treatment with β-blockers is controversial since their use has been associated with sudden cardiac arrest and unresponsive hypotension. Esmolol, because it is short acting, may be the most suitable drug in this class.
- Other general ICU measures include nutritional support and thromboprophylaxis.
- Mortality, even with supportive intensive care, is around 11%
- Patients die from aspiration, hypoxia, respiratory failure and cardiac arrest.

Bibliography

Cook TM, Protheroe RT, Handel JM. (2001). Tetanus: a review of the literature. *British Journal of Anaesthesia*, **87**(3), 477–87.
Thwaites CL. (2005). Tetanus. *Current Anaesthesia in Critical Care*, **16**, 50–7.

Thyroidectomy

What are the anaesthetic problems of a patient who is thyrotoxic with a large goitre presenting for thyroidectomy?

These may be divided into the effects of thyrotoxicosis and those of the goitre on the airway and surrounding structures.

Thyrotoxicosis

Cardiovascular	Tachycardia
	Arrhythmias (esp. AF)
	Congestive cardiac failure
	Ischaemic heart disease
	May be chronically hypovolaemic and vasodilated causing hypotension on induction
	Exaggerated response to laryngoscopy and surgical stimulation with tachycardia, hypertension and ventricular arrhythmias
Thyroid storm	See below
Eyes	Lid retraction, exophthalmos, conjunctivitis
Other	Proximal myopathy
	Anaemia
	Thrombocytopaenia
	Hypercalcaemia
	Abnormal glucose tolerance
	Associated auto-immune disease, e.g. diabetes, myasthenia

Effects of goitre

- ▓ **Compression**

Airway	May be worse in supine position, eased on side or prone
	Tracheomalacia (especially post-operatively)
SVC	Retrosternal extension
	Oedematous face and airway
	Engorgement of nasopharyngeal veins (epistaxis with fibre-optic intubation)
	Poor venous return therefore place i.v. line in lower extremity (IVC territory)
Recurrent laryngeal nerve	1% have involvement pre-operatively. This causes cord adduction leading to a hoarse voice.
	Bilateral nerve involvement causes stridor.

- ▓ **Tumour invasion of local tissues**

How would you assess her thyroid status?

- ▓ **Symptoms**
  - Weight loss, diarrhoea, vomiting
  - Restlessness, tremor
  - Palpitations
  - Heat intolerance
  - Eye complications (Graves' disease)
- ▓ **Signs**
  - Tachycardia
  - Atrial fibrillation
  - Cardiac failure
  - Warm, vasodilated peripheries
  - Goitre with bruit
  - Hyperkinesis
- ▓ **Investigations**
  - TSH ↓
  - T3 ↑
  - T4 ↑
  - Free T4 ↑
  - Thyroid scan (^{131}I) – 'hot' or 'cold' spots

Which drugs are used to manage thyrotoxicosis?

- ▓ **Carbimazole**
  - Inhibits hormone synthesis.
  - Takes 4–8 weeks to work.
  - Major side effect is depression of the white cell count.
  - Agranulocytosis in 1/1000 after 3 months.
- ▓ **Propylthiouracil**
  - Inhibits hormone synthesis.
  - Also inhibits peripheral conversion of T4 to more active T3.
  - Given if sensitive to carbimazole.
  - Takes 4–8 weeks to work.
  - Side effects include leucopaenia, aplastic anaemia, lupus-like syndrome.

▨ **Iodine**	(Lugol's solution) Traditionally given for 10 days prior to surgery to reduce the vascularity of the gland. This practice is now less common because the thyroid gland is dissected without transection.
▨ **β-blocker**	Propranolol controls cardiovascular effects and decreases peripheral conversion of T4 to more active T3 Heart rate of less than 85 has been recommended Atenolol or nadolol (both longer acting) may achieve better control of symptoms.

How would you assess the airway?

▨ **Symptoms**	Positional dyspnoea (esp supine with retrosternal goitre). Dysphagia
▨ **Signs**	Stridor
	Routine assessment of expected difficulty with intubation.
▨ **Investigations**	Indirect laryngoscopy or fibre-optic nasendoscopy by ENT surgeon will give clues as to whether the larynx is likely to be easily visualized at direct laryngoscopy.
	Chest X-ray/lateral thoracic inlet – tracheal compression/deviation.
	CT scan – extension of retrosternal goitre and site/degree of tracheal compression. Diameter of airway at narrowest point can also be measured.

This patient was euthyroid with no clinical or radiological evidence of obstruction. How would you anaesthetise them?

▨ Pre-medication	Benzodiazepine
	β-blocker continued

- ▨ Standard i.v. induction and muscle relaxation is acceptable.
- ▨ Care to obtund pressor responses.
- ▨ Armoured tube – well secured
- ▨ Attention to eye protection
- ▨ Sandbag between shoulder blades
- ▨ Head-up (reduces bleeding) and extended
- ▨ Arms by the side therefore long drip extensions
- ▨ Check cords at the end when breathing spontaneously – bilateral recurrent laryngeal nerve damage will cause bilateral cord adduction and stridor.
- ▨ Extubate 'awake'.
- ▨ Post-operative care to include attention to oxygenation, fluid balance, analgesia, airway monitoring for signs of obstruction – clip remover immediately available.
- ▨ Check serum calcium and have i.v. calcium by the bedside.
- ▨ Continue β-blocker.

What is thyroid storm and how is it managed?

This is a life-threatening syndrome seen in hyperthyroid patients typically 6–24 hours post-operatively, although it may occur intra-operatively. It is characterized by hyperpyrexia, tachycardia, hypotension and altered consciousness. It may initially mimic malignant hyperthermia, but is not associated with muscle rigidity or a rise in CK. Other factors such as labour or severe infection may also precipitate the syndrome.

Treatment consists of:

- Antithyroid drugs   Propylthiouracil – orally or N/G
  Iodide – inhibits release of hormone from gland
  Dexamethasone – inhibits synthesis, release and peripheral conversion
- β-blocker   Propranolol – combined β_1 and β_2 preferable
  β_1 Cardiovascular effects
  β_2 Suppresses metabolic effects
  Reduces muscle blood flow and therefore heat production
- Active cooling
- i.v. fluids
- Paracetamol
- Invasive monitoring and inotropic/vasopressor therapy as indicated

Bibliography

Craft T, Upton P. (1995). *Key Topics in Anaesthesia*. Bios Scientific Publishers.
Deakin CD. (1998). *Clinical Notes for the FRCA*. Churchill Livingstone.
Farling PA. (2000). Thyroid disease. *British Journal of Anaesthesia*, **85**(1), 15–28.
Goldstone J, Pollard B. (1996). *Handbook of Clinical Anaesthesia*. Churchill Livingstone.
Hagberg CA. (2000). *Handbook of Difficult Airway Management*. Churchill Livingstone.
Kumar P, Clark M. (2002). *Clinical Medicine*, 5th edition. WB Saunders.
Malhotra S, Sodhi V. (2007). Anaesthesia for thyroid and parathyroid surgery. *CEACCP*, **7**, 55–8.
Marshall P. (2002). *Oxford Handbook of Anaesthesia*. Oxford, UK: Oxford University Press.
Morgan GE, Mikhail MS. (1996). *Clinical Anaesthesiology*, 2nd edition. Appleton and Lange.

Trauma

You are called to casualty to assess a 25-year-old male pedestrian who has been hit by a car at unknown speed. He was unconscious at the scene and has an obvious compound fracture of his right tibia and fibula. His foot is cool and dusky. He is agitated and his GCS is now 14. The orthopaedic surgeons want to fix his leg as soon as possible.

How would you assess this patient?

This is a **major trauma** case and he should be **assessed** and **resuscitated** according to the **ATLS guidelines**. From the history he may have sustained occult life-threatening injuries such as a fractured pelvis, intra-abdominal or intra-cerebral haemorrhage.

Assessment
- **Airway and cervical spine**
  Look for evidence of airway obstruction, especially facial fractures and foreign bodies in the mouth.
- **Breathing**
  Expose the chest and examine for adequacy of ventilation:
  Inspection, palpation, percussion, auscultation
  Measure SaO_2 and respiratory rate.

Beware at this point:

- Tension pneumothorax
- Flail chest
- Open pneumothorax
- Massive haemothorax.

- **Circulation**
  Skin colour and capillary refill
  Pulse, ECG
  Blood pressure
  Level of consciousness
  This patient is likely to have sustained a head injury. It is therefore vital to maintain mean arterial pressure in order to optimize cerebral perfusion pressure
- **Dysfunction**
  AVPU
  GCS
- **Exposure**
  To complete the primary survey.

After a thorough assessment of his injuries in casualty, it is important to prioritise his further management, e.g. potential life-threatening haemorrhage from his abdomen takes precedence over a potential head injury.

What investigations would you like before taking him to theatre?

- Cervical spine, chest and pelvis X-rays.
- Haemoglobin and cross-match, urea, electrolytes and glucose.
- If there is any cardiovascular instability with no obvious cause or there are positive abdominal signs, then further investigation of the abdomen is indicated. This may take the form of diagnostic peritoneal lavage, ultrasound or CT scan. A general surgeon should be present from the outset as part of the trauma team.

■ In view of the history, a CT scan of his head is indicated to exclude intracranial pathology such as haemorrhage or oedema.

The patient is too agitated to tolerate a CT scan. How would you manage this situation?

This patient now requires a general anaesthetic for his CT scan. (He also needs an anaesthetic for his tibia and fibula fracture. Although a regional technique would be ideal for his lower limb surgery, it is not practical because of his agitation. A central neuroaxial block may also have detrimental effects on cerebral blood flow due to the fall in mean arterial pressure. In addition to this, there is the theoretical risk of coning associated with dural puncture.)

He should be anaesthetised in casualty with a rapid sequence induction and intubation with C-spine immobilisation (either by hard collar or manual in-line stabilisation). It is important to pay careful attention to measures that help prevent a rise in intracranial pressure (see question on raised intracranial pressure).

If there is vascular compromise in the leg, then manipulation and temporary stabilisation could be performed after the patient has been anaesthetised and is being prepared for transfer to the CT scanner.

The further management of the fracture will depend on the result of the CT scan and whether any other life-threatening injuries require treating first.

Bibliography
American College of Surgeons (2004). *Advanced Trauma Life Support Course for Physicians*, 7th edition. American College of Surgeons.

Trigeminal neuralgia

What are the clinical features of a patient with trigeminal neuralgia?

Sudden, usually unilateral, severe brief stabbing recurrent pain in the distribution of one or more branches of the trigeminal nerve. The most common sites are the mandibular and maxillary branches together (42%). The pain is usually unilateral but may be bilateral in 3%–5% of cases. The patient typically has a trigger zone.

What is the differential diagnosis?

■ **'Primary'** trigeminal neuralgia (more than 90% of cases) is caused by an abnormal vascular loop (usually arterial) in contact with the nerve at the **dorsal root entry zone** as it exits the pons. It is unclear how this contact with the nerve results in the characteristic clinical features however abnormalities of the somatosenory evoked response as well as sensory malfunction have been demonstrated. It may be detected by magnetic resonance imaging.
■ **Post-herpetic neuralgia**
■ **Atypical facial pain**

■ **Cluster headache**
■ **Temperomandibular joint dysfunction**
■ **Lesions by site**:

Brainstem	Tumour
	Multiple Sclerosis (18% of bilateral cases have MS)
	Infarct
	Syringobulbia
Cerebellopontine angle	Acoustic neuroma
	Meningioma
Apex of petrous temporal bone	Middle ear infection
Cavernous sinus	ICA aneurysm
	Tumour
	Cavernous sinus thrombosis

What features suggest primary trigeminal neuralgia?

■ **Asymptomatic between attacks.** Patients with another aetiology as listed above may complain of persistent pain.
■ **Absence of neurological signs.** The presence of <u>any</u> neurological signs suggests a secondary cause and should be investigated as such.
■ **Pain is usually unilateral.**

What treatment options are available?

Treatment will be determined by the cause and the suitability for surgery.

■ **Surgical** — **Microvascular decompression** (MVD) involves craniotomy and the associated anaesthetic and surgical risks. If an artery is found to be the cause of the compression it is dissected away and held clear of the nerve using Ivalon sponge or teflon. Veins may be ligated or coagulated. 'Minor' surgical interventions include radiofrequency rhizolysis and glycerol rhizolysis.
■ **Pharmacologica** — Usually involves the use of anti-convulsants such as Carbamazepine (NNT 2,6), phenytoin or sodium valproate.

Signs of complete trigeminal nerve lesion:

■ Loss of corneal reflex.
■ Unilateral sensory loss of face, tongue and buccal mucosa.
■ Mouth opening leads to deviation of jaw to the side of the lesion.

Bibliography

Grady KM, Severn AM. (2007). *Key Topics In Chronic Pain*, 3rd edition. Bios Scientific Publishers.
Nurmikko TJ, Eldridge PR. (2001). Trigeminal neuralgia – pathophysiology, diagnosis and current treatment. *British Journal of Anaesthesia*, **87**, 117–32.

Unconscious patient

An adult male is found collapsed at home with a decreased level of consciousness. He is brought to the accident department where his Glasgow Coma Score is 5/15.

What are the possible causes of his comatose state?

An exhaustive list will not be required, but a sensible and systematic approach looked for. Have a system for categorising your answer. Listed below is one method. Another would be:

- Trauma
- Infection
- Metabolic
- Tumour
- Drugs
- Vascular – Ischaemia/haemorrhage.

Consciousness depends on:

- **Intact cerebral hemispheres**
- A functioning **reticular activating system** in the **brainstem, the midbrain, the hypothalamus and the thalamus.**

NB: Focal damage to the cortex *does not* affect conscious level.

Diffuse brain insult
- Diabetic coma
- Hyponatraemia
- Hypoxia (due to respiratory insufficiency or blood loss, etc.)
- Uraemia
- Hepatic encephalopathy
- Infection, e.g. meningitis
- Post-ictal state

Brainstem pathology
- Subarachnoid haemorrhage
- Ischaemic event
- Intra-cerebral bleed
- Drugs (hypnotics / sedatives)
- Tonsillar herniation
- Compression by tumour

Midbrain pathology
- Compression by supratentorial mass

Trauma leads to loss of consciousness by global ischaemic damage (e.g. extradural haematoma causing raised ICP and decreased CPP) or by pressure on the brainstem.

How would you manage this patient in the accident department?

- ABC approach to **resuscitation**
  With a GCS of 5, the patient is comatose (GCS$\leq$8) and not able to protect his airway. He should therefore be intubated and ventilated. Treatment should aim to prevent any secondary brain injury.
- **History** from any family/paramedics/nursing staff. Ask about:
    Speed of onset (sudden onset suggests vascular cause)
    Self-poisoning
    Trauma
    PMH, e.g. epilepsy or diabetes
- **Examination**
General	Pulse
	Blood pressure
	Respiratory rate
Neurological signs	Lateralising signs
	Pupillary responses
Infection	Temperature
	Neck stiffness
	Rash
- **Investigations** will be directed by the history and examination
Trauma	$\rightarrow$	CT scan
Self-poisoning	$\rightarrow$	Toxicology screen
Metabolic cause	$\rightarrow$	Urea and electrolytes
		Blood glucose
		Arterial blood gases
		Blood cultures
Infection	$\rightarrow$	Lumbar puncture

  The diagnosis may not be immediately obvious and further tests for unusual conditions may be needed (e.g. thyroid function tests, porphyrins, serum calcium).
  This will not alter resuscitation and supportive treatment.

Uncontrolled hypertension

A 48-year-old male patient presents for day-case inguinal hernia repair. On arrival on the ward, his blood pressure is 220/130.

What would you do?

The patient's blood pressure **should be rechecked** ensuring that the cuff size is correct. Ascertain whether he is usually normotensive. A blood pressure this high is pathological and not likely to be due to anxiety (white coat hypertension). However, it could be rechecked following an anxiolytic if it is deemed appropriate. It may be that he is already on anti-hypertensives, but has not taken them recently.

This blood pressure is extremely high and raises the (rare) possibility of **malignant hypertension**. Other features of this include papilloedema, encephalopathy and end-organ damage. If these features were present, then it would be a medical emergency and necessitate admission to hospital and urgent anti-hypertensive therapy.

On rechecking, the BP is 200/120. Will you anaesthetise this patient?

No. The surgery should be postponed until the blood pressure is under control and an explanation given to the patient. He needs to understand the implications of having uncontrolled hypertension both in terms of having an anaesthetic and also the long-term health risks. A systematic review and meta-analysis of hypertensive disease and peri-operative cardiac events demonstrated a statistically but not clinically significant association. There is little evidence suggesting that patients with systolic pressures <180 mmHg and diastolic pressures <110 mmHG have an increased risk of peri-operative complications. The situation is less clear in patients with values above the aforementioned levels. These patients are at more risk of the complications listed below. However, this may relate to the presence of end-organ damage due to hypertension rather than the presenting blood pressure values. There is no evidence that postponing surgery reduces risk.

A medical history with regard to his hypertension, particularly looking for an underlying medical cause (found in less than 10% of cases) and symptoms of target organ damage should be taken. The condition should be investigated and treatment commenced. This would need to be co-ordinated through his primary care physician.

Routine investigation of hypertensive patients:

- **Urine strip test for blood and protein**
- **Blood electrolytes and creatinine**
- **Blood glucose – preferably fasted**
- **Serum Total:HDL cholesterol ratio**
- **12-lead ECG.**

(British Hypertensive Society guidelines)

What are the problems of anaesthetising a patient with uncontrolled hypertension?

- Cardiac ischaemic events (especially if LVH present on ECG)
- Arrhythmias
- Cerebral autoregulation reset (shifted to the right)
- Exaggerated cardiovascular responses
- Poor left ventricular relaxation (diastolic dysfunction)
- Renal failure
- Bleeding

How soon do you think you would be happy to anaesthetise this patient?

Treatment needs to be established and continued for **several weeks** with thorough pre-operative evaluation of end-organ damage. The numbers may 'normalise' quickly, but several weeks of therapy are needed to reduce the abnormal vessel reactivity. The patient could then be anaesthetised when the diastolic pressure is **controlled** at or below 90 – 110 mmHg and maintained within 20% of pre-operative levels during surgery.

The treatment target BP should be <140 mmHg systolic and <85 mmHg diastolic in non-diabetics.

Which anti-hypertensive medication would you prescribe?

For each major class of anti-hypertensive drug, compelling indications and contraindications exist for use in specific groups of patients. First-line treatment in this patient would be an ACE inhibitor, probably with the addition of a calcium channel blocker.

Anti-hypertensive therapy recommendations:

Agent	Compelling indication
α-blocker	Prostatism
ACE-Inhibitor	Heart-failure, LV dysfunction
	Type-1 diabetic nephropathy
Angiotensin II antag.	Intolerance to ACE-I
	Hypertension with LVF
β-blocker	MI, angina
Ca²⁺ antagonist (dihydropyridine)	Isolated systolic HT in elderly pts
Ca²⁺ antagonist (rate-limiting)	Angina
Thiazide	Elderly patients, secondary stroke prevention

British Hypertension Society and NICE Guidelines – which drugs?

- Aged 55 and over, or Black patients of any age:
  - **Calcium channel blocker** or a **thiazide-type diuretic**
    (Black patients are those of African or Caribbean descent, and not mixed race, Asian or Chinese patients.)
- Younger than 55:
  - **ACE inhibitor** or an **angiotensin receptor blocker** (if ACE inhibitor not tolerated).

If a second drug is required:

- If initial therapy was with a calcium channel blocker or thiazide-type diuretic, add an **ACE inhibitor** (or an angiotensin receptor blocker if ACE inhibitor not tolerated).
- If initial therapy was with an ACE inhibitor, add a **calcium channel blocker** or a **thiazide-type diuretic**.

If a third drug is required:

- Combination of **ACE inhibitor** (or an angiotensin receptor blocker if an ACE inhibitor is not tolerated), **calcium channel blocker** and **thiazide-type diuretic** should be used.

The decision not to recommend β-**blockers** for first-line therapy is based on evidence that suggests they perform less well than other drugs, particularly in the elderly, and the increasing evidence that the most frequently used β-blockers at usual doses carry an unacceptable risk of provoking **type 2 diabetes**.

Bibliography

Brown MJ, Cruickshank JK, Dominiczak AF. *et al.* (2003). Executive Committee, British Hypertension Society. Better blood pressure control: how to combine drugs. *Journal of Human Hypertension*, **17**, 81–6.

Howell SJ, Sear JW, Foëx P. (2004). Hypertension, hypertensive heart disease and perioperative cardiac risk. *British Journal of Anaesthesia*, **92**, 570–83.

Williams B, Poulter NR, Brown MJ. *et al.* (2004). British Hypertension Society guidelines for hypertension management 2004: summary. *British Journal of Anaesthesia*, **328**, 634–40.

www.bhsoc.org/NICE_BHS_Guidelines.stm (2008).

Unexpected difficult intubation

You are asked to anaesthetise a 35-year-old, 110 kg man who has been involved in a road traffic accident. He sustained mild facial trauma when he hit the steering wheel and has a bruised chest. He has a fracture–dislocation of the ankle that the surgeons want to operate on urgently as the foot is dusky. Primary and secondary surveys did not reveal anything else of concern.

How would you assess his airway?

Bedside tests should be used in combination with each other and include

- Mallampati score of the view of the pharynx
- Calder scale looking at the mobility of the lower jaw
- Thyromental or sternomental distance indicating mandibular space compliance, mouth opening and neck movements
- His weight of 110 kg can contribute to a difficult airway.

What else would you want to know prior to anaesthetising him?

- A full medical and anaesthetic history
- Clinical examination
- Chest x-ray and ECG – he has sustained blunt chest trauma
- Timing of his last meal prior to the RTA is important.
- Any opioids in A&E
- Spinal anaesthesia could be considered provided there are no contraindications.
- If regional anaesthesia is contraindicated, then the method of securing the airway would be influenced by the predicted difficulty of laryngoscopy and intubation.
- If a difficult airway is predicted, then awake fibre-optic intubation would be an appropriate technique.
- If the airway looks OK, then i.v. induction would be reasonable. If there is any doubt about his stomach being empty, a rapid sequence induction should be performed.

What drugs would you use for a rapid sequence induction?

- Keep it simple!
- Thiopentone 5–7 mg/kg and suxamethonium 1.5 mg/kg

He refuses a spinal and awake fibre-optic intubation.

Let's assume that you proceed to a rapid sequence induction and after pre-oxygenation and the application of cricoid pressure, you give your drugs. What laryngoscope blade would you use initially?

- Usually a Macintosh size 3 or 4 blade
- McCoy blade is an alternative.

Unfortunately, you cannot see the epiglottis at your first attempt. What do you do?

- Check that the head is extended and the neck is flexed (should be optimally positioned prior to induction!).
- Check that the larynx position is not distorted by the cricoid pressure.

- No more than three attempts
- Use an alternative blade such as straight or McCoy or use a bougie.

What would you do if the oxygen saturation starts to fall?

- **Call for help.**
- It is essential to **maintain oxygenation.**
- This should be done with a bag and mask initially.
- Ensure that cricoid pressure remains applied.

Would you give any other drugs?

- **No**. Further doses of muscle relaxant or induction agent are contra-indicated in a rapid sequence induction.
- There is no **'Plan B'** for alternative intubation techniques during RSI.
- The patient should be woken up with oxygenation maintained until the effects of the anaesthetic and muscle relaxant have worn off.

What would you do if you could not ventilate him?

- Standard airway manoeuvres such as head tilt and jaw thrust.
- Try two hand technique.
- Reduce the cricoid pressure slightly.
- Oropharyngeal and/or nasopharyngeal airway.
- LMA.

What if you couldn't ventilate through an LMA and the saturation continued to fall?

- This is a **'Can't intubate, can't ventilate'** scenario.
- **Rescue techniques** are needed.
- Laryngospasm should not be a problem after an adequate dose of muscle relaxant and induction agent but should be considered.
- If you cannot ventilate through a facemask or LMA, the saturation continues to fall beyond 85% and the patient is not waking up, then an **emergency cricothyroidotomy** needs to be performed.

Describe to me how you would do that?

- Identify the cricothyroid membrane.
- Pierce it with a cannula, aspirating air through a 5 ml syringe with saline or water in it.
- Confirm entry into the trachea by easy aspiration of air via the cannula after the needle has been removed.
- An assistant should hold the cannula in place.
- The kits can usually be connected to a high pressure jet ventilation system or a standard breathing circuit connector.
- This is an emergency technique to maintain oxygenation and 'buy time'.
- A definitive airway should be sought as soon as possible.

> **Cricothyroidotomy**
>
> ■ There are pre-packed kits for cricothyroidotomy.
> ■ It is essential that you are familiar with the one in your theatre suite.
> ■ There are many different types available on the market.
> ■ Needle cricothyroidotomy is considered to be quicker and safer than a surgical cricothyroidotomy in providing emergency oxygenation.
> ■ If you still can't ventilate or if surgical emphysema develops, then you should proceed to a surgical cricothyroidotomy.
> ■ A stab incision is made in the membrane.
> ■ Enlarged by blunt dissection.
> ■ A small 5 or 6 mm cuffed endotracheal tube is inserted.

Assuming the patient was successfully woken up from this, how would you proceed with his anaesthetic for his operation?

■ The surgery cannot be delayed.
■ An alternative technique to RSI is needed.
■ Regional anaesthesia such as a spinal should be reconsidered.
■ Awake fibre-optic intubation.

Any other regional techniques that you could use?

■ Combined spinal epidural
■ Femoral and sciatic nerve blocks
■ This would need to be discussed with the surgeon to take account of
  ● Nature and extent of the proposed surgery
  ● Potential for a compartment syndrome post-operatively
  ● (May be masked by a block.)
■ Combined femoral and sciatic blocks alone may prove to be inadequate for surgical anaesthesia.

What about an awake fibre-optic intubation?

■ This is an option for the patient with a known or suspected difficulty airway, especially if there is a risk of reflux.
■ If this patient had just undergone a cricothyroidotomy and extensive airway manipulation, then this might prove difficult.

> See also Long Case 1 'The one about the woman with a goitre for an emergency laparotomy' and the Short Question 'Airway blocks in the context of awake fibre-optic intubation'.

Bibliography

The Difficult Airway Society Guidelines. 2006. www.das.uk.com/guidelines

Universal precautions

A 25-year-old, HIV-positive, intravenous drug user presents for incision and drainage of an abscess. The theatre sister is concerned about transmission of the virus.

What do you understand by the term universal precautions?

Universal precautions as defined by the Center of Disease Control (CDC) in Atlanta are: 'A set of precautions designed to prevent the transmission of pathogens via blood and other body fluids that may be considered potentially infectious to healthcare workers.'

What do you understand by the term standard precautions?

The term universal precautions is now being replaced with the term standard precautions. Standard precautions include precautions to prevent the transmission of infections by other transmission routes, i.e. airborne precautions, droplet precautions and contact precautions.

What are the advantages of this change in approach?

Standard infection control precautions, as well as protecting healthcare workers, could prevent the transmission of many other pathogens and make a major contribution to the reduction of healthcare-associated infection (HCAI). Simplification of the traditional approach to isolation of infectious patients is accomplished if the same precautions are taken with all body fluids.

There is no need to identify different levels of protection for different infectious diseases.

The use of standard precautions, however, does not eliminate the need to isolate some potentially infectious diseases, e.g. tuberculosis or enteric infections.

Can you give examples of body fluids considered to be high risk in terms of transmitting pathogens?

- Blood
- Vaginal secretions
- Semen
- Synovial fluid
- Cerebrospinal fluid
- Pericardial fluid
- Pleural fluid
- Breast milk
- Amniotic fluid
- Any fluid that contains blood or has the potential for containing blood: saliva during dental procedures is therefore considered high risk.

What are the components of standard infection control precautions?

- Handwashing
- The wearing of protective clothing, including gloves
- Safe handling and disposal of sharps
- Dealing with blood spills promptly
- Decontamination of equipment
- Disposal of waste
- Disposal of linen
- Personal health and hygiene of staff
- Patient placement/isolation

Why are needlestick injuries important?

Needlestick injuries are common and affect some people more than others: nurses are the largest single group, and have high rates of injury. Over a lifetime, the risk for an individual is finite and measurable. In some high-risk specialties the risk is appreciable. In a study of French surgeons with a working lifetime estimate of 210 skin punctures, the individual cumulative risks of contamination were calculated to be 6.9% for hepatitis C and 0.15% for HIV. For hepatitis C that is a 1 in 14 chance (of a needlestick with contaminated blood), and for HIV it is a 1 in 660 chance. The figure for HIV is similar to estimates for US surgeons.

The risk is one of transmission of blood-borne viruses, HBV, HCV and HIV being the most important. The risk is dependent on the prevalence of the viruses in the population and on the transmission rate – higher with HBV and HCV than HIV.

The literature rates of seroconversion are 10%–30% for HBV, 1–10% for HCV and 0.1%–0.3% for HIV. Hollow bore needles with appreciable amounts of blood (and virus) carry the most risk. Prophylaxis and vaccination may help in some cases.

Bibliography
Caillot J-L, Voigloi EJ, Gilly FN, Fabry J. (2000). The occupational viral risk run by French surgeons: a disturbing perspective. *AIDS*, **14**, 2061–2.
Wilson J. (2001). *Infection Control in Clinical Practice*. London: Baillière-Tindall.
www.eBandolier.com. Needlestick injuries. July 2003.

Valvular heart disease

> **Preoperative evaluation of valvular heart disease**
>
> - Determine severity of lesion – history, examination and investigations.
> - Haemodynamic significance – e.g. echocardiogram, cardiac catheterization.
> - LV function
> - Degree of end-organ dysfunction – pulmonary, renal, hepatic
> - Concomitant ischaemic heart disease.

What are the principles of anaesthetising a patient with aortic stenosis?

- Maintain myocardial oxygen supply (maintain SVR with α-agonist).
- Maintain normal sinus rhythm.
- Maintain heart rate at 60–90 bpm.
- Maintain intra-vascular volume.
- Give SBE prophylaxis.
- Appropriate monitoring – arterial BP, ST changes (CMV_5), ?PAFC, ?TOE.
- Avoid hypotensive drugs, neuro-axial blocks.
- 'Slow and tight'.

Critical aortic stenosis exists when the orifice is less than 0.5–0.7 cm^2 (normal is 2.5–3.5 cm^2). This correlates with a trans-valvular gradient of >50 mmHg with a normal cardiac output. Note that a low gradient may indicate LV failure.

In aortic stenosis the left ventricle is **hypertrophied** (concentric) and **poorly compliant** resulting in diastolic dysfunction.

LVH increases myocardial oxygen demand while the supply is decreased as a result of high ventricular wall pressures compressing intramyocardial coronary vessels. Aortic diastolic pressure and normal heart rate must be maintained to promote coronary blood flow.

The poorly compliant left ventricle causes elevated LVEDP which impairs ventricular filling. Patients are therefore very sensitive to changes in intravascular volume. Filling by atrial contraction is extremely important (contributes 40% of ventricular filling). Loss of atrial systole may cause heart failure or hypotension. Avoidance of arrhythmias is essential (consider immediate cardioversion).

Patients may behave as though they have a fixed stroke volume. Cardiac output is thus dependent on heart rate. Bradycardia is poorly tolerated.

> **Principles of anaesthesia for aortic incompetence ('fast and loose')**
>
> - Eccentric hypertrophy, dilated left ventricle.
> - ↑Oxygen demand due to dilated ventricle and ↑ work.
> - GA generally well tolerated as ↓ afterload → ↓ regurgitation.
> - Watch diastolic (coronary perfusion pressure) – tends to be low.

- Keep HR 80–100.
- Avoid bradycardia as ↓ HR → ↑ LVEDP which may → failure.
- Avoid ↑ SVR as →↑ regurgitation.
- Dopamine/dobutamine preferable to vasoconstrictors.
- Keep the patient 'fast and loose'.

Principles of anaesthesia for mitral incompetence ('fast and loose')

- Eccentric hypertrophy, dilated left ventricle.
- Proportion regurgitated depends on LV afterload.
- Dilated left atrium.
- GA generally well tolerated as ↓ afterload → ↓ regurgitation.
- Keep preload ↓ (keeps LV volume ↓).
- Keep HR 80–100.
- Avoid bradycardia as → ↑ regurgitation.
- Avoid ↑ SVR as → ↑ regurgitation.
- Keep the patient 'fast and loose'.

Mitral stenosis is covered in a separate short question.

Bibliography
Brown J, Morgan-Hughes, NJ. (2005). Aortic stenosis and non-cardiac surgery *CEACCP*, **5**, 1–4.
Deakin CD. (1998). *Clinical Notes for the FRCA*. Churchill Livingstone.
Goldstone JC, Pollard BJ. (1996). *Handbook of Clinical Anaesthesia*. Churchill Livingstone.
Morgan GE, Mikhail MS. (1996). *Clinical Anaesthesiology*, 2nd edition. Appleton and Lange.

Vomiting and day surgery

A 32-year-old female patient presents for a day case laparoscopy as part of investigation of infertility. She has a previous history of vomiting after anaesthetics.

Is providing anti-emesis important?

- Post-operative nausea and vomiting (PONV) may be the most unpleasant memory that a patient remembers about their operation. The incidence of PONV in adults is approximately 25%, ranging from 5%–75% in the literature.
- Severe cases can lead to
  - Increased length of hospital stay
  - Aspiration pneumonia
  - Retching resulting in increased bleeding and incisional hernias.

- Prolonged vomiting results in loss of hydrogen ions, chloride, potassium, sodium and water.
- Dehydration, metabolic alkalosis and total body potassium depletion may occur.

What factors pre-dispose to Post-Operative Nausea and Vomiting?

This can be divided into patient, surgical and anaesthetic-related factors (see box at the end of the question for more detail).

The commonest factors are:

- Children
- Female sex
- Previous history of PONV
- History of motion sickness
- Opioids
- Sympathomimetics
- Gynae/ear/squint/laparoscopic surgery.

In principle, how would you reduce the risk of emesis?

- Think in terms of the patient factors, surgical factors and anaesthetic factors (see box).
- Laparoscopy is not suitable for a regional technique.

Pre-operatively

- Ensure adequate hydration
- Keep fasting times to the minimum
- Normalise electrolytes and glucose if necessary.

Induction

- Avoid etomidate and keep opioid use as low as possible.
- Avoid hypotension, coughing and straining.
- Avoid inflating the stomach with gas.
- Avoid tracheal intubation if possible (physical stimulation and drugs required).
- Avoid volatile anaesthetics (if particularly high risk) and nitrous oxide, i.e. use TCI propofol.
- Give anti-emetics in combination, based on risk factors.

Intra-operatively

- Ensure adequate hydration.
- Minimise visceral traction/distension.
- Encourage the surgeon to use minimal access surgery and ensure the abdomen is deflated as much as possible to reduce pain post-op.

- Give paracetamol and NSAIDs as opioid sparing agents if appropriate.
- Use local infiltration.

Emergence

- Avoid neostigmine if possible.
- Consider emptying the stomach if it is likely to be full of gas.
- Avoid rapid movements and turns on the way to recovery.

Post-operatively

- Regular anti-emetics.
- Avoid opioids if possible, with regular adjuvant analgesia.
- Avoid rapid oral intake.

Is this lady at risk of PONV?

She is a middle-aged female with a history of PONV undergoing gynaecological laparoscopic surgery, so she is high risk.

Discuss your anaesthetic technique.

- Use a TCI Propofol technique.
- Following a standard general and anaesthetic assessment and assuming routine preparation of the patient, theatre and equipment, give fentanyl 1 mcg/kg and commence TCI Propofol after pre-oxygenation.
- Paralyse the patient with Atracurium 0.5 mg kg and ventilate in oxygen (taking care not to over-inflate with the bag-valve-mask) until intubating conditions are achieved. Intubate carefully.
- Give paracetamol 1g, parecoxib 40 mg with ondansetron 4 mg and dexamethasone 8 mg as anti-emetics.
- Intravenous Hartmann's solution throughout.
- Reserve morphine for pain in recovery.
- Neuromuscular monitoring will guide the need for reversal. It should ideally be avoided.

- Some anaesthetists use LMAs or Proseal LMAs for laparoscopies, usually in thin patients.
- In the exam it is best to stick to the safe bet of intubating a head down patient with a pneumoperitoneum (in order to guard against aspiration) and accept that this may not be the ideal anaesthetic for preventing emesis.

Which volatile anaesthetic is most likely to cause emesis?

All of the volatile agents are likely to cause emesis in a dose-dependent manner.

Volatiles and emesis

- A randomised controlled trial of 1180 patients at high risk for PONV found that, in the early post-operative period (two hours or less), the leading risk factor for vomiting was dose-dependent use of volatile anaesthetics.
- Similar odds ratios found for isoflurane (odds ratio 19.8).
- Enflurane (16.1)
- Sevoflurane (14.5)
- Desflurane has been shown to have similar rates in other studies.
- Nitrous oxide probably causes PONV.

Name some anti-emetic agents. Where do they act?

Anticholinergics	which cross the blood-brain barrier can reduce the vestibular component of PONV. An example would be hyoscine. **Cyclizine** has anticholinergic and central antihistamine activity.
Dopamine antagonists	D_2 antagonists act on central (and some peripheral) dopamine receptors. Examples are **prochlorperazine, metoclopramide and droperidol.**
5HT$_3$ antagonists	Act on receptors found in the chemoreceptor trigger zone (CTZ) and peripherally in gut. **Ondansetron** is an example.
Dexamethasone	is a **corticosteroid** and may reduce 5HT$_3$ secretion in the gut, but its mechanism of anti-emesis is unknown.

- **Benzodiazepines** and **cannabinoids** also have actions on the CTZ.

When would you admit someone overnight with vomiting post-op?

1. Persistent nausea/vomiting despite multi-modal treatment.
2. Unable to tolerate oral intake.
3. Still requiring intravenous anti-emetics.
4. If it is felt that intravenous fluids may be necessary to correct electrolyte imbalance and provide hydration.

Factors pre-disposing a patient to PONV

Patient factors

- Children – risk of PONV is almost twice that for adults with an equal distribution between boys and girls until puberty.
- Adults – female sex ($3\times$ more likely).
- Incidence increases during menstruation and decreases after the menopause.
- After 70 years of age, both sexes are equally affected.

- Previous history of PONV or motion sickness.
- Smokers have 0.6× risk of non-smokers.
- Early ambulation.
- Early post-operative eating and drinking.
- Intestinal obstruction.
- Metabolic, e.g. hypoglycaemia, uraemia.
- Hypoxia.

Surgical factors

- Intra-abdominal-laparoscopic.
- Intracranial (especially posterior fossa).
- Middle ear.
- Squint surgery (highest incidence of PONV in children).
- Gynaecological, especially ovarian.
- Tonsillectomy and adenoidectomy.
- Prolonged surgery.

Anaesthetic factors

- Opioids (untreated pain is also emetogenic).
- Sympathomimetics.
- Inhalational agents.
- Etomidate and ketamine (compared with propofol and thiopentone).
- Neostigmine.
- Nitrous oxide (GIT distension/expansion of middle ear cavities).
- Prolonged anaesthesia.
- Hypotension.
- Intra-operative dehydration.
- Inexperienced bag and mask ventilation (gastric dilatation).
- GA has 11× risk of regional technique

Bibliography

Anaesthesia UK website. www.FRCA.co.uk [Resources, clinical anaesthesia, nausea and vomiting].

Apfel CC, Kranke P, Katz MH et al. (2002). Volatile anaesthetics may be the main cause of early but not delayed postoperative vomiting: a randomized controlled trial of factorial design. *British Journal of Anaesthesia*, **88**, 659–68.

Fisher DM. (1997). The 'big little problem' of postoperative nausea and vomiting: do we know the answer yet? *Anesthesiology*, **87**, 1271–3.

Wolff–Parkinson–White syndrome

A 22-year-old woman is admitted for a routine hysteroscopy. She has a history of being admitted to casualty six months ago with palpitations.

This is her ECG at the time of admission to casualty. What does it show?

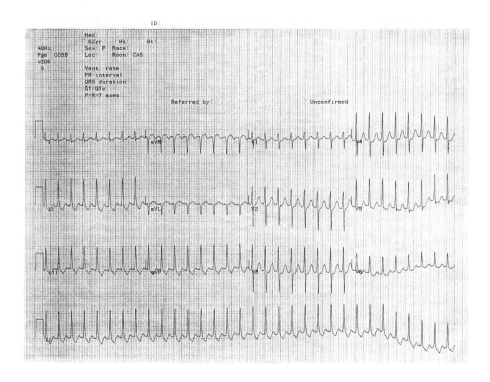

The ECG shows a supraventricular tachycardia. The rate 190 beats per minute.

What would be suitable initial management if her blood pressure was stable?

- ABC, oxygen, etc.
- Check electrolytes (including Mg^{2+}).
- Carotid sinus massage.
- Adenosine – caution in asthma and if taking dipyridamole (prolongs half-life).

This is her resting ECG. What does it show?

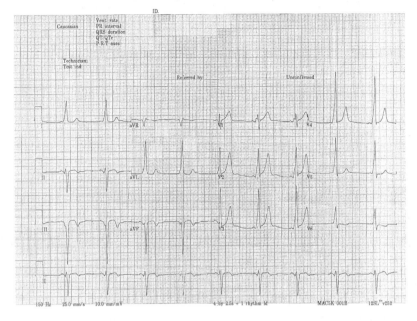

It shows sinus rhythm at a rate of 74 bpm. The axis is normal. The P-R interval is shortened (normal is 110 – 210 ms) and there are delta waves present. The diagnosis is Wolff–Parkinson–White syndrome. The ventricular complex is predominantly positive in lead V₁ suggesting Type-A WPW syndrome.

(Type-B has predominantly negative ventricular complex in lead V₁.)

What is the 'delta wave'?

There is an **accessory atrio-ventricular pathway** (formerly called the bundle of Kent), which conducts the atrial impulse to the ventricles much faster than the A–V node. This results in the start of ventricular depolarisation sooner than normal, hence the short P-R interval. That initial ventricular depolarisation takes place in normal ventricular tissue (i.e. not specialised conducting tissue). The initial rate of depolarisation is therefore slower, hence the slurred, delta wave. When the rest of the impulse finally arrives through the A–V node, the specialised conducting tissue continues, the ventricular depolarisation as normal, so the rest of the QRS complex looks normal.

What are the implications for anaesthesia?

These patients may develop paroxysmal tachyarrhythmias during anaesthesia.
Patients who have a history suggestive of frequent arrhythmias should ideally be investigated by a cardiologist and put on appropriate therapy. Those with infrequent episodes may not require any treatment.

What types of arrhythmia do they develop?

There are **two common arrhythmias in WPW**. These are **atrial fibrillation** (AF) and **A-V nodal re-entrant tachycardia**.

- **Atrial fibrillation** Patients with WPW who develop atrial fibrillation are at risk of very rapid ventricular responses as the accessory pathway does not provide any 'protective delay' like the A-V node. This may result in heart failure or may even deteriorate into ventricular fibrillation. In AF, most conducted impulses reach the ventricles via the accessory pathway, so **delta waves are seen on the ECG**.
- **Re-entrant tachycardia** A re-entry circuit is set up. After transmitting an atrial impulse, the A–V node usually recovers before the accessory pathway. If an atrial ectopic occurs at the right time, it will transmit through the A–V node while the accessory pathway is still refractory. By the time it has done this, the accessory pathway may have recovered and the impulse will then pass through it back into the atria. As the impulses are all reaching the ventricles via the A–V node and not the accessory pathway, there are **no delta waves on the ECG**.

How would you manage an intra-operative tachycardia?

- **Treat possible triggers of rhythm disturbance** such as hypoxia, hypercarbia, acidosis, electrolyte disturbance or any cause of sympathetic stimulation.
- **Assess the degree of cardiovascular compromise**. If there was significant compromise, then **synchronised DC cardioversion** starting at 25–50 J would be the treatment of choice. If the blood pressure was stable, then the management would depend on the rhythm.
- **Pharmacological therapy**: For re-entrant tachycardia, adenosine would be the first choice. Class 1a drugs such as procainamide (5–10 mg/kg) and disopyramide prolong the refractory period, decrease conduction in the accessory pathway and may terminate both re-entrant tachycardia and AF. More conventional drugs such as amiodarone, sotalol and other beta-blockers such as esmolol may also be useful.

Are there any drugs you should not use?

Verapamil and **digoxin** are contra-indicated as they both preferentially block A–V conduction thereby increasing conduction through the accessory pathway. Although verapamil could, in theory, be used to terminate a re-entrant tachycardia, its use is not advisable, because these patients may then revert to AF or flutter. A further hazard with verapamil is that a tachyarrhythmia that *looks* like re-entrant tachycardia may actually be VT.

Adenosine would preferentially block the A–V node and therefore should not be used in AF.

Bibliography

Bennett D. (1994). *Cardiac Arrhythmias*. Butterworth-Heinemann.
Goldstone JC, Pollard BJ. (1996). *Handbook of Clinical Anaesthesia*. Edinburgh, UK: Churchill Livingstone.
Morgan GE, Mikhail MS. (1996). *Clinical Anaesthesiology*, 2nd edition. Appleton and Lange.

Chapter 3

The Long Cases

Long Case 1

'The one about the woman with a goitre for an emergency
laparoscopy'

*A 75-year-old woman was admitted 24 hours ago with
right-sided abdominal pain, nausea and vomiting over the last
week. She has a past medical history consisting of a right total
hip replacement 10 years ago and a CVA with right hemiparesis 4
years ago.*

The surgeons wish to perform an urgent laparoscopy.

Drugs	Amiodarone 200 mg o.d.
	Frusemide 20 mg b.d.
	ISMO 60 mg b.d.

O/E	Height 1.60 m, Weight 80 kg
	Large diffuse goitre
	HR 94 regular
	BP 110/80 mmHg
	HS I + II + 0
	Chest clear

Investigations	Hb	9.7 g/dl	Na	132 mmol/l
	WCC	13.5×10^9/l	K	3.3 mmol/l
	Plt	189×10^9/l	Urea	12.2 mmol/l
	MCV	78 fl	Creat	110 µmol/l

The Clinical Anaesthesia Viva Book, Second edition, ed. Julian M. Barker, Simon L. Maguire and
Simon J. Mills. © J. M. Barker, S. L. Maguire, S. J. Mills 2009.

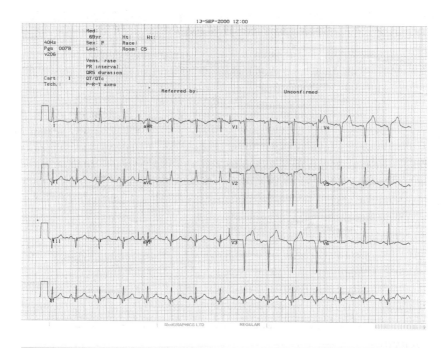

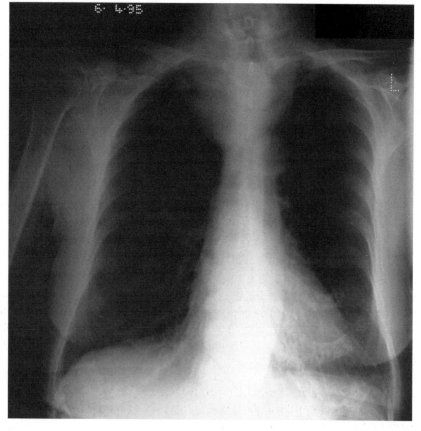

Questions

1. Summarise the case and the problems presenting to you as the anaesthetist.

This is an elderly lady presenting for emergency surgery with a significant cardiovascular history and a potentially difficult airway. She has been ill for the last week and may well be significantly dehydrated and septic. She will need careful resuscitation before surgery and a detailed assessment of her airway including imaging. The potential for a difficult airway and intubation is compounded by the high risk of aspiration. Surgery is urgent but not an emergency and these issues should be addressed before taking her to theatre.

2. Interpret the ECG.

The ECG shows sinus rhythm at a rate of 90 beats per minute. There are Q waves in leads II, III and a VF, suggesting a previous inferior myocardial infarction. There are also Q waves in V_2, V_3 and V_4 indicating an old anterior infarction.

3. What does the CXR show?

This is a PA chest X-ray showing a large retrosternal mass with evidence of tracheal deviation to the left. The heart is not enlarged and the lungs are clear. Thoracic inlet views may help to image the lesion further, but a CT scan would be ideal.

4. What is the mechanism of action of each of the drugs she is taking?

Amiodarone is an agent used to treat atrial and ventricular arrhythmias. It works by prolonging the repolarisation phase of the action potential (Vaughan-Williams Class III). It also possesses some α- and β-receptor blocking activity.

Frusemide acts at the thick ascending limb of the loop of Henle. It inhibits the co-transport of sodium, potassium and chloride into the medulla. The reduction in tonicity in the medulla results in the production of hypotonic or isotonic urine.

Isosorbide mononitrate is probably being used in this patient as anti-anginal therapy. It causes venous and arterial vasodilatation (venous>arterial especially at lower doses). Its mechanism of action is via the production of nitric oxide in the endothelial cells. This diffuses into the smooth muscle cells, activating guanylyl cyclase to convert GTP to cyclicGMP. The cGMP stimulates a reaction through protein kinases resulting in dephosphorylation of the myosin light chain and subsequent muscle relaxation (this may be by decreased free calcium concentration in the cytosol). The ultimate effects of nitrates are to reduce myocardial oxygen demand by reducing left ventricular end-diastolic pressure and wall tension. Coronary blood flow is also redistributed to the subendocardium.

5. Would you like any further investigations?

A CT scan of the neck and thoracic inlet is required to assess further the degree of encroachment on the airway. This will have significant implications for the conduct of anaesthesia.

Thyroid function tests (in particular TSH and free T4) would exclude thyrotoxicosis and the associated risk of thyroid storm under anaesthesia.

Given that the ECG suggests an old inferior MI and possible subendocardial ischaemia, an echocardiogram may be useful to establish the resting ejection fraction. However, an echocardiogram gives no information about cardiac reserve. For example, a resting ejection fraction of 60% does not give any information about the ability to increase cardiac output. Of the numerous cardiac investigations available, there are no consistently reliable indicators of cardiac risk for non-cardiac surgery except perhaps angiography. CPEX testing may give information about functional reserve and assist with risk stratification but is impractical in this situation.

6. How would you resuscitate her?

She has features that put her at high risk for post-operative mortality:

- Age > 65
- Presence of co-morbid disease
- Emergency presentation

Fluid resuscitation should be implemented and may best be performed with invasive monitoring in a critical care environment. As she is probably septic, a mixed central venous oxygen level (<70%) and blood lactate (>4 mmol/l) may be helpful in detecting organ hypo-perfusion and the need for goal-directed resuscitation. There is no compelling evidence on whether crystalloid or colloid resuscitation is preferable in this situation and resuscitation should be aimed at restoring adequate tissue perfusion. Many resuscitation goals have been quoted, but correction of tachycardia, hypotension, and restoration of normal urine output (0.5 ml/h) are good starting points. CVP targets are contentious but 8–12 mmHg is often quoted (Rivers *et al.* **Early Goal Directed Therapy**). If flow monitoring is available, fluid boluses may be monitored to ensure increasing cardiac output.

7. Are you aware of any publications concerning pre-optimisation of surgical patients?

There have been a number of publications looking at the pre-operative optimisation of oxygen delivery for high-risk patients. They are based on studies showing that high-risk patients surviving major surgery achieved consistently higher postoperative oxygen delivery and cardiac index compared with non-survivors.

- **Shoemaker** showed the following values to be associated with survival:

Cardiac index (CI)	4.5 l/min/m^2
Oxygen delivery (DO$_2$)	600 ml/min/m^2
Oxygen consumption (VO$_2$)	170 ml/min/m^2

- **Shoemaker** et al. in 1987 and **Boyd** et al. in 1993 showed that producing supranormal values of oxygen delivery (>600 ml/min per m^2) resulted in a reduction in post-operative mortality in high risk surgical patients.
- **Wilson** et al. (BMJ, April 1999) studied pre-operative optimisation of oxygen delivery in major elective surgery. Three groups: conventional pre-operative care, fluid + adrenaline, fluid + dopexamine. Patients in the treatment groups were taken to ICU/HDU at least 4 hours pre-operatively and arterial and pulmonary artery lines inserted. Fluids were given to increase the PAWP to 12 (average total fluid given = 1500 ml) after which adrenaline or dopexamine were commenced and increased until the target oxygen delivery was achieved (>600 ml/min per m^2). They showed a reduction in hospital mortality from 17% to 3% (no difference between adrenaline and dopexamine groups) and a reduction in morbidity in the dopexamine group compared with adrenaline and control (fewer infective complications).
- A paper in *Critical Care Medicine* in 2000 (prospective, randomised controlled trial of 412 patients undergoing major abdominal surgery in 13 hospitals from 6 European countries) compared the effects on morbidity/mortality of dopexamine infusion or placebo on fluid resuscitated patients. Patients were taken to ICU pre-operatively, invasive monitoring inserted and fluids given until set criteria met. Randomisation to dopexamine 0.5 mcg/kg per min, 2 mcg/kg per min or placebo followed. There was no statistically significant difference in 28-day mortality in the three groups, although the authors speculated a trend towards lower mortality in the low-dose dopexamine group.
- **Consensus meeting: management of the high-risk surgical patient, April 2000**
  - Increasing global oxygen delivery in high-risk patients significantly reduces morbidity and mortality.
  - In patients with significant ischaemic heart disease, care needs to be taken to minimise oxygen demand.
  - The earlier the intervention, the better the outcome.
  - Strategy should be as defined by Shoemaker's criteria for CI, DO$_2$ and VO$_2$.
  - Low-dose dopexamine *may* have additional benefits.
- A meta-analysis of fluid optimisation by **Kern and Shoemaker** in *Critical Care Medicine* in 2002 concluded that patients at high risk (predicted mortality >20% would benefit from fluid optimisation but not those with a predicted mortality <15%.

'Meta-analysis of the 14 published and three unpublished RCTs of peri-operative optimisation of high-risk patients indicates that, were the strategy generally adopted, 11 lives could be saved for every 100 operations performed.' **Dr Owen Boyd**

■ On the flip side of the coin, **excessive fluid resuscitation** has been shown to worsen outcome in abdominal surgery (Brandstrup *et al.*, 2003).

8. How would you assess her airway?

Standard bedside tests for airway assessment such as the Mallampati score and thyromental distance need to be taken into consideration, along with the CT scan appearances. An indirect laryngoscopy or fibre-optic nasendoscopy should be performed by an ENT surgeon to assess the likelihood of a good view of the larynx at direct laryngoscopy. However, an expected easy laryngoscopy does not imply a straightforward intubation in the presence of a large goitre. The site and severity of any obstruction should be established on CT scan (retrosternal goitre is midtracheal). The narrowest part of the trachea can be measured to guide the choice of tube size. It will also demonstrate exactly how far down the trachea the obstruction extends so that it will be known whether an endotracheal tube or tracheostomy will be able to get below it or not. In most cases it is possible to pass a size 7.0 tube beyond the obstruction and allow both the tube bevel and cuff to sit above the carina in a conventional way.

9. How would you manage her airway?

This woman is likely to have a full stomach even if starved and thus presents considerable aspiration risk.

If there is no evidence of tracheal compression on CT scan and clinically the intubation looks straightforward, then a conventional rapid sequence induction and intubation could be performed. If the goitre is compressing the airway, then a rapid sequence induction may be hazardous, potentially leading to loss of the airway in the event of a failed intubation. If there was no risk of aspiration, then a gas-induction might be considered, but this would not be appropriate here. An awake fibre-optic intubation, although not always the first choice technique, might be the technique of choice in this case.

10. What technique of awake fibre-optic intubation would you use?

There are many ways to perform awake fibre-optic intubation. Having your own chosen technique and sticking to it will confirm to the examiners that you have performed the procedure many times before!

The procedure should be explained to the patient in an attempt to minimise anxiety (!). Intravenous access and standard monitoring is established. Pre-medication with an antisialogogue and a benzodiazepine/opioid would be given if necessary according to the clinical state of the patient. Supplementary oxygen should be administered via a face mask or nasal catheter. The patient may prefer the semi-upright position to being totally supine. Note that, if there is a significant risk of loss of the airway, then a surgeon experienced at rigid bronchoscopy should be present.

The nasal route is chosen in this patient for the sake of this question.

Five sprays of 10% aerosolised lignocaine are directed into the oropharynx at the start of the procedure (the nasal route should not stimulate the gag reflex).

The more patent nostril is chosen (ask the patient). The ET tube is lubricated and 'loaded' onto the bronchoscope. Topical anaesthesia and vasoconstriction of the nose can be achieved using 4% cocaine applied with cotton buds. The bronchoscope is advanced through the nose and pharynx with a 'spray as you go' technique using aliquots of 4% lignocaine injected through the working channel of the scope (alternatively, the ET tube may be passed through the nose before the scope). A jaw thrust manoeuvre will help to lift the tongue forward if it is obstructing the view. The cords and trachea are both visualized and sprayed sequentially. After a pause of 30–45 seconds, the bronchoscope may be advanced into the trachea and the tube railroaded carefully over it. (Trans-tracheal injection can be used to anaesthetize the trachea but may not be feasible or advisable in the presence of a large goitre.) The bronchoscope is withdrawn under direct vision to confirm the position of the ET tube above the carina. Once the tube is in place, the induction agent can be given.

11. What are the risks of laparoscopic surgery?

These have been discussed in the short case on laparoscopic cholecystectomy.

12. How would you manage gas embolus?

The surgeon should be informed and the abdomen deflated. Nitrous oxide, if used, should be discontinued. 100% oxygen should be administered and fluid given to increase central venous pressure. The patient may be turned into the left lateral and head down position and the central venous line aspirated to try to remove gas.

Bibliography
Boyd O, Grounds RM, Bennett ED. (1993). A randomised clinical trial of the effect of the deliberate perioperative increase of oxygen delivery on mortality in high-risk patients. *Journal of the American Medical Association*, **270**(22), 2699–707.

Brandstrup B, Tonnesen H, Beier-Holgersen R *et al*. (2003). Effects of intravenous fluid restriction on postoperative complications: comparison of two perioperative fluid regimens: a randomized assessor-blinded multicentre trial. *Annals of Surgery* **238**, 641–8.

Diprose P, Deakin MA. (2001). Fibreoptic bronchoscopy for emergency intubation. *International Journal of Intensive Care*,

Farling PA. (2000). Thyroid disease. *British Journal of Anaesthesia*, **85**(1), 15–28.

Hagberg CA. (2000). *Handbook of Difficult Airway Management*. Churchill Livingstone.

Kern J, Shoemaker W. (2002). Meta-analysis of hemodynamic optimization in high-risk patients. *Critical Care Medicine*, **30**, 1686–92.

Mason RA. (1999). The obstructed airway in head and neck surgery. *Anaesthesia*, **54**, 625–8.

Report of consensus meeting: Management of the High Risk Surgical Patient, *International Journal of Critical Care Medicine*, 13–14 April 2000.

Rivers E, Nguyen B, Havstad S. (2001). Early goal-directed therapy in the treatment of severe sepsis. *New England Journal of Medicine*, **345**, 1368–77.

Shoemaker WC, Appel PL, Kram HB, Waxman K, Lee TS (1998). Prospective trial of supranormal values of survivors as therapeutic goals in high-risk surgical patients. *Chest* **94**(6), 1176–86.

Takala J, Meier-Hellmann A, Eddleston J, Hulsaert P, Sramek V. (2000). Effect of dopexamine on outcome after major abdominal surgery: A prospective, randomised, controlled multicentre study. *Critical Care Medicine*, **28**(10), 3417–23.

Wilson J, Woods I, Fawcett, J *et al.* (1999) Reducing the risk of major elective surgery: randomised controlled trial of preoperative optimisation of oxygen delivery. *British Medical Journal* **318**, 1099–103.

Long Case 2

'The one about the man with pneumonia who needs a laparotomy'

A 42-year-old man presents with a short history of upper abdominal pain, vomiting and shortness of breath. The pain radiates to his right shoulder. The surgeons wish to perform a laparotomy.

PMH	Peptic ulcer disease His brother was admitted to intensive care with a high temperature following an appendicectomy
O/E	Sweaty, Cyanosed Temp 38.2 °C HR 120 SR BP 105/45 mmHg RR 25 bpm Reduced air entry at the right base with bronchial breathing

Investigations				
	Hb	15 g/dl	Na	149 mmol/l
	WCC	14 × 10⁹/l	K	4.5 mmol/l
	Plt	380 × 10⁹/l	Urea	11 mmol/l
	PCV	0.46 l/l	Creatinine	124 μmol/l
	Blood gas on 40% oxygen:		pH	7.28
			PCO₂	31 mmHg
			PO₂	63 mmHg
			SBC	19 mmol/l
			BE	−5 mmol/l

LFTs normal

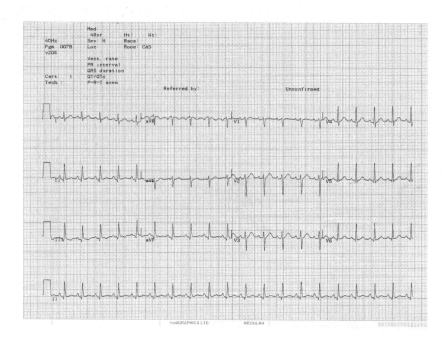

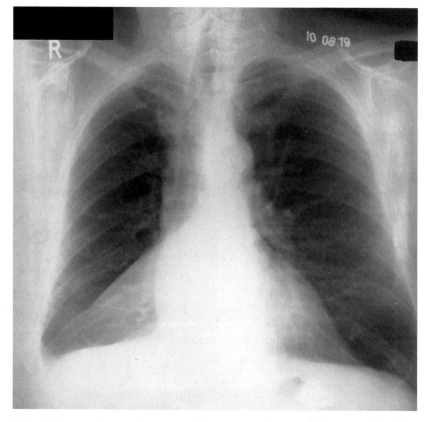

Questions

1. Can you summarise the case?

This man presents with a short history of abdominal pain and vomiting with a history of peptic ulcer disease but also has significant signs suggestive of an acute respiratory illness. There may be dual pathology. He appears septic, dehydrated and hypoxaemic. Of note in the anaesthetic history is what may have been a malignant hyperthermia reaction occurring in his brother and this should be thoroughly explored in the history and in his brother's case notes if necessary.

2. What do you think about the chest X-ray and ECG?

This is a PA chest X-ray. There is shadowing in the right lower zone. There is also loss of definition of the right hemidiaphragm. The horizontal fissure is pulled down. These appearances are suggestive of right lower lobe collapse/consolidation. Given the clinical history, this is most likely to represent pneumonia.

The ECG shows a sinus tachycardia of 120 beats per minute. There are no other abnormalities.

> **X-ray features of right lower lobe collapse**
> ■ Well-demarcated shadowing/opacity in right lower zone.
> ■ Loss of right medial hemidiaphragm behind the heart.
> ■ Horizontal fissure displaced downwards.
> ■ Right heart border still seen.

3. Tell me about the gases.

He is hypoxaemic on 40% oxygen. There is a metabolic acidosis with partial respiratory compensation.

4. What is meant by the term 'cyanosis'?

Cyanosis is a bluish discolouration of the skin (peripheral) or mucous membranes (central). It is seen when there are more than 5 g/dl of deoxygenated haemoglobin in the blood. Central cyanosis is caused by cardiac or respiratory disorders and may improve with the administration of oxygen (providing there is not a large shunt). Peripheral cyanosis is caused by vasoconstriction, stasis and increased oxygen extraction by the peripheral tissues.

5. What do you think about his volume status? Discuss.

As mentioned earlier, he is dehydrated. The evidence for this is the history of vomiting and the presence of tachycardia, high Na^+ and disproportionately high urea compared with creatinine. His clinical picture is one of sepsis (see box below) and this will cause a relative hypovolaemia. He needs fluid resuscitation before theatre. This would be best achieved in a high dependency or intensive care setting and may be guided by a CVP line, pulmonary artery catheter and cardiac output measurements if available.

SIRS and sepsis: systemic inflammatory response syndrome (SIRS) is a clinical condition with two or more of the following:

- Temperature $>38\,^{\circ}C$ or $<36\,^{\circ}C$
- HR >90 bpm
- RR >20 bpm or $PaCO_2$ <32 mmHg
- WCC $>12 \times 10^9/l$ or $<4 \times 10^9/l$

Sepsis is a cause of SIRS that requires the presence of infection.

---

6. What is the differential diagnosis of his upper abdominal pain?

Given his history of peptic ulcer disease, a perforated ulcer is an obvious suspect. Other causes might include pancreatitis, acute cholecystitis or a common bile duct stone, hepatitis, a subphrenic collection or even abdominal aortic aneurysm.

The abdominal symptoms may even be related to the lower lobe pneumonia.

7. What may be the cause of his shoulder pain?

This is likely to be due to referred pain from irritation of the right hemidiaphragm (C3, 4, 5). The origin of this irritation could be above or below the diaphragm.

8. Are there any other problems of note from the history?

A major issue if he requires surgery is the suspicion of a malignant hyperthermia reaction in his brother. The management would be greatly influenced by knowledge of what took place. Therefore, a thorough review of his brother's case notes and a discussion with his brother and the primary care physician if necessary is warranted. The MH unit at Leeds holds a database of all the patients tested for MH susceptibility. His brother's name may be on this list.

The suspicion is high from the history, so if the diagnosis cannot be excluded it would be wise to assume the family to be MH susceptible and anaesthetise this man as such.

9. Summarize your anaesthetic technique for laparotomy in this man.

During the period of resuscitation, preparations should be made to provide a safe anaesthetic for a patient at risk of developing MH. This will include a vapour-free machine and circuit and the avoidance of known triggers such as suxamethonium and volatile agents. An epidural would have been ideal for analgesia and to help with post-operative respiratory function, but it should probably be avoided in this case as he is septic. He is at risk of aspiration at induction but suxamethonium cannot be used. The airway could be secured either by a modified rapid sequence with rocuronium (only if expected easy intubation) or awake fibre-optic intubation. Thiopentone, etomidate, propofol and ketamine are all safe induction agents. Anaesthesia can be maintained with a propofol infusion and opioids such as fentanyl, morphine or remifentanil.

Dantrolene should be immediately available.

10. *Where would you send him post-operatively?*

Post-operatively he should be nursed on intensive care. He has multi-organ failure (respiratory, cardiovascular, renal and gastrointestinal) and is likely to become more septic following the 'second hit' of surgery. He will also need to be monitored closely for the development of malignant hyperthermia.

Long Case 3

'The one with the woman with a melanoma on her back'

A 60-year-old woman presents for wide excision of a malignant melanoma in the middle of her back. The surgeons would like her to be prone. She is hypertensive, a heavy smoker and has a chronic cough. She had breast surgery for carcinoma 10 years ago.

Drugs	Enalapril 5 mg OD			
O/E	Temperature 36.8 °C HR 72 regular BP 165/105 mmHg HS I+II+0 BS		Widespread crackles and wheeze	
Investigations	Hb	11.6 g/dl	Na^+	143 mmol/l
	WCC	10×10^9/l	K^+	4.1 mmol/l
	Plt	260×10^9/l	Urea	8.9 mmol/l
			Creatinine	148 μmol/l
PFTs				Post-salbutamol
	FEV_1	1.5 l	(predicted 2.6)	1.7
	FVC	2.3 l	(predicted 3.5)	2.5
	FEV_1/FVC	65%	(predicted 74%)	68%

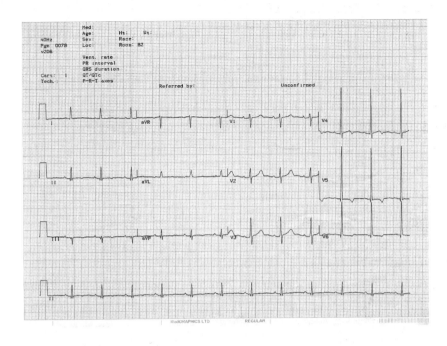

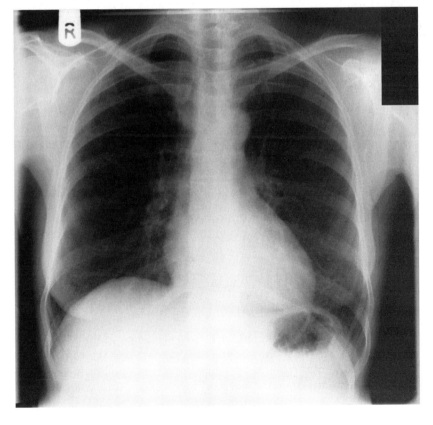

Questions

1. Can you summarise the case?

This lady presents for urgent cancer surgery that presumably cannot be performed under local anaesthetic for surgical reasons. She is hypertensive and has evidence of chronic obstructive pulmonary disease with a reversible component. She also has renal impairment. The pre-operative assessment should concentrate particularly on optimising her chest and blood pressure before theatre.

2. Does the hypertension worry you? Why?

Yes. There is evidence of end-organ damage with the ECG showing left ventricular hypertrophy with strain pattern and the creatinine is raised at 148. Cardiac ischaemic events are more common in hypertensive patients with ECG changes of LVH.

3. What do you think about the chest X-ray?

This is a PA chest X-ray. There is asymmetry of the breast shadows in keeping with the previous left-sided breast surgery, the heart size appears normal and the lungs are clear. No metastases are seen.

4. What about the ECG?

The ECG shows sinus rhythm and a normal axis. There is left ventricular hypertrophy (sum of deflections in V2 + V5 >35 mm) and T wave flattening/inversion in the lateral leads suggesting left ventricular strain. This is likely to be due to long-standing hypertension.

5. What do you think about the creatinine?

As mentioned before, this could be due to long-standing hypertension. It could also be due to enalapril if there is an element of renal artery stenosis. This should be investigated.

6. How would you interpret the pulmonary function tests?

There is a reduction in FEV_1 and FVC but also a reduction in the FEV_1/FVC ratio. This suggests an obstructive pattern of airway disease and the results after the administration of salbutamol show an element of reversibility. It is noteworthy that she is not currently on any respiratory medications such as a beta-agonist or steroid inhaler. She is also on enalapril, which could be contributing to her chronic cough.

7. *How would you anaesthetise her?*

> Do not expect to be able to persuade the examiners that this can be done under local anaesthetic.
> That would make for a very short long case!
> Mention it in passing to make them aware you are thinking of the options.

Her chest disease and hypertension do not appear to be well controlled at present. Although her surgery is for cancer and therefore not truly elective, she would benefit from being postponed until better control of her chest and blood pressure have been achieved. A balance must be struck between the risk of postponing surgery and the risks of continuing when she is poorly controlled. Her chest could potentially be improved over a period of a few days by simple measures. She could be referred to a respiratory physician to optimise her chest with β-agonists, physiotherapy, steroids and antibiotics if necessary. The hypertension may require an increase in the dose of enalapril or the addition of another agent. Whilst it is recognised that, under normal circumstances, a period of several weeks is necessary to reduce the abnormal vascular reactivity associated with hypertension, she is only mildly hypertensive and it would not be appropriate to wait 4–6 weeks in a patient with a malignant melanoma.

On the day of surgery, her ACE inhibitor should be omitted. A benzodiazepine such as temazepam 20 mg and nebulised salbutamol 5 mg would be appropriate pre-medication. In addition to standard monitoring, intra-arterial blood pressure monitoring could be instituted before induction. Following pre-oxygenation and careful induction to minimise fluctuations in blood pressure, an armoured ET tube is inserted and secured. Anaesthesia is maintained with nitrous oxide and isoflurane in oxygen. Her baseline respiratory function is relatively poor and the prone position will restrict lung expansion and increase airway pressures if not managed properly. Post-operative analgesia could be provided by combinations of paracetamol and morphine (via PCA if felt appropriate, e.g. large resection). Non-steroidals may be best avoided, given that her renal function is not normal and she is already on an ACE inhibitor.

8. *What are the important aspects of prone positioning?*

- Plenty of people to perform the manoeuvre – control of head, feet and two people on each side means a minimum of six required to turn the patient.
- Patient is rolled with arms by the side onto the arms of 2 assistants.
- Chest and pelvis are supported by rolls. Abdomen left free.
- Respiration may be severely impeded if the abdomen is not free to move though respiratory function is often improved in correct prone position (increased FRC and VQ matching).
- Head may be facing directly down or turned to the side, but ensure the neck is not hyperextended.
- Eyes should be padded and taped.

- Care to avoid pressure on the eyes (blindness and supraorbital nerve compression reported) and downside ear.
- Avoid pressure over pre-auricular area (facial nerve).
- Arms secured either by the side or in front. Both arms should be moved together and positioned slightly flexed, abducted, and rotated by 90 degrees.
- Avoid brachial plexus damage by not turning the head too much, keeping the arms in a 'relaxed' position, not over-abducted at the shoulder. Protect the radial and ulnar nerves at the elbow.
- Adequate padding of the feet, knees, and pelvis should be applied to prevent pressure necrosis.
- Avoid excessive compression of genitalia and breasts.
- CVS effects – usually well tolerated, may kink jugular vein. Obstructed IVC or femoral vein may lead to vertebral venous engorgement (problem in spinal surgery).
- ET tube must be well secured as must all lines.

Bibliography

Knight D, Mahajan R. (2004). Patient positioning in anaesthesia. *BJA CEACCP* **4**(5), 160–3.

Stone D, Sperry R, Johnson J, Spiekerman B, Yemen T. *The Neuroanaesthesia Handbook*, 1996. Louis, USA: Mosby

Long Case 4

'The one about the man with hypertension and AF who needs a total hip replacement'

A 75-year-old man is scheduled for left total hip replacement. He was diagnosed with hypertension 2 years ago and recently developed dyspnoea on mild exertion. He takes dyazide, aspirin and digoxin.

O/E	Looks well for his age
	Weight 68 kg Height 5′ 7″
	HR 80 irregular
	BP 180/105 mmHg
	Apex 5th intercostal space lateral to mid-clavicular line
	Ejection systolic murmur heard over precordium
	Breath sounds vesicular

Investigations

Hb	12.3 g/dl	Na	138 mmol/L
WCC	8.9×10^9/L	K	3.6 mmol/L
Plt	287×10^9/L	Urea	12.6 mmol/L
		Creat	170 μmol/L
		Glucose	7.8 mmol/L

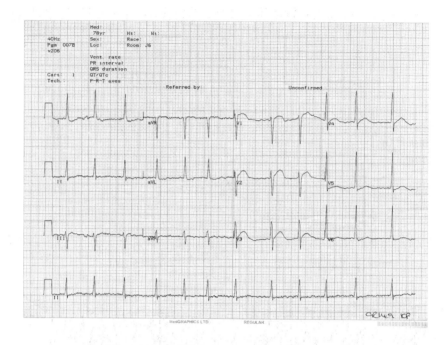

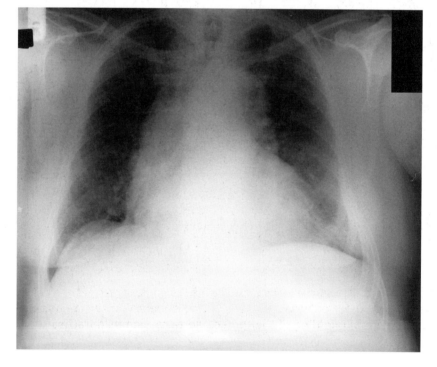

Questions

1. Summarise the case.

This elderly man presents for elective surgery with significant medical problems. He has hypertension, atrial fibrillation and evidence of left ventricular enlargement on the chest X-ray. He also has renal impairment. These problems need further investigation and optimization before he can be safely anaesthetised.

2. Is he hypertensive? Is it controlled?

His blood pressure is 180/105. The British Hypertension Society (BHS) recommends that this level of hypertension is treated, as there are established cardiovascular effects. It is not adequately controlled as it is higher than would be recommended by the BHS, and he has evidence of end-organ damage in the heart and kidneys.

See the short question on uncontrolled hypertension.

3. Why does he get short of breath on exertion?

This may be due to left ventricular dysfunction secondary to long-standing hypertension. It may also be due to reduced cardiac output as a result of loss of diastolic filling secondary to the onset of atrial fibrillation (recent onset AF would account for the relatively new symptoms). Symptoms such as orthopnoea or paroxysmal nocturnal dyspnoea might give extra clues and should be sought. Left ventricular failure has a poor prognosis in terms of post-operative cardiac events. The presence of an ejection systolic murmur may be significant. It could be a flow murmur related to the hypertension, but it would be wise to exclude significant aortic stenosis (although this would usually produce a lower pulse pressure). The shortness of breath could of course be related to another pathology such as COPD.

4. Look at the chest X-ray. Does he have pulmonary oedema?

The chest X-ray shows an enlarged heart with a cardiothoracic ratio of >0.5. There are prominent pulmonary vessels but no evidence of frank pulmonary oedema. There is unfolding of the thoracic aorta causing mild tracheal deviation.

5. Why is he on a diuretic?

This is most likely to have been commenced as first-line treatment of hypertension by his GP.

6. How does dyazide work?

Dyazide is a thiazide diuretic that works by inhibiting the sodium chloride cotransporter in the distal tubule. Excretion of sodium, chloride and consequently water is increased. Some of the sodium is reabsorbed from the distal tubule by exchange with potassium and hydrogen ions (hence the side effects of hypokalaemia and metabolic alkalosis). The exact mechanism by which thiazides exert their anti-hypertensive effect is not known. They do, however, cause a reduction in plasma volume, systemic vascular resistance and cardiac output.

7. Would that be your first choice of anti-hypertensive agent in this situation?

Thiazides are still the current first-line treatment of hypertension particularly in elderly patients but, given that the control is poor, the treatment should be re-evaluated. In the presence of cardiac failure an ACE-inhibitor would normally be justified, but his renal function is abnormal. Renal artery stenosis would need to be excluded.

8. Why is he on aspirin?

This may have been commenced to reduce the risk of stroke as he is in atrial fibrillation and hypertensive.

9. Is that the most appropriate 'anticoagulant'?

No. For a man of this age in chronic atrial fibrillation, the most effective treatment to reduce the incidence of stroke is warfarin.

10. Why is he on digoxin? How does it work?

He is in atrial fibrillation.

Digoxin has direct and indirect actions:

It acts *directly* by inhibiting $Na^+K^+ATPase$ in the sarcolemma cell membrane causing increased intracellular sodium and decreased potassium concentrations. The decrease in intracellular potassium causes a slowing of A/V conduction and pacemaker cell activity. The increased sodium concentration results in decreased extrusion of calcium and therefore a rise in intracellular calcium with a positive inotropic effect.

It acts *indirectly* by increasing central vagal activity.

> **Digoxin and hypokalaemia:** Digoxin *competes* with K^+ for a $Na^+K^+ATPase$ receptor on the outside of the muscle membrane, therefore hypokalaemia potentiates digoxin toxicity.

11. *Have a look at the ECG. What makes you say AF?*

The rhythm is irregularly irregular and there are no discernible P waves. There is also evidence of left ventricular hypertrophy. The ST segments are depressed in leads I, aVL, V_5 and V_6 and the T waves are flattened. This may indicate left ventricular strain or may be a digoxin effect (not a typical 'reverse tick' appearance).

12. *Is it controlled? How could you check?*

The ventricular rate is around 70 beats per minute, which appears to be controlled. However, resting heart rate is a poor predictor of rate control during exertion in atrial fibrillation. To assess the degree of control ambulatory ECG, monitoring would be useful.

13. *Would you anaesthetise him today? Why not?*

No.
He is listed for an *elective* major operation. His hypertension is not well controlled and he requires further investigation and management of possible left ventricular failure and his atrial fibrillation. Although the blood pressure 'numbers' may come down quickly, the abnormal vascular reactivity associated with hypertension takes several weeks to settle down. The operation should therefore be delayed for this length of time.

A cardiology opinion and an echocardiogram may be beneficial to guide management.

14. *What do you want an echocardiogram for?*

An echocardiogram will help to assess his resting left ventricular function (not necessarily representative of cardiac reserve) and will exclude significant aortic stenosis or mitral valve disease. It may also reveal the presence of atrial thrombus secondary to atrial fibrillation. Formal anticoagulation followed by elective cardioversion to return him to sinus rhythm may significantly improve function.

15. *His medical condition is optimised. He has no evidence of aortic stenosis. How would you anaesthetise him?*

> As in many of the long cases, there is probably no definite right or wrong answer here. You need to use a safe technique and provide sound reasons for choosing it.

If the atrial fibrillation is controlled (or ideally cardioverted to sinus rhythm) and his hypertension is controlled, then the operation could be performed safely under regional or general anaesthesia. A spinal anaesthetic is appropriate if the surgeon is known to be quick enough. However, an epidural would be preferred, as it is less likely to result in marked swings in blood pressure, it will allow for prolonged surgery and it will provide ideal post-operative analgesia, thereby reducing the stress response. There is now compelling evidence for the use of regional techniques where possible.

The evidence for regional versus GA

1. A paper in *Anesthesia and Analgesia* in November 2000 entitled 'Outcomes Research in Regional Anaesthesia and Analgesia' looked at a meta-analysis of 142 trials (9553 patients) comparing regional with GA for various types of surgery before 1997.

   Regional associated with:
   - 30% reduction in overall mortality
   - 44% reduction in DVT
   - 55% reduction in PE
   - Reduction in graft thrombosis
   - Earlier return to normal GI function
   - 39% reduction in post-op pneumonia (48 RCTs)
   - MI reduced by 1/3 in 30 RCTs

2. **A review in the *BMJ* in December 2000** looked at 141 trials including 9559 patients (before Jan 1997) where patients were randomised to receive intra-operative neuraxial block (epidural or spinal) or not.

   The authors concluded that:
   - Mortality was reduced by 30% in those allocated neuraxial blockade.
   - The reduction in mortality was not affected by surgical group, type of blockade or where neuraxial blockade was combined with GA.
   - There is a reduction in DVT, PE, transfusion requirements, pneumonia, respiratory depression, myocardial infarction and renal failure when neuraxial blockade is used.

3. A **clinical review in the *BMJ*** April 2001 looked at interventions in *fractured hip*:
   - One systematic review of 15 RCTs (Cochrane review, 2000) showed reduced mortality at 1 month in the 'regional' group (borderline statistical significance). Not possible to conclude 1 year mortality.
   - May be a reduction in DVT.
   - Longer operating time with regional technique.
   - Summary... 'regional anaesthesia may reduce mortality in the short term after hip fracture surgery in comparison to general anaesthesia and may be associated with a lower rate of deep venous thrombosis.'

Bibliography

Gillespie WJ. (2001). Extracts from 'Clinical evidence': hip fracture. *British Medical Journal*, **322**, 968–75.

Rodgers, Walker N, Schug S. *et al.* (2000) Reduction of postoperative mortality and morbidity with epidural or spinal anaesthesia: results from overview of randomised trials. *British Medical Journal*, **321**, 1493–7.

Wu CL, Fleisher LA. (2000). Outcomes research in regional anesthesia and analgesia. *Anesthesia and Analgesia*, **91**, 1232–42.

Long Case 5

'The one about the young, thyrotoxic woman listed for a thyroidectomy'

A 31-year-old woman presents for a thyroidectomy. Three years ago she presented with tachycardia, heat intolerance and exophthalmos. She was diagnosed as having Graves' disease that proved to be unresponsive to radioactive iodine. She was therefore treated with carbimazole.

O/E	HR 120 regular
	BP 138/84 mmHg
	HS normal
	Chest clear

Investigations	Hb	13 g/dl
	WCC	$15 \times 10^9/l$
	Plt	$170 \times 10^9/l$
	Urea and electrolytes normal	
	Albumin	37 g/l
	Calcium	2.23 mmol/L (corrected)
	TSH	0.17 mU/l (0.3 – 3.5 mU/l)
	Free T4	64 pmol/l (13 – 30 pmol/l)
	Thyroid scintogram – nodular thyroid	

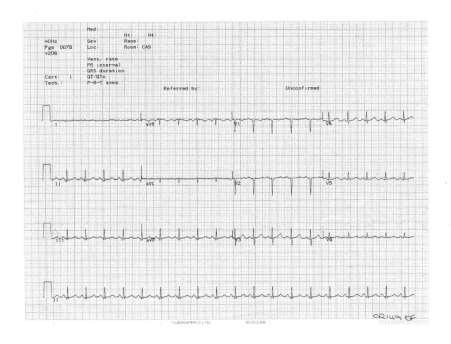

Questions

1. Tell me about the case.

This is a young woman presenting for elective thyroidectomy after failed medical treatment. There are two major issues that need addressing in the preoperative assessment.

She has been treated for Graves' disease but remains thyrotoxic. The operation must be postponed until she is euthyroid to minimise the risk of developing thyroid storm peri-operatively. In addition, there is no comment in the history regarding the presence of a goitre and there has been no imaging of the thyroid to assess the airway such as a CT scan, chest X-ray or lateral thoracic inlet views.

2. Do you want any other investigations?

She should have the airway imaged as above. A plain chest X-ray will show lateral tracheal deviation or compression. Lateral thoracic inlet views will show compression in the AP plane. A CT scan will show both of the above and give additional information concerning the exact level at which the compression is occurring and should be performed where >50% compression is seen on plain X-ray. It is especially useful with retrosternal extension of a goitre. Magnetic resonance imaging can give views in the saggital and coronal planes if required. A nasendoscopy should be performed routinely by the ENT surgeon pre-operatively. It will give information on the quality of laryngeal view likely to be obtained at direct laryngoscopy and whether there is any evidence of recurrent laryngeal nerve palsy. Unilateral palsy results in ipsilateral cord adduction. This is associated with glottic incompetence, hoarseness, poor cough and aspiration.

Respiratory function tests (flow-volume loops) are of debatable value.

3. What are the symptoms and signs of Graves' disease?

> Signs of thyrotoxicosis have been described in the short case on thyroidectomy.

The signs of particular importance to the anaesthetist are atrial fibrillation, cardiac failure and cardiac ischaemia.

Signs unique to Graves' disease include the eye signs, pre-tibial myxoedema and thyroid acropachy.

The eye signs of Graves' disease are due to specific antibodies causing retro-orbital inflammation. The extra ocular muscles are affected leading to a reduction in the range of movement. There may be exophthalmos, lid lag, lid retraction, conjunctival oedema and corneal scarring. These signs may be present even if the patient is euthyroid.

Pre-tibial myxoedema is a skin infiltration over the shins and thyroid acropachy consists of clubbing, swollen fingers and periosteal new bone formation.

4. *How do thyroid hormones exert their effects?*

The thyroid hormones T_3 and T_4 are transported in the blood mainly bound to plasma proteins. Their mechanism of action is thought to involve specific receptors bound to the plasma membrane, mitochondria and nucleus. The hormones enter the cell by a carrier mechanism, after which most of the T_4 is converted to T_3. Binding of T_3 to specific receptors results in alterations in DNA transcription and thus protein synthesis and energy metabolism.

5. *What do you think of the white cell count?*

The white cell count is high. The differential count would help to distinguish the many causes. It would be important to exclude acute infection, the source of which should be found and treated before surgery.

Causes of a neutrophil leukocytosis:

- Bacterial infection
- Inflammation/tissue necrosis
- Metabolic disorders
- Neoplasms
- Haemorrhage/haemolysis
- Myeloproliferative disorders
- Drugs, e.g. steroids

6. *How does carbimazole work? What are the side effects?*

Carbimazole is the pro-drug, the active compound is methimazole. It acts by inhibiting iodine incorporation and the coupling of iodotyrosines, it also has immunosuppressive properties. It may take up to 8 weeks to render the patient euthyroid, after which it is continued at a reduced dose for about 18 months. Side effects include rashes, pruritis, headache, nausea and arthralgia. The most serious side effect is agranulocytosis (1/1000 after 3 months).

7. *Would the surgeon be happy if the carbimazole had been continued up until the day of surgery?*

No. Carbimazole increases the vascularity of the gland making surgical conditions more difficult.

8. *Would you anaesthetise this lady today?*

No. She should be rendered euthyroid before surgery and the rest of her investigations need addressing. She should also have the raised white cell count investigated and any infection treated.

9. What could be done to improve her pre-operative state?

She could be changed to propylthiouracil for several weeks to see if she responds. In any case, she should be commenced on a beta-blocker to control the cardiovascular symptoms and signs. Corticosteroids inhibit the conversion of T4 to T3 and are sometimes used short term to prepare patients for surgery.

10. Which beta-blocker would you use and why?

Propranolol is the traditional beta-blocker used to control the symptoms of thyrotoxicosis. It controls the cardiovascular complications and also reduces the peripheral conversion of T_4 to T_3. A heart rate of less than 85 has been recommended. Atenolol or nadolol are other suitable beta-blockers.

11. She returns in 1 month well controlled. How would you anaesthetise her?

She should continue her beta-blocker on the day of surgery and an anxiolytic such as a benzodiazepine would also be reasonable.

The technique for securing the airway would be determined by the clinical findings and the results of the investigations of her airway. If a difficult intubation is expected, then either gas induction or awake fibre-optic intubation is appropriate (intubation is difficult in 6% of cases of thyroidectomy). If there is serious concern that the airway may be lost after induction, then awake fibre-optic intubation is the method of choice, though care should be taken as complete obstruction by the fibre-optic scope can occur if severe stenosis. If complete obstruction occurs after induction of anaesthesia and attempts to pass an endotracheal tube fail, ventilation via a rigid bronchoscope may be necessary. An awake surgical tracheostomy may be considered, but could be technically difficult.

> The general principles of anaesthesia for thyroidectomy have been described in the short question on thyroidectomy.

12. She is on the femodene OCP. Would you stop it?

When a patient who is taking a combined oral contraceptive stops it, there is a period of hypercoagulability before a return to baseline. It should ideally be stopped 4 weeks before surgery.

13. What else could you do to reduce the risk of thromboembolism?

The use of heparin and graduated compression stockings is recommended in the British National Formulary for women still taking the combined OCP and undergoing major elective surgery (and all surgery to the legs). In addition, pneumatic calf compressors should be used in theatre.

Bibliography

Bent G. (2008). Graves' disease. *New England Journal of Medicine*, **358**(24), 2594–605.

Farling PA. (2000). Thyroid disease. *British Journal of Anaesthesia*, **85**(1), 15–28.

Hagberg CA. (2000). *Handbook of Difficult Airway Management*. Edinburgh, UK: Churchill Livingstone.

Malholta S, Sodhi V. (2007). Anaesthesia for thyroid and parathyroid surgery. *BJA CEACCP*, **7**, 55 – 8.

Morgan GE, Mikhail MS. (1996). *Clinical Anaesthesiology*, 2nd edition. Appleton and Lange

Long Case 6

'The one about the RTA with a flail chest'

A 35-year-old male has sustained multiple injuries in an RTA. He was the driver of a car hit by a lorry and the fire brigade spent some time extracting him from the vehicle. You are called to A+E to assist with the resuscitation and assess him for theatre.

Examination	Complaining of pain in right hip and chest		
	GCS 15		
	Intravenous fluids running, oxygen 15l/m via facemask		
	CVS	Pulse	115/min
		BP	85/40 mmHg
	Resp	Rate	40/min
		Paradoxical chest movement on the right	
		Chest drains in situ	
	Positive DPL		
Investigations	C-spine X-ray normal		
	Hb	11.0 g/dl	
	PCV	0.31	
	WCC	$14.2 \times 10^9/l$	
	Sodium	138 mmol/l	
	Potassium	4.2 mmol/l	
	Urea	6.2 mmol/l	
	Creatinine	64 μmol/l	
	Glucose	11.4 mmol/l	
	Arterial gas on 15 l/min O_2	pH	7.20
		PO_2	9 kPa
		PCO_2	7 kPa
		BE	−11
		HCO_3^-	19 mmol/l

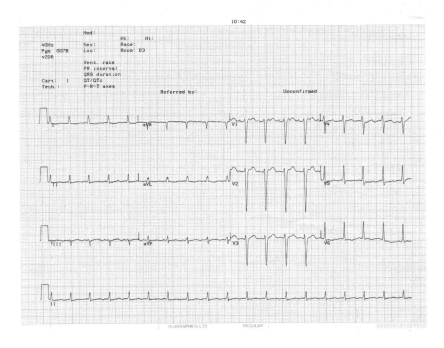

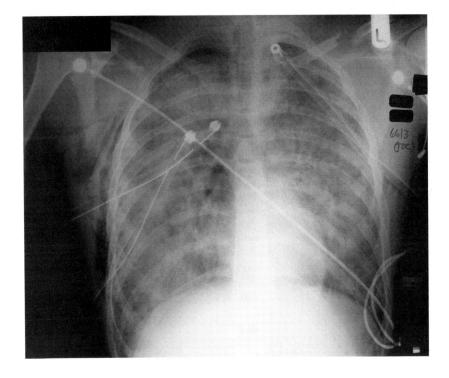

Questions

1. Can you summarise the case?

This is a 35-year-old man with severe multiple trauma who is still shocked and in need of further resuscitation. In particular, he has severe chest injuries with a flail segment, evidence of intra-abdominal haemorrhage, significant blood loss and a metabolic acidosis.

2. Tell me about the full blood count and arterial blood gases.

The full blood count shows anaemia with a low haematocrit suggesting there has been blood loss with (non-blood) fluid resuscitation. The white cell count is raised secondary to haemorrhage, acidosis and/or the stress response.

The arterial blood gases show a mixed respiratory and metabolic acidosis, in keeping with the clinical picture of a chest and lung injury along with untreated shock.

3. What are the causes of a metabolic acidosis?

The causes can be categorised according to the anion gap.

Anion gap = $(Na^+ + K^+) - (HCO_3^- + Cl^-)$

Normal anion gap is 10–18 mmol/l

Metabolic acidosis – normal anion gap

- GI bicarbonate loss
- Renal tubular acidosis
- Ingestion of chloride containing acids

Chloride tends to be retained as bicarbonate is lost

Metabolic acidosis – high anion gap

- Drugs*
- Lactic acidosis
- Ketoacidosis
- Uraemic acidosis

Bicarbonate is used to maintain normal pH

*The drugs responsible for a high anion gap include salicylates, paraldehyde, methanol and ethylene glycol.

Lactic acidosis is an important and common cause of acidosis. Normal blood lactate is 0.6–1.2 mmol/l and levels above 5 mmol/l cause significant acidosis. Concentrations greater than 9 mmol/l carry an 80% mortality rate.

Lactic acidosis can be subdivided into type A and type B:

Type A lactic acidosis is the more common form, resulting from poor tissue perfusion and anaerobic glycolysis, e.g. shock, severe hypoxia, post-epileptic convulsion or exercise. The liver becomes unable to metabolise the high amount of lactate. Treatment is aimed at restoring the peripheral perfusion and oxygen supply/demand ratio.

Type B lactic acidosis is not directly caused by poor tissue perfusion. It is normally drug-related (biguanides, ethanol, paracetamol), but can be due to rare metabolic defects. These patients present with hyperventilation, vomiting, abdominal pain, drowsiness and coma.

4. Where is lactate made?

Lactate is made in skeletal muscle and red blood cells. When oxygen supplies are limited, pyruvate is reduced by NADH to form lactate, the reaction being catalysed by lactate dehydrogenase. The importance of this reaction is twofold. It produces 2 ATP molecules and regenerates NAD^+ which sustains continued glycolysis in skeletal muscle and erythrocytes under anaerobic conditions. The limiting factor is the liver, which must oxidise lactate back to pyruvate for subsequent gluconeogenesis. This pathway merely 'buys time' during times of stress.

5. Why is acidosis undesirable?

Acidosis (respiratory or metabolic) is negatively inotropic and causes dilatation of systemic and cerebral arterioles. There will be a reduction in cardiac output and blood pressure.

Respiratory effects include hyperventilation (initially driven by the peripheral aortic and carotid chemoreceptors) and a right shift of the oxygen dissociation curve – Bohr effect). The latter will improve the unloading of oxygen to tissues but may impair uptake in the lungs.

Other effects include inhibition of glycolysis, hyperkalaemia, reduced consciousness and a leukocytosis.

6. Tell me about the ECG and chest X-ray.

The ECG shows a sinus tachycardia with a rate of about 110 beats per minute. There is minor ST depression in the lateral leads with T wave flattening. This may represent ischaemia related to cardiac trauma or secondary to severe hypotension.

The chest X-ray shows bilateral pneumothoraces with two chest drains on the right and one on the left. There are fractures of the third, fourth, fifth and sixth ribs on the right and there is bilateral surgical emphysema with mediastinal emphysema visible at the upper right heart border. There is also a fractured clavicle and scapula on the left. The lungs are severely contused. Although it is not possible to demonstrate ribs fractured in two places on the X-ray, there may be injury through the costochondral joints which would result clinically in a flail segment.

7. What is a flail segment?

This is due to severe chest trauma and occurs when a segment of the chest wall does not have bony continuity with the rest of the thoracic cage. The fractures at either end of the flail segment may be through rib or costal cartilage and therefore the diagnosis may be overlooked if chest X-rays are relied upon. The clinical signs are tachypnoea and asymmetrical chest wall movement with paradoxical excursion of the flail segment. Palpation may aid the diagnosis, feeling for abnormal movement and crepitus of rib or cartilage fractures.

Hypoxia results from a number of factors. Normal chest wall movement is disrupted, pain may limit tidal ventilation and there may be extensive underlying lung damage.

8. Why is he tachypnoeic?

He has a raised PCO_2, which is a potent respiratory stimulant.

Tachypnoea is also a response to shock as the body attempts to increase oxygen delivery to the tissues.

He has sustained a major chest injury with rib fractures, a flail chest and probable underlying lung injury. His lung mechanics will be altered, ventilation ineffective and gas exchange reduced leading to hypoxia. These will cause an increase in respiratory rate to try and compensate. In addition to this, pain will limit his chest wall movement forcing him to take rapid, shallow breaths.

9. How would you manage his fluid resuscitation?

This man is still shocked, most likely haemorrhagic in nature given the extent and detail of his injuries. He is tachycardic and hypotensive indicating that he has lost 30–40% of his blood volume (1.5–2 l).

ATLS classification of haemorrhagic shock

■ Class I	up to 15% loss	Few clinical signs, replace primary fluid loss
■ Class II	15–30% loss	Tachycardia, tachypnoea, decreased pulse pressure, BP low OR normal Use crystalloid initially.
■ Class III	30–40% loss	As above plus low BP, anxious/confused Crystalloid + blood
■ Class IV	>40% loss	Life-threatening, rapid transfusion and surgical intervention

Reproduced with permission from the American College of Surgeons.

He needs swift assessment and management of Airway (with C-spine control), Breathing and Circulation, some of which has already been initiated.

Two large bore (at least 16-gauge) cannulae should initially be inserted with rapid infusion of 1–2 litres of crystalloid or colloid. Obvious bleeding from any external wounds should be controlled by direct pressure. Further management will depend on the response to fluid administration.

This man requires:

- Blood cross-matched (type-specific if necessary)
- Central line
- Arterial line
- Urinary catheter
- Active warming and warmed fluids
- Cardiothoracic assessment
- General surgical assessment – he has a positive DPL
- Regular blood and blood gas analysis

Types of shock

- Haemorrhagic
- Cardiogenic   Myocardial damage, cardiac tamponade, tension pneumothorax
- Neurogenic   Often no tachycardia and normal pulse pressure
- Septic   Uncommon immediately after injury

---

10. Is he ready for theatre?

No.

He is still hypotensive and requires on-going resuscitation with repeated reassessment to address this. If, however, his condition were to deteriorate, he may need a thoracotomy or early laparotomy as part of the resuscitation process.

Bibliography

American College of Surgeons. (2004). *Advanced Trauma Life Support Course for Physicians*. 7th edition.

Stryer L. (1988). *Biochemistry*. 3rd edition. Freeman.

Weatherall DJ, Ledingham JGG, Warrell DA. (1996). Oxford Textbook of Medicine. 3rd edition. Oxford Medical Publications.

Long Case 7

'The one about the chesty, obese man having a laparotomy'

A 60-year-old retired miner presents on your list for resection of a sigmoid carcinoma. He has long-standing COAD with shortness of breath after walking 50 metres on the flat. He has had previous general anaesthetics with no problems.

Medication	Salbutamol nebuliser		
	Salmeterol nebuliser		
	Pulmicort inhaler		
	Prednisolone – reducing regimen, currently on 2.5 mg qds		
Examination	Obese		
	Unable to lie flat		
	CVS	Pulse	120 bpm
		BP	150/90 mmHg
	HS	muffled	
	Resp	Central trachea	
		Hyperinflated chest	
		Widespread wheeze	
		Basal crepitations	
Investigations	PFTs	FEV_1	0.88
		FEV_1/FVC	36% predicted
		PEFR	128 (predicted 439)
	ABGs on air	pH	7.32
		pO_2	7.7 kPa
		pCO_2	6.8 kPa
		SBC	28
		BE	−1.2
		SaO_2	91% (air)

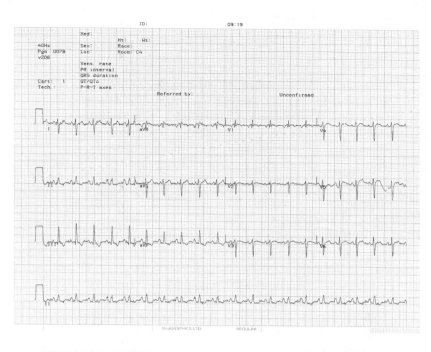

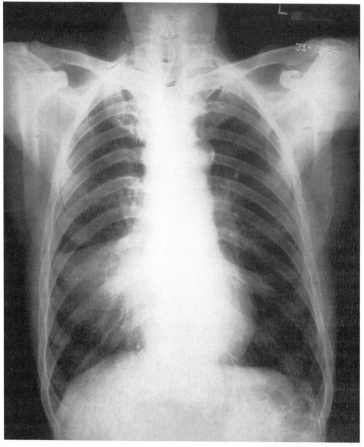

Questions

1. Can you summarise the main points in this case?

This is an elderly man with significant lung disease presenting for scheduled cancer surgery. His long-standing lung disease has resulted in concurrent cardiac changes and is compounded by a possible infective lobar consolidation. He is presenting for major abdominal cancer surgery and is at high risk of developing post-operative respiratory failure.

2. How would you differentiate between cardiac and respiratory causes of breathlessness?

A history of smoking or occupational risk factors with progressive breathlessness, cough and sputum production would suggest a respiratory cause, while recurrent acute chest pain, palpitations, orthopnoea and paroxysmal nocturnal dyspnoea might suggest a cardiac cause.

Examination may reveal clubbing, wheeze and hyper-resonance (respiratory) or cardiomegaly, murmurs and a third heart sound (cardiac). Raised jugular venous pressure and other signs of right heart failure may occur with both aetiologies.

Signs of right heart failure

- Raised JVP
- Tender smooth hepatic enlargement
- Dependent pitting oedema
- Free abdominal fluid
- Pleural transudates

Investigations may give further clues and should include ECG, chest X-ray, pulmonary function tests and echocardiography. If the diagnosis remains unclear, some form of cardiovascular stress testing may be indicated.

3. Can you comment on the ECG and chest X-ray?

The ECG shows a sinus tachycardia of 120 beats per minute and features consistent with right atrial and ventricular hypertrophy. (Right atrial hypertrophy results in tall, peaked P waves in II, III and aVF. Right ventricular hypertrophy results in right axis deviation, a dominant R wave with T wave inversion in V1 and a persisting S wave in V6.)

The chest X-ray shows large volume lungs consistent with long-standing chronic obstructive airways disease. In addition, there is right middle lobe consolidation suggested by airspace shadowing in the region of the right middle lobe with loss of the right heart border and sharp demarcation of the horizontal fissure.

> **X-ray features of right middle lobe collapse**
> ▪ Shadowing/opacity in right middle zone
> ▪ Loss of the right heart border
> ▪ Horizontal fissure displaced downwards
> ▪ Diaphragm still seen behind heart

4. Tell me about the PFTs and ABGs.

The FEV_1 is severely reduced and the FEV_1/FVC ratio suggests an obstructive picture. There is no information about his effort during the pulmonary function tests. An FEV_1 of less than 1 litre is likely to result in post-operative respiratory difficulties such as sputum retention particularly as he will be having a laparotomy incision. His chest may be partially improved with treatment of the pneumonia.

The blood gas shows hypoxaemia with a mixed metabolic and respiratory acidosis. The bicarbonate is high-normal but may be higher than that when he is 'well'.

5. Are there any problems with steroids?

Yes.
There are known side effects from long-term steroid administration including:

▪ Osteoporosis
▪ Hypertension
▪ Peptic ulcer disease
▪ Pancreatitis
▪ Growth retardation
▪ Central obesity
▪ Cataracts
▪ Easy bruising
▪ Thin skin
▪ Psychiatric effects (especially mania).

Particular side effects of interest around the time of surgery and anaesthesia are immunosuppression, diminished wound healing, interaction with non-depolarising muscle relaxants (resistance to pancuronium), altered glucose tolerance, fluid retention and myopathy.

The other consideration with steroids is the peri-operative regimen to use. A review article in *Anaesthesia* in November 1998 gave suggested treatment regimens:

> **Peri-operative steroid regimes:**
>
> **Patient currently on steroids**
> ▪ <10 mg/day   no additional cover
> ▪ >10 mg/day + minor surgery   25 mg hydrocortisone on induction

▪ >10 mg/day + moderate surgery	above plus 100 mg/day for 24 hours
▪ >10 mg/day + major surgery	above plus 100 mg/day for 72 hours
Patient stopped taking steroids	
▪ <3 months	Treat as if on steroids
▪ >3 months	No peri-operative steroids required

6. Will you anaesthetise this patient on your list today?

No. His lung function should be improved as much as possible prior to surgery. He has right middle lobe consolidation, which needs treatment and further investigation to exclude a primary bronchial neoplasm or metastatic deposit. He also requires further basic investigations including a full blood count, urea and electrolytes.

7. How might you improve his condition prior to surgery?

He needs oxygen and regular physiotherapy with sputum sent for culture and antibiotic sensitivities. He should then be treated with appropriate antibiotics for a community acquired pneumonia (determined by the hospital policy). He may require a flexible bronchoscopy by a respiratory physician.

A CT scan of his chest would help to exclude pulmonary metastases or a second primary.

8. All the above is done, no underlying lung tumour is found and his right middle lobe consolidation is treated. How would you anaesthetise him?

Oxygen and nebulizers should be prescribed pre-operatively with careful consideration given to the potential side effects of an anxiolytic pre-med. An intensive care bed should be booked for the post-operative period. Blood must be cross-matched and available in theatre.

With standard monitoring instituted in the anaesthetic room, an arterial line and epidural catheter should be sited prior to anaesthesia. The epidural may be commenced to ensure the block is both working and adequate for the proposed surgery.

The patient is pre-oxygenated and anaesthesia induced with propofol, alfentanil and vecuronium. An endotracheal tube is inserted and anaesthesia maintained with isoflurane, oxygen and air. A central line and urinary catheter are inserted.

In theatre, important considerations are oxygenation (ventilator settings, FiO_2, regular blood gas analysis), fluid status (CVP, urine output, pulse, blood pressure, blood loss), temperature control (warm fluids, HME, warm air blower) and maintenance of anaesthesia and analgesia.

9. At what level would you place an epidural?

This needs some discussion with the surgeon to establish what incision they intend to make. The epidural catheter should be sited near the dermatomal level of the midpoint of the incision, often lower thoracic. The choice may be limited by technical difficulties of siting a thoracic epidural.

10. What would your post-operative care focus on?

This patient is at high risk of developing post-operative respiratory failure and therefore needs close monitoring on high dependency or intensive care. The most important aspect of post-operative care is ensuring adequate gas exchange. Attention should be paid to:

- Humidified oxygen
- Analgesia without respiratory depression, optimally provided by an epidural. This should allow good tidal volumes and coughing to help prevent sputum retention and maintain gas exchange.
- Physiotherapy
- Bronchodilators
- Antibiotics.

Other important elements include thromboprophylaxis, careful fluid balance and an assessment of nutritional status with total parenteral nutrition if required.

Bibliography
Kumar P, Clark M. (2000). *Clinical Medicine*, 5th edition. W B Saunders.

Nicholson G, Burrin JM, Hall GM. (1998). Perioperative steroid supplementation. *Anaesthesia* **53**, 1091–4.

Long Case 8

'The one about the old lady with a fractured humerus'

An 81-year-old lady is admitted to A&E with a supracondylar fracture of her right humerus. The orthopaedic surgeons have put her on the emergency list for an open reduction and internal fixation.

Past medical history	Hypertension for 10 years. Mastectomy 8 years ago for carcinoma of the breast. Diagnosed as hypothyroid 6 months ago. For the past 3 weeks she has complained of severe back pain radiating to the right side of the chest and is due to be seen by a pain specialist.		
Medication	Atenolol 50 mg/day Thyroxine 100 mcg/day		
On examination	She is conscious but breathless and pale. Temperature 36.6 °C		
	CVS:	Pulse 85/min, regular BP 110/70 mmHg Apex not easily palpated HS quiet Mild ankle oedema	
	Chest:	reduced air entry on the left side	
Investigations	Hb	9.9 g/dl	Sodium	137 mmol/L
	MCV	90 fl	Potassium	3.9 mmol/L
	WCC	7.3×10^9U/l	Urea	10.7 mmol/L
	Platelets	208×10^9U/l	Creatinine	57 μmol/L
			Glucose	8.0 mmol/L

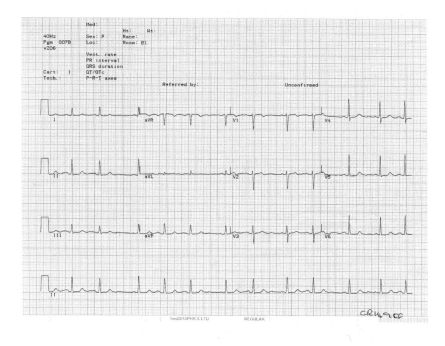

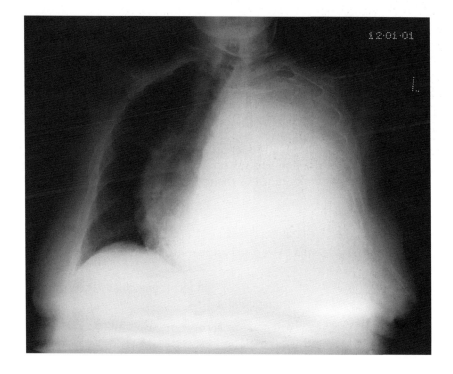

Questions

1. Can you summarise this case?

This is an elderly lady with a huge left-sided pleural effusion, possibly secondary to a recurrent breast carcinoma. She is also anaemic and hypertensive. She has presented with a supracondylar fracture, which may require urgent reduction and fixation if there is associated neurovascular injury.

2. What are the main problems this lady presents?

The main concern with this lady is her respiratory disease and the aetiology of her pleural effusion. She is breathless with reduced air entry on the left side and the chest X-ray shows a massive left pleural effusion with mediastinal shift.

She has a normocytic anaemia, which may be due to an underlying malignancy (pleural effusion, possible pathological fracture and previous mastectomy), hypothyroidism or may be from acute blood loss following the fracture.

The other concern with this lady is her cardiovascular status. She is a known hypertensive on anti-hypertensive therapy.

Supracondylar fractures are associated with neurovascular problems. The brachial artery together with the median and ulnar nerves are at risk of injury and this may warrant urgent exploration. The need for urgent surgery may not give sufficient time for further investigations of her concurrent medical problems.

3. What are the causes of anaemia and how can you differentiate between them?

Anaemia occurs when there is a reduction in haemoglobin in the blood below the reference level for the age and sex of the individual. The aetiology may be classified either by the appearance of the red cells or by the underlying disease process.

Classification of anaemia by red cell appearance

1. **Hypochromic) microcytic (low MCH, MCHC, MCV)**
   Classically iron deficiency
   ?occult GI or gynaecological loss
   Thalassaemia

2. **Normochromic normocytic (normal MCV)**
   Anaemia of chronic disease
   Acute blood loss
   Hypothyroidism
   Bone marrow failure
   Haemolysis

3. **Macrocytic** (high MCV)	Megaloblastic	B_{12}, folate deficiency (MCV >110 fl)
	Non-megaloblastic	pregnancy, alcohol, drugs (MCV 100–110 fl)
	(a megaloblast is a cell in which cytoplasmic and nuclear maturation are out of phase)	

Classification of anaemia by disease process

1. **Deficiency**	Iron Folic acid B_{12}	
2. **Haemolysis**	Intrinsic	sickle cell, thalassaemia, G6PD, hereditary sphereocytosis
	Extrinsic	immune, e.g. SLE, lymphomas non-immune, e.g. DIC, drugs, infection
3. **Marrow failure**	Aplasia Suppression, e.g. malignancy, drugs, infection Dyserythropoesis, e.g. myelodysplastic syndrome	

General symptoms of anaemia include tiredness, fatigue and dyspnoea but in this age group it can manifest as angina, heart failure and confusion.

The various forms of anaemia can be distinguished by history, examination (glossitis, angular stomatitis, koilonychia, lymph nodes, splenomegaly, hepatomegaly) and investigations.

Look at the degree of anaemia on the FBC, together with the MCV, MCH and MCHC. The FBC will also show the white cell and platelet counts which, if normal, suggest the anaemia is not due to leukaemia or marrow failure. Haemolysis and haemorrhage will produce a reticulocytosis (check haptoglobins, bilirubin, urobilinogen). Examination of the peripheral blood film may give further information. Other investigations may include serum folate, B_{12}, iron, ferritin, or haemoglobin electrophoresis but will be dictated by the clinical findings.

4. Would you request any further investigations?

The extent of investigation into this lady's medical problems will, in the acute setting, be dictated by the degree of urgency of surgery.

Although the ECG is normal (sinus arrhythmia), there is little evidence available to estimate her exercise tolerance or response to cardiovascular stress. Ideally, these should be tackled before anaesthesia. Any symptoms of ischaemic heart disease such as chest pain, shortness of breath, reduced exercise tolerance and palpitations should be specifically asked for. After the effusion is drained, a repeat chest X-ray would be needed to assess her heart size. If her heart was enlarged, then echocardiography would give some indication of the (resting) left ventricular ejection fraction.

Ideally, her thyroid function tests should be checked and thyroxine dose adjusted if necessary (although the results are unlikely to be available prior to surgery).

Of major concern is the cause of the pleural effusion and a CT scan may help identify whether she does indeed have metastatic disease in her chest.

5. Would you want to drain the pleural effusion before surgery/anaesthesia?

Yes. This is a large pleural effusion causing mediastinal shift and clinical symptoms. Draining the effusion will improve her respiratory function in the short term and may give a further clue to the underlying diagnosis. A chest drain should be inserted and connected to an underwater seal. The drain should be intermittently clamped after each litre has drained to prevent re-expansion pulmonary oedema. Pleural effusions may be divided into transudates or exudates according to the protein and lactate dehydrogenase content of the fluid.

Causes of transudates
(protein <30 g/l and LDH <200 i.u./l)

- Heart failure
- Hypoproteinaemia
- Hypothyroidism
- Constrictive pericarditis
- Meig's syndrome.

Causes of exudates
(protein >30 g/l and LDH >200 i.u./l)

- Pneumonia
- Bronchial carcinoma
- Pulmonary infarction
- TB
- Others, e.g. SLE.

---

6. How would you anaesthetise this lady?

Brachial plexus block using the interscalene approach would be a reasonable technique in this lady.

The **advantages** of this technique are that it avoids the need for general anaesthesia and ventilation, provides excellent intra- and post-operative analgesia (a catheter can be used), avoids excessive movement of the painful arm (compared with the axillary approach) and should have minimal impact on her cardiovascular system.

The **disadvantages** of this technique are the potential complications, i.e. vertebral artery puncture, pneumothorax, phrenic nerve palsy, subarachnoid puncture, recurrent laryngeal nerve palsy and Horner's syndrome. Not all anaesthetists perform this block regularly and therefore they may choose a different technique.

7. How would you perform the block?

Informed consent should be obtained. Full monitoring should be established and an intravenous cannula sited.

The patient is positioned supine with the head turned slightly away from the side to be blocked. Gown and gloves are worn and the skin is cleaned. The interscalene groove is located at the midpoint of the posterior border of sternomastoid, at the level of the cricoid cartilage. The patient may be asked to sniff to make the scalene muscles more prominent.

The skin is anaesthetised at this point and the block needle inserted, aiming slightly dorsal. An ultrasound machine is used to locate the appropriate site. A 'pop' may be felt as the fascial sheath is entered (1–2.5 cm). The syringe is aspirated and the local anaesthetic solution injected slowly with regular aspiration.

Bibliography
Kumar P, Clark M. (2002). *Clinical Medicine*, 5th edition. W B Saunders.
Pinnock CA, Fischer HBJ, Jones RP. (1996). Peripheral nerve blockade. Churchill Livingstone.

Long Case 9

'The one about the obese woman with a fractured neck of femur'

A 76-year-old woman (height 148 cm, weight 87 kg) is awaiting a left hip hemiarthroplasty following a fractured neck of femur. She has osteoarthritis and a history of chronic obstructive airways disease having smoked most of her life.

She also gives a history of recent onset of chest pain, relieved by GTN spray.

She is complaining of pain in her hip.

Medications	Ibuprofen 1600 mg/day Moduretic GTN spray			
O/E	Temp	38 °C		
	Pulse	90 bpm, regular		
	BP	160/95 mmHg		
	Apex impalpable			
	Quiet heart sounds			
	RR	20 bpm		
	Bilateral basal crepitations			
Investigations	Hb	8.4 g/dl	Sodium	132 mmol/l
	Plt	190 × 10⁹/l	Potassium	5.1 mmol/l
	WCC	5.8 × 10⁹/l	Urea	12 mmol/l
	MCV	105 fl	Creatinine	137 μmol/l
			Calcium	2.1 mmol/l (corrected)

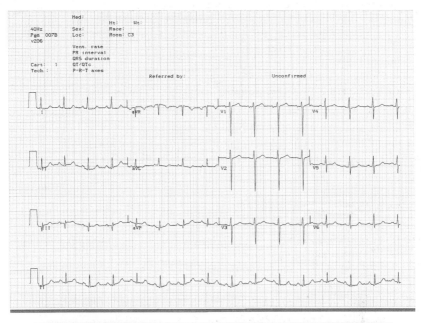

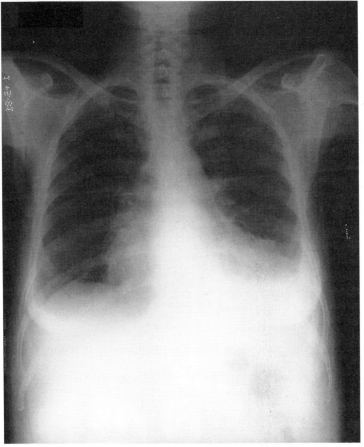

Questions

1. Can you summarise the case?

This is a 76-year-old morbidly obese lady with severe intercurrent medical problems who requires urgent surgery for a fractured neck of femur.
The medical problems include:

- Ischaemic heart disease with currrent undiagnosed chest pain
- Possible cardiac failure
- Hypertension
- Renal impairment
- Chronic obstructive airways disease
- Macrocytic anaemia.

These are the issues that need addressing during the pre-operative assessment.

2. Would you like to comment on the chest X-ray and the ECG?

The ECG shows sinus rhythm with Q waves in the inferior leads, suggestive of an old inferior myocardial infarction.
The chest X-ray is a PA film. The heart is enlarged and there are bilateral pleural effusions. The features are those of congestive cardiac failure.

3. What do you think about her weight? Can you classify obesity?

She is morbidly obese with a body mass index of nearly 40.
A commonly used measure of obesity is the body mass index. This is defined as the weight (in kilograms) divided by the height (in metres) squared.
Morbidly obese is defined as a BMI > 35.
The Broca index provides another measure of the degree of obesity.

See short case on obesity.

4. Tell me about her anaemia. What are the causes of a raised MCV?

She has a macrocytic anaemia, the more common causes of which would be vitamin B12 or folate deficiency, alcohol excess or liver disease.

> **Causes of raised MCV**
>
> ■ Megaloblastic B_{12} deficiency (commonly pernicious anaemia)
>   Folate deficiency (commonly nutritional)
> ■ Non-megaloblastic   Alcohol
>   Liver disease
>   Hypothyroidism
>   Reticulocytosis
>   Aplastic anaemia.

5. Would you transfuse this lady pre-operatively?

Her haemoglobin is 8.5 g/dl and, although there is evidence that a haemoglobin of above 8 g/dl is acceptable, this is urgent surgery with a high likelihood of significant blood loss in a lady with known ischaemic heart disease. It would therefore be reasonable to transfuse her pre-operatively being careful to avoid precipitating pulmonary oedema.

Hard evidence around the appropriate 'trigger' haemoglobin level for transfusion is lacking and haemoglobin-based transfusion triggers do not take in to account the ability of individual patients to compensate for anaemia. The **ASA Task Force on Blood Component Therapy** issued some recommendations in 1996. They suggested that transfusion is rarely indicated when the haemoglobin is >10 g/dl but almost always indicated when <6 g/dl. Patients in the grey area (haemoglobin concentrations between 6 and 10 g/dl) should have their transfusion need assessed on an individual basis, weighing up the risks of transfusion against inadequate oxygenation. There is general agreement now that an assessment of global and regional oxygen requirements should inform the need for transfusion with numerical triggers used where there is insufficient information regarding oxygenation.

A **paper published in *JAMA* in 1998** studied 8787 consecutive patients over the age of 60 years with hip fractures. Peri-operative transfusion in patients with haemoglobin levels of 8 g/dl or higher did not appear to influence the risk of 30- or 90-day mortality in this elderly population. At haemoglobin concentrations of less than 8 g/dl, 90.5% of patients received a transfusion, preventing meaningful interpretation of this data.

6. What do you think might be the cause of her abnormal urea and electrolytes?

There is renal impairment with a disproportionately raised urea compared to creatinine suggesting a pre-renal cause. Likely causes include dehydration or hypovolaemia secondary to haemorrhage. This could have been exacerbated by the use of non-steroidal anti-inflammatory drugs (inhibition of renal prostaglandin synthesis resulting in sodium retention and reduced renal blood flow).

The sodium may be low secondary to her diuretic therapy or could be due to cardiac or renal failure.

> **Common causes of hyponatraemia:**
>
> ▪ Excess water   Renal impairment
>   Cardiac failure
>   Liver failure – hypoalbuminaemia
>   Inappropriate ADH
> ▪ Sodium depletion Intrinsic renal disease
>   Mineralocorticoid deficiency
>   Diuretics

7. Do you think her recent chest pain is significant?

Although the chest pain could be related to the ingestion of regular NSAIDs, the possibility of a cardiac origin cannot be excluded in view of her past history of myocardial infarction. The fact that the pain is relieved by GTN is not pathognomonic of a cardiac origin as oesophageal pain is also sometimes relieved by GTN.

A careful history must be elicited and may give further clues to the origin of the pain. Investigations such as exercise stress testing to differentiate between the aetiologies is clearly not an option in this case.

8. Are there any other investigations you would like?

An echocardiogram will give some information about resting left ventricular function and the risk of post-operative cardiac events. A low ejection fraction (<35%) combined with a cardiac history and an abnormal resting ECG is predictive of post-operative cardiac mortality and would help determine the need for peri-operative intensive care. A normal resting echocardiogram, however, gives no information about cardiac reserve.

Although this lady has bilateral pleural effusions which could explain her tachypnoea, she also has a history of chronic obstructive airways disease. Pulmonary function tests will give an indication of the severity of her underlying lung disease as well as the degree of reversibility with bronchodilators.

In view of the raised MCV and hyponatraemia, it would be worth checking her liver function tests and coagulation profile, particularly if a regional block is being considered. She may have liver disease.

Morbid obesity is associated with a higher than normal incidence of difficult airway, which will need a full assessment and possibly further investigations.

9. How would you anaesthetise this lady?

This lady is a high-risk patient. She would benefit from pre-optimisation with invasive monitoring, fluids (including blood) and possibly inotropes before theatre. However, there is also evidence to support the use of regional techniques at least in terms of short-term mortality and peri-operative events such as blood loss and DVT . . .

Choose your technique and back it up.

Two of the authors were examined on this long case. One gave a spinal anaesthetic and the other a general anaesthetic after pre-operative optimisation with invasive monitoring. Both passed.

Bibliography

Carson JL et al. (1998). Perioperative blood transfusion and postoperative mortality. *Journal of the American Medical Association*, **279**, 199–205.

Chen AY, Carson JL. (1998). Perioperative management of anaemia. *British Journal of Anaesthesia*, **81**, Suppl. 1, 20–4.

Kumar P, Clark M. (2002). *Clinical Medicine*, 5th edition. W B Saunders.

Louridas G, Clinton CW, Olver P. (1992). *et al.* The value of the ejection fraction as a predictor of postoperative cardiac mortality in patients undergoing peripheral vascular surgery, *SA Journal of Surgery*, **30**, 12–14.

Madjdpour C, Spahn DR. (2005). Allogeneic red blood cell transfusions: efficacy, risks, alternatives and indications *British Journal of Anaesthesia*, **95**, 33–42.

Long Case 10

'The one about the asthmatic child with torsion'

A 7-year-old boy presents with severe testicular pain (6-hour history) requiring urgent surgical intervention. He has been nil-by-mouth for 5 hours but has vomited in the last hour.

He has asthma with several previous hospital admissions for this. For the past 10 days he has had a cough.

Medication	Becloforte and salbutamol inhalers	
Examination	Weight 30 kg	
	Pale, in pain and frightened	
	Pulse	145/min
	BP	105/60 mmHg
	Resp	widespread expiratory wheeze
Investigations	Hb	12.4 g/dl
	WCC	15.7×10^9/l
	PCV	0.38 l/l
	Sodium	137 mmol/l
	Potassium	4.1 mmol/l
	Urea	5.9 mmol/l
	Creatinine	54 μmol/l

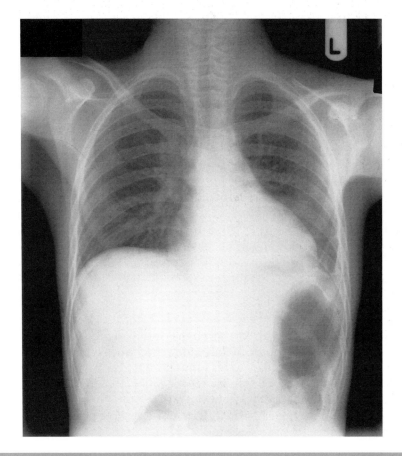

Questions

1. Can you summarise the case?

This case is a 7-year-old asthmatic boy presenting for urgent surgery. The important anaesthetic considerations are that this is an urgent paediatric case in which the child has symptomatic asthma, possible left lower lobe collapse/consolidation and requires a rapid sequence induction.

2. What is the differential diagnosis of testicular pain in this age group?

■ Testicular torsion	This results from rotation of the testis with interference of the blood supply and is usually associated with some abnormality. Venous compression from the torsion leads to congestion and eventual venous infarction unless corrected.

■ Acute epididymo-orchitis
■ Testicular trauma
■ Strangulated inguinal hernia
■ Idiopathic scrotal oedema

It is often impossible to differentiate between the first two diagnoses.

3. How urgent is surgery?

Surgery is urgent if testicular torsion is diagnosed or suspected. The torsion is corrected and the testicle fixed with anchoring sutures at the upper and lower poles. The other testicle is always explored and fixed in a similar fashion as this can occur bilaterally.

4. How would you assess the severity of asthma?

The history will elicit the duration of asthma symptoms, precipitating factors, frequency of attacks, increasing need for treatment and hospital admissions. The child's normal peak flow rate should be asked for.

On examination the respiratory rate, ability to speak, pulse rate and peak flow rate should be noted. The chest X-ray may reveal some pathology as in this case.

> See short case on asthma.

This child has significant asthma given the history of previous hospital admissions and a recent cough. He has widespread wheeze, a raised white cell count (which may be secondary to his surgical condition or from a chest infection) and left lower lobe collapse/consolidation on his chest X-ray. His respiratory rate, peak expiratory flow rate and response to bronchodilators need to be measured. He may benefit from pre-operative physiotherapy if time permits.

5. Take me through the chest X-ray.

The chest X-ray shows blunting of the left costophrenic angle and loss of the left hemi-diaphragm behind the heart. Although there is not a classic 'sail sign' behind the heart, the features are consistent with collapse of the left lower lobe.

> **X-ray features of left lower lobe collapse**
>
> ■ Triangular opacity behind the heart (sail sign)
> ■ Loss of medial part of hemidiaphragm

6. What are the other important issues in the pre-operative preparation of this child?

The important pre-operative considerations in addition to assessment of respiratory function are:

▦ The pre-operative visit which should focus on the parental anxieties as well as those of the patient.

▦ This boy has been vomiting and therefore fluid and electrolyte status is important. An intravenous cannula should be in situ with appropriate fluid therapy commenced.

▦ The patient's airway needs careful assessment as anaesthesia will involve a rapid sequence induction.

▦ In addition to this, pre-operative questions such as previous anaesthesia, allergies and loose dentition should be asked.

▦ The patient and parents should be informed of the proposed method of induction and post-operative analgesic regimen.

▦ Pre-medication may include bronchodilators and topical local anaesthetic cream if required.

7. How do you assess and treat dehydration in children?

Distribution of water as a percentage of body weight

	Premature	Neonate	Infant	Adult
ECF	50	35	30	20
ICF	30	40	40	40
Plasma	5	5	5	5
Total	85	80	75	65

Dehydration is commonly defined as mild ($<$5%), moderate (5%–10%) or severe ($>$10%) and assessed clinically by decreased urine output, dry mouth, decreased skin turgor, sunken fontanelle (in babies), sunken eyes, tachypnoea, tachycardia, drowsiness and irritability.

Dehydration is treated by calculating the fluid deficit from reduced intake and insensible losses (vomiting, respiratory losses, sweating) and replacing the fluid and electrolytes needed. The hourly maintenance requirements should be calculated and added into the equation.

8. How would you anaesthetise this child?

In the anaesthetic room, ECG, blood pressure and pulse oximetry monitoring should be established. An intravenous cannula should be in situ. All drugs doses must be calculated for a 30 kg boy and drawn up. The child's blood volume should be estimated (approximately $75 \times 30 = 2250$ ml for this boy) so that if blood loss is greater than 10% (225 ml), it can be replaced with blood. Appropriately sized endotracheal tubes must be available.

Following pre-oxygenation for 3 minutes, a rapid sequence induction is performed with thiopentone 150 mg and suxamethonium 60 mg. The trachea is intubated (6–6.5 mm ETT) and, when the position is confirmed and the tube secured, cricoid pressure is removed. Anaesthesia is maintained with a volatile agent in oxygen and nitrous oxide or air. A non-depolarising neuromuscular blocking agent is added when the suxamethonium induced block is wearing off.

A caudal epidural block can then be performed with the patient in the left lateral position and paracetamol suppositories inserted. For the caudal block, 0.5–0.8 ml/kg of 0.25% bupivacaine would be suitable.

In theatre, anaesthesia is maintained as above. The boy should have core temperature measured with a nasal or rectal probe and should be actively warmed with a warm air blower. A suitable HME filter and warming blanket should also be used.

At the end of surgery, neuromuscular blockade is reversed and the patient extubated awake in the left lateral position.

Paediatric formulae:

Weight in kg	(Age + 4) x 2
Tracheal tube internal diameter (mm)	Age/4 + 4.5 (if >2 yrs)
Oral tracheal tube length (cm)	Age/2 + 12 (if >2 yrs)

Maintenance fluid requirements (4+2+1 regimen)

0–10 kg	4 ml/kg per hour
10–20 kg	40 ml + 2 ml/kg per hour for each kg over 10 kg
Over 20 kg	60 ml + 1 ml/kg per hour for each kg over 20 kg

---

9. What are the options for post-operative analgesia?

The options are opioids, local anaesthetic block, NSAIDs and paracetamol. Opioids may be given intra-operatively and continued post-operatively as an infusion or PCA if the child is old enough to manage it.

Morphine doses:

Child <6 months	i.v. loading dose	25–75 mcg/kg
	i.v. infusion dose	0–20 mcg/kg per hour
Child >6 months	i.v. loading dose	100 mcg/kg
	i.v. infusion dose	0–25 mcg/kg per hour

Diclofenac suppositories (1 mg/kg) are commonly used for post-operative analgesia but caution must be exercised in patients with asthma.

Paracetamol suppositories (initial dose of up to 40 mg/kg, then 15 mg/kg 6-hourly thereafter) are also used as co-analgesics with opioids.

Perhaps the best form of post-operative analgesia is from a local anaesthetic block, in this case a caudal epidural.

A caudal block is performed as an aseptic technique with gown, gloves and mask. The patient is positioned in a lateral position with the hips and knees flexed. The sacral hiatus is identified, flanked by the sacral cornua, and a needle is introduced through the skin and sacrococcygeal membrane. A 22-gauge needle or cannula-over-needle technique can be used. Once identified and after aspiration, the solution can be injected. It should inject with little resistance and there should be no subcutaneous swelling. The complication of dural puncture is more likely in children as the spinal cord ends at L3 but the dura ends at S3–4.

Long Case 11

'The one about the man for a total hip replacement with a history of previous DVT'

You are asked to anaesthetise a 62-year-old male for a right total hip replacement. He has been a smoker for 30 years and has ignored advice to stop. Consequently, he has a long history of respiratory and cardiac problems. He has had three admissions to hospital in the last year for chest pain and he becomes short of breath after walking 30 yards. He had a DVT 6 months ago, treated with warfarin for 3 months. He also has a small hiatus hernia diagnosed on CT scan.

Current medication	GTN tablets prn	
	Oxivent inhaler	
On examination	Weight	85 kg
	Height	5' 8"
	BP	140/80 mmHg
	HR	80 bpm
	HS	normal
	Auscultation of chest — widespread fine expiratory crepitations	
Investigations	Hb	15.0 g/dl
	WCC	$7.0 \times 10^9/l$
	Plt	$386 \times 10^9/l$
	Sodium	138 mmol/l
	Potassium	3.9 mmol/l
	Urea	5.2 mmol/l
	Creatinine	85 μmol/l
PFTs		

Spirometry

		Ref	Pre Meas	Pre % Ref
FVC	Liters	4.00	3.21	80
FEV1	Liters	3.15	(1.01)	(32)
FEV1/FVC	%	76	(32)	
FEF25-75%	L/sec	3.40	(0.37)	(11)
FEF50%	L/sec	4.29	(0.30)	(7)
PEF	L/sec	8.12	(3.29)	(40)
MVV	L/min			

Diffusion

		Ref	Pre Meas	Pre % Ref
DLCO	mmol/kPa.min	9.1	(2.2)	(24)
DL Adj	mmol/kPa.min	9.1	(2.2)	(24)
DLCO/VA	DLCO/L	1.75	(0.51)	(29)
DL/VA Adj	DLCO/L		0.51	
VA	Liters		4.27	

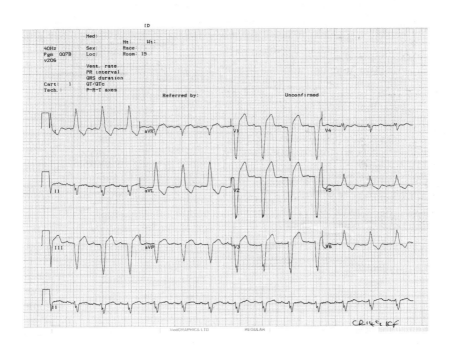

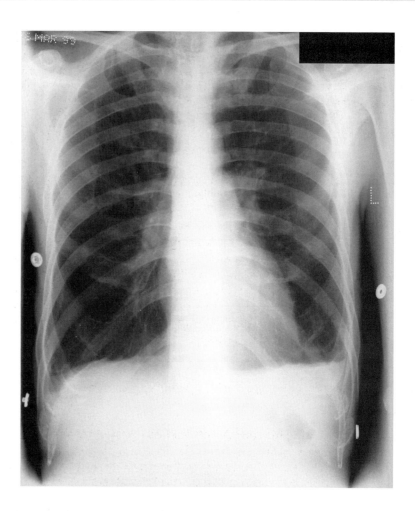

Questions

1. Present the history.

This 62-year-old smoker with severe COAD requires anaesthesia for a total hip replacement. He also has severe uncontrolled ischaemic heart disease and a history of DVT. This is an elective case, and because his symptoms are poorly controlled at present, he needs investigation and treatment of his cardiorespiratory problems before he is anaesthetised. He will also require attention to anti-thrombotic prophylaxis because the operation will put him at further risk of DVT and PE.

2. Discuss the significant findings.

The ECG shows left bundle branch block. This is likely to be due to severe ischaemic heart disease

> **Causes of left bundle branch block**
>
> ■ Severe ischaemic heart disease
> ■ Hypertension
> ■ Aortic stenosis
> ■ Acute myocardial infarction
> ■ Cardiomyopathy.

The chest X-ray shows hyperinflated lungs, flattened hemidiaphragms and generally coarse lung markings in keeping with long standing COAD. The heart is not enlarged.

The PFTs show an obstructive picture with a markedly reduced FEV_1, a reduced FVC and a ratio of 32% suggesting severe airways disease. The reduced FEF_{25-75} is also in keeping with small airways obstruction. The transfer factor is only 24% of normal. He therefore has a diffusion problem and, although the transfer factor corrected for lung volume is not much higher (as one would normally expect with emphysema), the clinical picture of many years of smoking combined with an obstructive picture on the other PFTs makes emphysema the likely diagnosis.

3. Is there anything else you would like to do before you anaesthetise him?

Further history regarding his episodes of chest pain would be very important in this case. If his pain was due to angina, he should be referred to a physician to improve his condition prior to elective surgery. He is not currently taking any anti-anginal medication apart from GTN tablets for symptomatic relief.

The presence of left bundle branch block on the ECG precludes further analysis. It is therefore impossible to say from the ECG whether or not he has suffered a previous myocardial infarct. An echocardiogram would show any wall motion abnormalities that might indicate previous myocardial infarction. It would also give an idea of his resting ejection fraction. If the ejection fraction is normal, however, this does not necessarily imply good cardiac reserve. An exercise ECG would not be possible in this patient, so a dobutamine stress test or a thallium scan with dipyridamole would be more useful for assessing the potential for increasing cardiac output.

Arterial blood gas analysis on air would be helpful to further delineate his respiratory function and as a baseline with which to compare post-operative results.

It would also be important to establish the circumstances surrounding his previous DVT. If it was totally out of the blue, he may require a thrombophilia screen (protein C, protein S, lupus anticoagulant, antithrombin III and test for factor V Leiden mutation).

4. *How do you distinguish cardiac from non-cardiac chest pain?*

This is distinguished on the basis of the **history, examination and investigations**. Features of the pain that should be ascertained in the history are:

- Site and radiation
- Character (e.g. burning, stabbing, etc.)
- Duration
- Severity
- Precipitating factors (e.g. exercise, emotion, movement or related to breathing or eating)
- Relieving factors (e.g. rest, antacids, GTN, etc.)
- Previous episodes
- Associated symptoms (e.g. sweating, palpitations, shortness of breath)

When attempting to diagnose the cause of a patient's chest pain, the history is likely to give the most clues. Further points that may be noted in the examination include:

- General features of vascular disease, e.g. hypertension, poor peripheral pulses, atrial fibrillation, etc.)
- Chest wall tenderness
- Pericardial or pleural rubs
- Pneumothorax

Investigations will be dictated by the preceding history and examination. Possibilities are (ranging from the simple to the more complex):

- ECG
- Chest X-ray
- Serial cardiac enzymes
- Troponin T
- Exercise ECG
- Gastroscopy
- V/Q scan
- Angiography

5. *Tell me about regional blockade and anticoagulants.*

The issue of central neuroaxial blocks and anticoagulation is one of risk versus benefit. Sometimes these risks and benefits are more quantifiable than others. Frequently, the case is clear-cut, but there is a grey area in between. However, some guidelines are applicable.

In this country, the use of low molecular weight heparins (LMWH) for thromboprophylaxis is now very common. These drugs have some advantages over standard heparin:

- Laboratory monitoring of the anticoagulant effect is unnecessary.
- No dosage adjustment is necessary.
- They can be administered subcutaneously once a day.

However, they also present some problems to the anaesthetist related to the timing of neuroaxial blocks. The half-life of LMWH is two to four times longer than standard heparin (and increases further with renal failure). This means that considerable anticoagulant effect may still exist in the 'troughs'. Relative overdosing of smaller patients could occur because the dose is not adjusted for the individual patient and the effect on Xa levels is not monitored.

The incidence of spinal haematomas has been greater in the US than in Europe. This may be a reflection of the fact that a twice-daily dosing regimen is used in the US (as opposed to once daily here) and therefore the troughs in plasma levels are not as deep.

Due to these factors, many studies have arrived at similar conclusions:

- Single daily dosing results in a true trough in anticoagulant level that permits the insertion of neuroaxial blocks and catheter removal.
- Risk of spinal haematoma is increased with concomitant anti-platelet or oral anticoagulant treatment.
- Needle placement should be delayed until 12 hours after LMWH.
- The risk of spinal haematoma in patients with an indwelling catheter is increased if they receive LMWH.
- Catheter removal should take place 12 hours after LMWH or 1–2 hours before the next dose.
- The neurological state of the patient must be monitored.

In this case, a regional technique would offer the advantages of improved outcome, reduced surgical blood loss, a decreased incidence of DVT and less interference with respiratory function. The patient is not anticoagulated at the present time and therefore a spinal or epidural is not contraindicated on this basis. The regional block must be appropriately timed between doses of prophylactic subcutaneous heparin in order to maintain adequate prophylactic cover whilst minimizing the risk of spinal/epidural haematoma.

> In the Final FRCA, questions about preoptimisation and the benefits of regional versus general anaesthesia have been asked in relation to this case. These topics are covered elsewhere in the long cases and are therefore not repeated here.

Bibliography

Horlocker TT, Wedel DJ. (1998). Spinal and epidural blockade and perioperative low molecular weight heparin: smooth sailing on the Titanic. *Anesthesia and Analgesia*. **86**, 1153–6.

Smetana G, Lawrence V, Cornell JE; American College of Physicians. (2006). Preoperative pulmonary risk stratification for noncardiothoracic surgery: systematic review for the American College of Physicians. *Annals of Internal Medicine* **144**(8), 581–95.

Long Case 12

'The one about the diabetic man for TURP'

A 70-year-old man presents for a TURP. He has a past history of a shadow on his lung treated with drugs and irradiation. He is an ex-smoker (smoked for 20 years), gets breathless on exertion and takes glibenclamide for NIDDM.

On examination	Heart rate	90 bpm
	BP	180/90 mmHg
	Chest clear	
	Bladder distended	
Investigations	Sodium	141 mmol/l
	Potassium	4.2 mmol/l
	Urea	10 mmol/l
	Creatinine	190 μmol/l
	Blood sugar (random)	10 mmol/l
	Hb	158 g/l
	WCC	8.3×10^9/l
	Platelets	240×10^9/l
	Calcium	normal
	LFTs	normal
PFTs	FEV_1	1.5 l (predicted = 3.0 l)
	FVC	2.8 l (predicted = 3.9 l)
	FEV_1/FVC	54%
	DL_{CO}	76% predicted
	K_{CO}	79% predicted

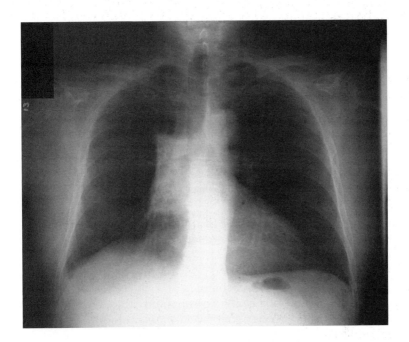

Questions

1. Summarise this patient's problems.

This elderly diabetic patient requires an anaesthetic for a TURP. He has significant respiratory pathology and renal impairment. As he is diabetic and has smoked heavily in the past, he may well have ischaemic heart disease (which may be covert due to diabetes), cerebral vascular disease and peripheral vascular disease.

2. What could account for the biochemical results?

The urea and creatinine are both raised, indicating renal impairment. His potassium and sodium are normal (important because of the risk of hyponatraemia due to TUR syndrome). The impaired renal function is most likely to be due to obstructive nephropathy secondary to prostatic hyperplasia. Other possible causes include diabetic nephropathy and end-organ damage from hypertension.

His random blood sugar of 10 mmol/l is not significantly elevated. The WHO currently recommends a diagnosis of diabetes mellitus if a random blood glucose is greater than 10.0 mmol/l. This gentleman is already diagnosed as diabetic and the concern now is the degree of control of his blood sugar.

3. What do you think of the pulmonary function tests?

The FEV_1 is decreased as is the FVC. However, the FEV_1 is decreased more and the FEV_1/FVC ratio is thus 54%. This suggests airflow obstruction. The transfer factor (DL_{CO}) is reduced, but not enough to suggest a major problem with diffusion. It may be related in part to the previous radiotherapy and chemotherapy. The fact that the transfer factor corrected for lung volume (K_{CO}) is not very different would support fibrosis rather than emphysema. Chemotherapy with agents such as bleomycin or mitomycin can result in generalised pulmonary fibrosis.

4. What other information might you want?

Further information from the **history** such as:

- Exercise tolerance/SOBOE
- Any change in respiratory symptoms recently, e.g. cough, haemoptysis or wheeze
- Symptoms suggestive of ischaemic heart disease (e.g. chest pain) or other vascular pathology such as peripheral vascular disease or cerebral vascular disease.
- History of hypertension. Is his blood pressure checked regularly?
- When was he diagnosed with diabetes?
- Usual blood sugar control including out-patient attendance, GP follow-up and method of testing blood sugar level (urine or blood)
- Haemoglobin A_{1c}
- History of postural hypotension (suggesting autonomic neuropathy)
- Previous anaesthetic history
- Whether the patient can recognize when his blood sugar is high or low.

The patient needs a **12-lead ECG** to look for evidence of previous myocardial infarction, ischaemia or LVH.

From the point of view of his pulmonary function tests, it would be helpful to know if he had any **reversibility of airflow obstruction with β-agonists**, and if he had cooperated well with the test. Depending on the degree of respiratory compromise, a set of **arterial blood gases** on air should be obtained.

His current chest X-ray should be compared to a **previous chest X-ray**.

A **coagulation screen** would be useful if a spinal anaesthetic was being considered because some prostatic tumours can produce clotting abnormalities.

Further investigations (e.g. echocardiography) would be guided by the history.

5. Describe the chest X-ray. What may account for this?

This is a PA film showing right sided perihilar shadowing. It is sharply demarcated in keeping with fibrosis secondary to radiotherapy. The heart is probably slightly enlarged as the CTR is just greater than 0.5.

We think the chest X-ray in the exam probably showed right upper lobe fibrosis compatible with previous radiotherapy.
Other causes of upper lobe fibrosis include:

- TB
- Sarcoidosis
- Silicosis
- Ankylosing spondylitis
- Chronic extrinsic allergic alveolitis
- Progressive massive fibrosis.

6. How would you manage anaesthesia for TURP in this patient? What drugs might you give intra-operatively?

Also see short case on anaesthetic management of the diabetic patient.

A spinal anaesthetic technique would be appropriate for this patient. The advantages of a spinal over a general anaesthetic in this situation are:

- Recent papers suggest reduced mortality with regional techniques when compared to general anaesthesia alone.
- Earlier detection of TUR syndrome or bladder perforation
- Superior analgesia
- Less detrimental effect on respiratory function post-operatively
- Decreased incidence of DVT
- Decreased surgical blood loss
- Earlier detection of hypoglycaemia
- Decreased stress response resulting in better control of blood sugar
- Decreased post-operative nausea and vomiting
- No hangover from a general anaesthetic
- Earlier resumption of oral intake (advantageous in a diabetic patient).

If he was keen to have pre-medication, care must be taken to avoid respiratory depression. Administration of oxygen would be prudent.

As the patient is diabetic, he should be first on the list having omitted his glibenclamide. This drug has a long duration of action and therefore the patient should have his blood sugar monitored regularly for hypoglycaemia. There is debate amongst anaesthetists about the best regimen for managing blood glucose in these patients. I would start a sliding scale of i.v. insulin pre-operatively.

Once in the anaesthetic room, monitoring should be established, a peripheral cannula (at least 16 gauge) sited and a crystalloid infusion started. Lactate and glucose containing fluids should be avoided. With full aseptic technique, I would use 3.0 ml of 0.5% heavy marcain for the spinal anaesthetic having first anaesthetised the skin with 1% lignocaine. Ephedrine and/or metaraminol should be drawn up ready to treat hypotension should it occur. A sensory level of T10 should be the aim.

Oxygen should be continued intra-operatively and gentamicin (or other prophylactic antibiotic) administered. If the surgical resection is prolonged or bloody, then intra-operative haemoglobin estimation will help to guide the need for blood transfusion.

Glycine irrigation fluid containing alcohol is available. An alcohol breath test can then be used to calculate the volume of irrigation fluid absorbed by the patient. Intra-operatively he may require some sedation depending on his level of anxiety. Propofol or midazolam may be titrated.

7. During the TURP the patient becomes confused. What may be causing this?

Possible causes are:

- TUR syndrome
- Hypoxia
- Haemorrhage
- Hypotension
- Cerebrovascular event
- Myocardial infarction
- Hypothermia
- Bladder perforation
- Septicaemia.

8. Tell me about TUR syndrome.

The TUR syndrome represents a group of symptoms and signs that occur as a result of the absorption of large amounts of irrigating fluid. This fluid is usually 1.5% glycine, which is slightly hypotonic and has good optical and electrical properties for transurethral surgery. During resection of the prostate, large numbers of venous sinuses may be exposed to the irrigating fluid, which is under pressure. The syndrome, which can be fatal, can present intra-operatively or post-operatively. The symptoms are due to fluid overload, water intoxication and sometimes solute toxicity.

Symptoms include:

- Headache
- Confusion
- Restlessness
- Dyspnoea
- Temporary blindness.

Signs include:

- Cyanosis/decreased O_2 saturation
- Arrhythmias
- Fitting
- Hypotension or hypertension (often hypertension initially followed by hypotension)

- Bradycardia
- Pulmonary oedema.

Symptoms of hyponatraemia are likely to develop if the serum sodium falls below 120 mmol/l. Haemolysis can occur due to very hypotonic plasma. Hyperglycinaemia can cause central nervous system toxicity and cardiovascular embarrassment. TUR syndrome is also more likely to occur if the irrigation fluid height is greater than 60 cm and/or the resection lasts longer than 45–60 minutes.

Treatment should be instituted as early as possible and therefore early recognition is vital. Hypoxia must be treated aggressively and may necessitate endotracheal intubation. This may also be required to prevent aspiration due to a decreased conscious level. Fluid restriction and loop diuretics are used to treat the fluid overload. If there are symptoms of hyponatraemia, then hypertonic saline may be required. However, it must be given slowly to avoid exacerbating fluid overload. Central pontine myelinosis can occur if correction of the serum sodium is too rapid. Diazepam or phenytoin may be required to treat convulsions.

References

Hahn R. (2006). Fluid absorption in endoscopic surgery (Review). *British Journal of Anaesthesia*, **96**(1), 8–20.

McAnulty GR, Robertshaw HJ, Hall GM. (2000). Anaesthetic management of patients with diabetes mellitus. *British Journal of Anaesthesia*, **85**(1), 80–90.

Shah T, Flisberg P. (2006). Early recognition of the two cases of TURP syndrome in patients receiving spinal anaesthesia. *Anaesthesia and Intensive Care*, **34**(4), 520–1.

Long Case 13

'The one with the stridulous woman for oesophagoscopy'

You are asked to anaesthetise a 65-year-old lady who has been admitted for an EUA, laryngoscopy, oesophagoscopy +/− biopsy. She has a 2-month history of dysphagia, stridor and a choking sensation when supine. She has recently lost 12 kg in weight, and now weighs 57 kg. She had a myocardial infarction 7 years ago but, apart from being a smoker (20 cigarettes per day), her other medical history is unremarkable. She is on no medication.

On examination	Mild inspiratory stridor	
	HR	80 bpm
	BP	170/100 mmHg
	HS	normal
Investigations	Sodium	148 mmol/L
	Potassium	3.9 mmol/L
	Urea	8.3 mmol/L
	Creatinine	119 μmol/L
	Hb	17 g/dL
	WCC	9.3×10^9/L
	Plt	236×10^9/L

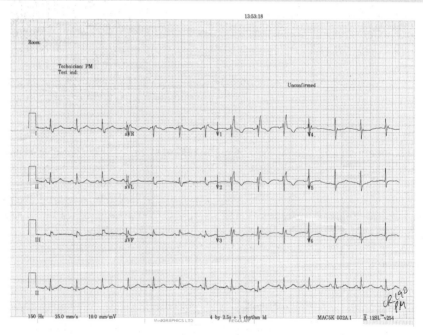

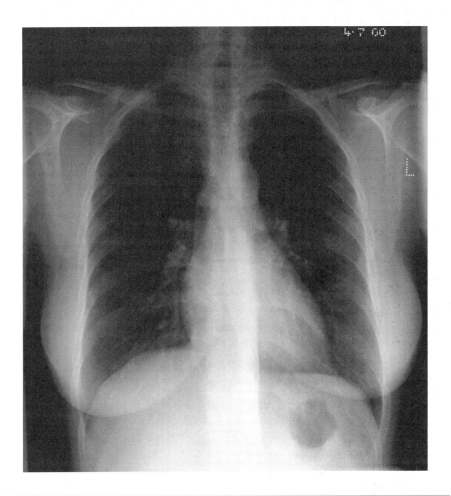

Questions

1. Can you summarise the case?

This 65-year-old lady, with a history of weight loss and stridor, has symptoms suggestive of a tumour that is partially obstructing her airway. The fact that she feels like she is choking when she lies flat suggests the obstruction is severe. She requires an EUA of her oesophagus and larynx +/− biopsy of any lesion found. She has ischaemic heart disease, hypertension, atrial fibrillation and is also likely to have lower respiratory tract pathology because she is a smoker. Management of her airway will need careful consideration and consultation with the ENT surgeon.

2. What further investigations would you like?

Further investigation is important to help define the nature and level of the obstruction. The results of these investigations will dictate the anaesthetic approach to managing her airway. Helpful investigations would be:

- **A CT scan of her upper airway**. This will define the size and level of the obstruction. It will also help to suggest a diagnosis which will be relevant when considering if she is likely to need further surgery such as a laryngectomy.
- **Nasal endoscopy**. If the glottis can be easily visualised in this manner, then there is a good chance of being able to visualize the cords with direct laryngoscopy (providing there is no other anatomical reason why laryngoscopy would be difficult, of course).
- **Arterial blood gases**
- **Pulmonary function tests** including a flow-volume loop.
- **X-rays of the thoracic inlet.** Not as useful as a CT scan.

3. What are the possible causes of her symptoms?

Inspiratory stridor occurs when there is something partially obstructing the lumen of the airway. This may be arising from the lumen or the wall of the airway, or it could be due to extrinsic compression. This lady is a smoker and has suffered with considerable recent weight loss making the diagnosis of a tumour more likely. The tumour could be pharyngeal, laryngeal or oesophageal in nature.

4. Tell me about her ECG.

The ECG shows sinus rhythm with a rate of around 80 beats per minute and a normal axis. There is right bundle branch block given by the QRS complex being wider than 3 mm and the typical RSR pattern in lead V_1. The corrected QT interval is also prolonged.

5. What are the causes of RBBB?

- Normal finding in 5% of elderly adults
- Congenital heart disease

  ASD
  Fallot's tetralogy
  Pulmonary stenosis
  VSD

- Respiratory disease

  Cor pulmonale
  Pulmonary embolism

- Cardiac disease

  Acute MI
  Cardiomyopathy
  Fibrosis of conducting system

- Other

  Hyperkalaemia
  Anti-arrhythmic drugs

6. How would you exclude a recent myocardial infarction?

A recent myocardial infarction may be identified by the history, examination and investigations available. This patient does not have hard ECG evidence of a past myocardial infarction (the exam ECG had inferior Q waves in addition to

RBBB). If there were Q waves without ST elevation or T wave inversion, it would only be possible to say that the infarct was older than a few days. ECG changes may have finished evolving after this time with Q waves developing and the ST segments returning to normal.

A recent history of sustained central crushing chest pain may help to date the infarct!

The cardiac enzyme changes may still be evident because the LDH can remain raised for 2 weeks. There are, of course, other explanations for a raised LDH.

Troponin T takes approximately 8 hours to begin rising and 12 hours to peak. It returns to normal within 5 days.

Recent onset of cardiac failure or an arrhythmia (e.g. atrial fibrillation) may have been precipitated by a myocardial infarct.

Other investigations such as echocardiography and thallium imaging can identify areas of abnormal movement or abnormal/absent perfusion, but these tests are unable to date a myocardial infarction.

7. What are the causes of polycythaemia?

The causes of polycythaemia can be primary, secondary or relative. The secondary causes can again be divided into those with an appropriate increase in erythropoietin and those with an inappropriate increase.

Primary
- Polycythaemia rubra vera.

Secondary – with an appropriate increase in erythropoietin
- High altitude
- Respiratory disease
- Cyanotic heart disease
- Heavy smoking.

Secondary – with an **in**appropriate increase in erythropoietin
- Renal cell carcinoma
- Hepatocellular carcinoma
- Cerebellar haemangioblastoma
- Massive uterine fibroma.

Relative
- Stress polycythaemia
- Dehydration
- Burns.

8. What are the anaesthetic problems associated with hypertension?

See short answer question on uncontrolled hypertension.

9. How would you anaesthetise this woman?

The way in which this patient should be anaesthetised depends very much on the results of the investigations listed above. The nature and level of the obstruction are critical to the planning of the anaesthetic. If we assume that she has an obstructive lesion in or around the larynx, then the first decision to be made is whether intubation is likely to be possible or whether the patient will require an awake tracheostomy under local anaesthesia. Whether or not the patient will ultimately require a tracheostomy for relief of symptoms will be an important consideration anyway.

These decisions should be made in collaboration with an experienced ENT surgeon who has performed a nasal endoscopic examination of the patient. This examination will show whether direct laryngoscopy is likely to be possible. If, with nasal endoscopy, the larynx is not visible and the anatomy is very abnormal, then an awake tracheostomy under local anaesthesia should be performed.

If intubation is considered likely to be possible, then an inhalational induction should be planned. This should take place in theatre with the ENT surgeon scrubbed to perform a tracheostomy if necessary. Other difficult airway equipment should be available to hand, including a rigid bronchoscope.

Sevoflurane or halothane could be used and laryngoscopy attempted when the patient is deep enough. It may still be prudent at this point to perform a tracheostomy if the patient is breathing spontaneously, but the larynx is not visible on direct laryngoscopy. Once intubation is confirmed, a neuromuscular blocker could be given.

For monitoring this patient, an arterial line would be useful because of her hypertension (which is not controlled and the surgery cannot be postponed for 6 weeks until it is) and ischaemic heart disease.

Fibre-optic intubation in the patient with an obstructed airway

This can be hazardous for several reasons:

- Altered anatomy causes loss of usual landmarks.
- Airway trauma can cause oedema and bleeding leading to total airway obstruction.
- Sedation and relaxation of the patient are difficult to achieve (and dangerous).
- Emergency tracheostomy in an awake but hypoxic patient is very difficult.

---

10. What would your maintenance technique be and how would you manage her post-operative care?

A remifentanil infusion may be useful for a stimulating procedure of short duration that is unlikely to require a large amount of post-operative analgesia. The rapid recovery from remifentanil is also desirable. In addition to this, sevoflurane in a mixture of oxygen and nitrous oxide could be used. This technique would hopefully give stable cardiovascular conditions. It is important to liaise with the surgeon during the procedure in order to know what the surgical findings were and what has been done to the airway.

Her post-operative care would depend on the operative findings and on the difficulties encountered with her airway on induction and emergence. These factors would dictate what level of nursing care (i.e. general ward, HDU or ICU) the patient required.

As with any patient in the post-operative period, it is important to pay attention to . . . *see box below*.

Questions on post-operative care

When answering questions on post-operative care, you should think about the following:

- Nursing dependency (ward, HDU or ICU)
- Pain-relief *and* anti-emetics
- Oxygen therapy
- Fluid therapy
- Physiotherapy
- Specific complications (e.g. post-thyroidectomy bleeding)
- Specific observations (e.g. neurological observations).

Bibliography

Kumar PJ, Clark ML. (2005). *Clinical Medicine*, 6th edition. W.B. Saunders.

Mason RA, Fielder CP. (1999). The obstructed airway in head and neck surgery. *Anaesthesia*, **54**, 625–8.

Long Case 14

'The one about the collapsed drug addict'

You are called to the accident and emergency department to see a 26-year-old male. He has been found semiconscious, complaining of weak legs. There is a past history of intravenous drug abuse, depression and alcohol abuse. There is a vague history of heroin overdose.

On examination	He is agitated	
	GCS	13/15 after naloxone
	BP	80/40 mmHg
	Heart rate	56 bpm
Investigations	Sodium	135 mmol/l
	Potassium	7.9 mmol/l
	Urea	30.1 mmol/l
	Creatinine	352 μmol/l
	CK	43 000 U/l
	Hb	14 g/dl
	WCC	15×10^9/l
	Plts	255×10^9/l
	Blood gases on air	
	pH	7.2
	pO_2	8.0 kPa
	pCO_2	6.0 kPa
	HCO_3^-	19 mmol/l
	BE	−6 mmol/l

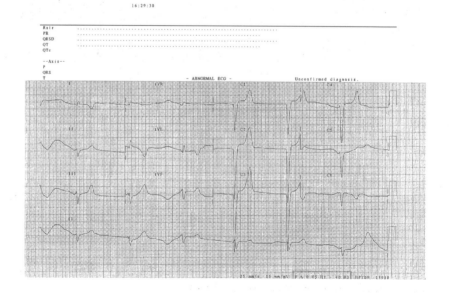

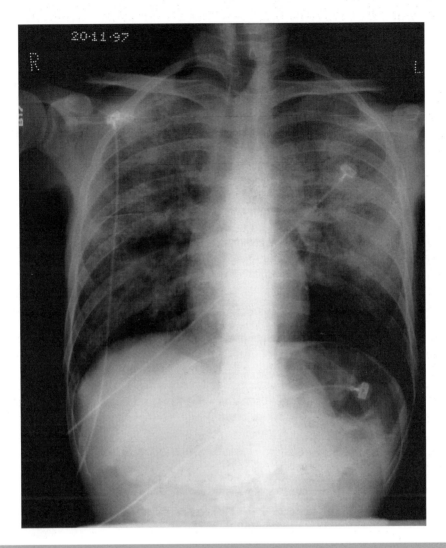

Questions

1. What are the possible causes of weak legs in such a patient?

The most likely cause of this patient's weak legs is muscle damage from rhabdomyolysis. Other possible causes are:

■ The extremely high serum potassium level
■ Polyneuropathy caused by drugs or alcohol
■ Vascular injury secondary to injection
■ Spinal cord damage from either compression (by tumour, blood clot or disc prolapse), infarction or trauma
■ Guillain–Barré syndrome
■ Vitamin deficiencies.

Important points in the history will be whether the onset was gradual or sudden, and whether the limbs are spastic or not.

2. What do you think of the blood results?

The urea and electrolytes show that the patient is in acute renal failure. Both the urea and the creatinine are more than trebled. The serum potassium is very high and needs immediate correction, as the patient is in imminent danger of suffering a cardiac arrest.

The creatine kinase is so high that this can only be caused by significant skeletal muscle damage (rhabdomyolysis). This destruction of muscle will have largely contributed to the raised potassium.

The full blood count is normal except for a raised white cell count. This suggests infection or an acute phase response.

The blood gases show a metabolic acidosis with poor respiratory compensation. The failure of the respiratory system to compensate may be due to a decreased conscious level and possible opioid intoxication. The metabolic component will be the result of rhabdomyolysis, sepsis (decreased perfusion) and renal failure. The patient is also hypoxaemic and this may be due to ARDS / sepsis.

3. What do you think the diagnosis is?

The diagnosis is rhabdomyolysis. High levels of myoglobin released from dead muscle have caused acute renal failure. Lying immobile on the floor for a long period of time may have caused the rhabdomyolysis. Hypotension and dehydration will exacerbate the damage. Other causes of rhabdomyolysis include cocaine abuse, alcohol (both chronic abuse and binge drinking), sepsis, prolonged fitting, electric shock or crush injury.

4. What effect does a raised K$^+$ have on the myocardium?

A raised extracellular potassium level causes a less negative resting membrane potential in the cardiac myocytes. The higher the potassium level the more fast Na$^+$ channels are inactivated. The action potential then becomes dependent on the slow (Ca^{2+}) channels, so the steepness and duration of the action potential upstroke become diminished.

The ECG changes include:

- Peaked T waves
- Widening of the QRS complex
- Bradycardia
- Atrial standstill
- Ventricular tachycardia and ventricular fibrillation can occur
- Sine-wave appearance
- Asystole.

5. What are the possible causes of the pulmonary oedema?

The pulmonary oedema could be cardiogenic (although the heart does not appear enlarged on the AP film) or non-cardiogenic. ARDS is the most likely cause of pulmonary oedema in this situation.

Cardiac causes could be secondary to an alcoholic cardiomyopathy or sepsis causing poor left ventricular function.

6. *What would be your immediate management?*

It should be recognised from the outset that this patient is critically ill. He should be nursed in a high-dependency or intensive care area, such as the accident and emergency resuscitation room. A defibrillator should be readily available. The patient should be given 100% oxygen and the hyperkalaemia must be given urgent attention, as this is immediately life-threatening.

Consideration should be given to intubation and ventilation (avoiding suxamethonium!) for the following reasons:

1. He is agitated and therefore may not tolerate the necessary treatment (dialysis, i.v. infusions, central venous catheterization and O_2 therapy).
2. He is hypoxaemic.
3. He is hypoventilating because his pCO_2 is inappropriately high in the face of a metabolic acidosis.

His haemodynamic state is complicated because he is hypotensive and bradycardic and has signs of left ventricular failure. The haemodynamic indices may be explained by the hyperkalaemia. Resolution of the hyperkalaemia may therefore produce a different haemodynamic picture. If the patient is still hypotensive, the cause of his shock could be septic or cardiogenic in nature. Cardiac output monitoring may be useful.

7. *How would you treat a high K^+?*

Immediate measures to prevent cardiac arrest would be:

- 10–15 units of soluble Insulin in 50 ml of 50% glucose i.v.
- 10 ml of 10% calcium chloride i.v. This stabilises the myocardium against arrhythmias.
- 50 ml of 8.4% sodium bicarbonate will help correct acidosis and reduce the potassium level. However, the high sodium load should be considered and the minute ventilation needs to be adequate to excrete the CO_2 load produced, otherwise intracellular acidosis may be worsened.
- Hyperventilation (if the patient is intubated) will also help reduce acidosis and therefore the hyperkalaemia.
- Nebulized β_2-agonists shift potassium into the cells.
- Avoidance of any potassium containing i.v. fluids, e.g. Hartmann's
- 15 g of calcium resonium qds p.o. (may take greater than 30 minutes to work). This acts as an ion exchange resin in the gut.

These measures temporarily push the potassium back into the cells. This patient will need renal replacement therapy (ideally haemodialysis) to remove the excess potassium.

8. Which methods of renal replacement therapy do you know?

Haemodialysis

- Efficient
- Specialist centres only
- A thin film of blood is passed by one side of a synthetic semi-permeable membrane, whilst on the other side dialysate fluid is passed in the opposite direction. This creates a constant diffusion gradient for electrolytes.
- The technique is performed intermittently for 4–6 hours.
- Anticoagulation is required.

Haemofiltration

- More cardiovascularly stable than haemodialysis.
- More widely available on intensive care units.
- Plasma water is removed by convection through a filter. The fluid is replaced with an appropriate electrolyte solution.
- Less efficient than haemodialysis.
- Can be combined with dialysis (haemodiafiltration).
- This technique is usually used continuously until the filter clots
- Anticoagulation is required.

Peritoneal dialysis

- No need for sophisticated equipment.
- Principle is the same as haemodialysis, but the membrane used is the peritoneal lining.
- 2 litres of sterile dialysate are placed into the peritoneal cavity via a catheter through the abdominal wall. In the acute situation this is drained out every hour. Electrolyte movement is by osmosis. Tonicity of the dialysate (and therefore degree of fluid removal) is determined by its glucose concentration.

9. Why is he hypotensive?

This could be due to:

- A cardiogenic cause, e.g. hyperkalaemia (causing bradycardia and myocardial dysfunction) or an alcoholic cardiomyopathy
- Septic shock
- Drug overdose

10. What about the treatment of rhabdomyolysis?

Treatment consists of management of the airway, breathing and circulation and correcting the underlying cause of the rhabdomyolysis. Further specific treatment of rhabdomyolysis is aimed at the prevention of renal failure.

The two factors that predispose to acute renal failure in the presence of myoglobinuria are **hypovolaemia** and **aciduria**. These two factors must therefore be addressed in the treatment:

- Aim for urine output of 100 ml/hour.
- Dip urine hourly for pH and myoglobin testing.
- If urine pH < 7.0 give 100 mmol of sodium bicarbonate (can be repeated). Studies have shown bicarbonate therapy may be of benefit.
- If urine pH < 7.0 give acetozolamide 500 mg i.v. (can be repeated 4-hourly). This has not, however, been shown to be of consistent benefit.
- Mannitol can be used to promote a diuresis.
- Loop diuretics should be avoided as they acidify the urine.
- The depletion of extracellular iron by desferrioxamine may be of benefit.
- Allopurinol (xanthine oxidase inhibitor) has been used to try to decrease the hyperuricaemia associated with increased muscle protein breakdown.

Mechanisms that underlie haem protein toxicity to the nephron

- **Renal vasoconstriction**. Severe muscle damage results in gross ECF volume contraction. There is strong evidence that early volume repletion decreases the incidence of renal failure.
- **Intraluminal cast formation**. Myoglobin combines with tubular proteins to form casts. Acid pH of the tubular fluid favours the formation of these complexes. Alkaline conditions help to stop myoglobin-induced lipid peroxidation by stabilizing the reactive ferryl myoglobin complex that is responsible for causing oxidative damage. If the urinary pH is below 6.0, ferrihaemate (nephrotoxic) dissociates from myoglobin.
- **Haem-protein induced cytotoxicity**. Haemoglobin and myoglobin are usually re-absorbed into the proximal tubular cells by endocytosis. Inside the cell, porphyrin is metabolised producing free iron, which is converted into ferritin. When this pathway is overwhelmed, the free iron builds up to levels that cause oxidant stress and cell damage.

---

11. Is there a need for surgery in these patients?

Yes. Compartment syndrome must be looked for and treated. If compartment syndrome is suspected, then the compartmental pressures should be measured. A normal pressure is less than 15 mmHg. A pressure of greater than 25 mmHg should trigger a surgical referral.

If compartment syndrome is diagnosed, urgent fasciotomies are indicated. Debridement of any necrotic tissue is also frequently required.

> ### Symptoms and signs of compartment syndrome
>
> ■ Pain – especially with passive flexion
> ■ A swollen, hard limb
> ■ Poor capillary refill
> ■ Pulses may be present.

Bibliography

Brown C, Rhee P, Chan L *et al.* (2004). Preventing renal failure in patients with rhabdomyolysis: do bicarbonate and mannitol make a difference? *Journal of Trauma*, **56**(6), 1191–6.

O'Connor G, McMahon G. (2008). Complications of heroin abuse. European *Journal of Emergency Medicine* **15**(2), 104–6.

Visweswaran P, Guntupalli J. (1999). Rhabdomyolysis. *Critical Care Clinics*, **15**(2), 415–28.

Long Case 15

'The elderly woman with kyphoscoliosis for an urgent cholecystectomy'

An 82-year-old lady is admitted to hospital with vomiting and jaundice. This is her second episode. She is known to have gallstones and the surgical team want to perform an open cholecystectomy.

She lives in a nursing home and has restricted mobility due to osteoarthritis. She is an ex-smoker and enjoys embroidery and knitting. Previous medical history includes post-herpetic neuralgia and mild Alzheimer's disease.

Medications		
	Ibuprofen	400 mg t.d.s.
	Bendrofluazide	5 mg o.d.
	Carbamazepine	200 mg b.d.

O/E

Mildly confused, frail, jaundiced, kyphoscoliosis,
Temperature 37.7 °C
Weight 75 kg
Pulse 100 irregular   Resp rate 16 bpm
BP 160/84 mmHg   Generally quiet breath sounds
HS normal   No wheeze audible
Abdomen: tender with guarding in the right upper quadrant.

Investigations

Hb	9.6 g/dl	Na 133 mmol/l	ALT 28 U/l(5 − 40)
WCC	14.3×10^9/l	K 3.3 mmol/l	AST 16 U/l(10 − 40)
Plt	187×10^9/l	U 11.6 mmol/l	Alk phos 238 U/l
MCV	84 fl	Cr 125 μmol/l	(25 − 115)
			GGT 475 U/l (7 − 32)
		Glucose	Bilirubin
		6.4 mmol/l	36 μmol/l (<17)

PFTs

FEV_1	1.8 l (2.3 − 3.6)
FVC	2.2 l (3.9 − 5.0)
FEV_1/ FVC ratio	82%
TLC	4.6 l (5.6 − 7.5)
DL_{CO}	7.8 mmol/kPa per min (8.2)

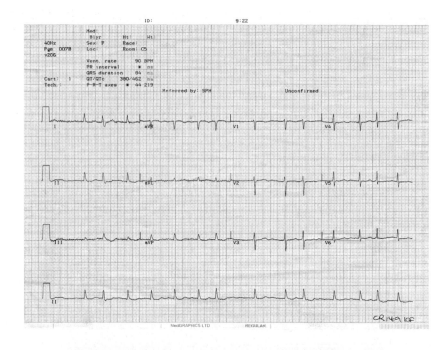

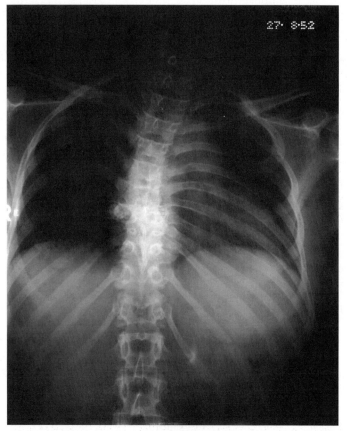

Questions

1. What do you think are the important features of this case?

This is an elderly lady with complex medical problems presenting for emergency upper abdominal surgery. The main issues of concern from the anaesthetic viewpoint are her atrial fibrillation, restrictive lung disease, fluid balance and post-operative analgesia.

2. What does the ECG show?

There is atrial fibrillation with a ventricular response of 90 beats per minute. The corrected QT interval is also slightly prolonged at 460 milliseconds, the normal being 420 milliseconds.

QT interval

- Measured from onset of QRS to end of T wave.
- Can be difficult to measure precisely.
- Normal QTc (corrected for heart rate) < 420 milliseconds.

Significance

- Pre-disposes to torsade de pointes ventricular tachycardia.

Some causes of prolonged QTc

- Congenital — Syndromes – Romano Ward, Jervell-Lange-Nielsen
- Acquired — Hypokalaemia, hypomagnesaemia, hypocalcaemia drugs, e.g. terfenadine, cisapride, erythromycin, amiodarone, amitriptyline, quinidine
  Severe bradycardia
  Acute MI.

Treatment

- Magnesium
- Overdrive pacing.

---

3. What does the CXR show?

There is significant kyphoscoliosis in keeping with the examination finding. A lateral chest X-ray would confirm this.

4. Would you like to comment on the pulmonary function tests?

All lung volumes are reduced, but the FEV_1/FVC ratio is raised. This suggests a restrictive defect. The diffusion capacity for carbon monoxide is normal so it is unlikely to be pulmonary fibrosis. These results are compatible with the severe kyphoscoliosis seen clinically and on the chest X-ray.

See appendix for interpretation of commonly occurring PFTs.

5. What do you think about the haemoglobin?

The haemoglobin is low, but the MCV is normal. If this was iron deficiency anaemia secondary to ibuprofen, one would expect the MCV to be low as well. It may be anaemia of chronic disease.

6. Would you transfuse the patient pre-operatively?

The haemoglobin is 9.6 g/dl. She does not have clinically overt ischaemic heart disease and is unlikely to have significant blood loss intra-operatively. There is no current evidence to show that pre-operative transfusion in patients with this level of anaemia has any effect on mortality. Blood transfusion is not without complications so, on balance, it would be reasonable to withhold transfusion. However, the surgeon should take extra care to avoid any unnecessary blood loss and blood should be available.

> See Long case 9 and Short case on massive blood transfusion.

7. Comment on the urea, electrolytes and liver function tests.

There is mild hyponatraemia and hypokalaemia, possibly secondary to bendrofluazide. The raised urea and creatinine suggest an element of dehydration as the urea is out of proportion to the creatinine. Although hepato-renal syndrome is another possibility the level of jaundice makes it unlikely to be the cause.

The liver function tests show a raised bilirubin, alkaline phosphatase and GGT in keeping with obstructive jaundice. This is most likely to be secondary to gallstones, although carbamazepine is also a recognized cause of an obstructive picture.

> **Causes of hypokalaemia**
>
> The list is enormous!
> Some of the more common causes to remember include:
> - Diuretics
> - Hyperaldosteronism   Liver failure
>   Heart failure
>   Nephrotic syndrome
> - GI losses

8. Are there any other investigations you might want?

Coagulation profile: this lady has poor respiratory function and the nature of the surgery will result in significant post-operative pain and difficulty with deep breathing and coughing. She would therefore benefit from a regional block for post-operative analgesia but the liver function tests are abnormal.

9. What anaesthetic technique would you use for this lady?

Although this operation could, in theory, be performed under purely regional anaesthesia, the height of the epidural block necessary to undertake the operation with the patient awake is likely to result in respiratory embarrassment.

General anaesthesia with some form of regional block would be an appropriate technique. She would require a rapid sequence induction and intubation.

The options for post-operative analgesia include:

- Systemic opioids and NSAIDs (care with renal impairment)
- Thoracic epidural sited prior to induction but likely to be difficult in view of the kyphoscoliosis. She is also septic. One would weigh up the pros and cons.
- Paravertebral block
- Intercostal blocks (risk of pneumothorax)
- Interpleural catheter.

> Preferably choose a regional technique that you have performed before and can describe in detail.

Post-operative care on a high dependency unit with careful attention to oxygenation, fluid balance and analgesia is important.

Bibliography
McCrossan L, Masterson G. (2002). Blood transfusion in critical illness. *British Journal of Anaesthesia*, **88**(1), 6–9.

Tziavrangos E, Schug S. (2006). Regional anaesthesia and perioperative outcome. *Current Opinion in Anaesthesiology*, **19**(5), 521–5.

Long Case 16

'The one about the elderly woman for cataract extraction'

A 77-year-old woman presents for cataract extraction and intra-ocular lens implant – she does not want a general anaesthetic.

PMH	Previous acute myocardial infarction – uncomplicated Infrequent angina Atrial fibrillation Deep vein thrombosis Previous mastectomy Five weeks ago she suffered with an episode of a cool mottled ischaemic left arm which resolved with heparin. Previous GA was uneventful.
O/E	Weight 50 kg, height 160 cm Ankle oedema BP 170/70 Pansystolic murmur at her apex radiating to her axilla Diastolic murmur Displaced apex Irregular pulse Fine bibasal crepitations
Medication	Digoxin 125 mcg daily Frumil Warfarin 8 mg/day GTN on a PRN basis
Investigations	Urea 10.8 mmol/l Na 137 mmol/l K 5.5 mmol/l Creatinine 144 µmol/l INR 1.6 FBC normal CXR shows cardiomegaly, pulmonary oedema, Kerley B lines and an enlarged left atrium.

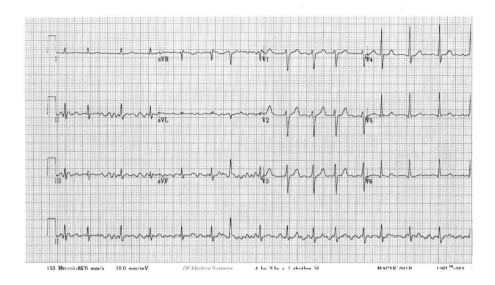

Can you summarise the case?

This elderly lady presents for elective surgery with significant medical problems. She has hypertension, ischaemic heart disease, atrial fibrillation and evidence of cardiac failure on CXR. Her cardiac examination indicates a possible valvular heart lesion. She also has renal impairment and has had a thromboembolic episode in the recent past.

Why might she be on digoxin and warfarin?

She is in atrial fibrillation, which is the most common arrhythmia in clinical practice and affects approximately 4.5 million people in the European Union. The primary objectives in patients with atrial fibrillation are rate control, prevention of thromboembolism and correction of the rhythm disturbance.

Oral digoxin is effective in the control of heart rate at rest in patients with atrial fibrillation and is indicated in patients with heart failure, left ventricular dysfunction or for sedentary individuals.

Anti-thrombotic therapy in patients with atrial fibrillation
One of every six strokes occurs in a patient with atrial fibrillation, which is associated with an increased long-term risk of stroke.

Weaker risk factors
- Female gender
- Age 65–74
- Coronary artery disease
- Thyrotoxicosis.

Moderate risk factors
- Age greater than or equal to 75
- Hypertension
- Heart failure
- LVEF 35% or less
- Diabetes mellitus.

High risk factors
- Previous stroke, TIA or embolism
- Mitral stenosis
- Prosthetic heart valve.

No risk factors	Aspirin 81–325 mg daily
One moderate risk factor	Aspirin 81–325 mg daily or warfarin (INR 2.0–3.0 target 2.5)
Any high-risk factor or more than one moderate risk factor	Warfarin (INR 2.0–3.0 target 2.5)

What are the symptoms and signs of digoxin toxicity?

Vomiting, confusion, delirium, hallucinations, blurred vision, disturbed colour perception (yellow vision) photophobia, all types of arrhythmias and all degrees of AV block. A shortened QT interval and the 'reverse tick' pattern may be seen on the ECG. The combination of supraventricular tachycardia and AV block suggests digoxin toxicity. Hyperkalaemia can occur with acute overdose and hypokalaemia with chronic intoxication.

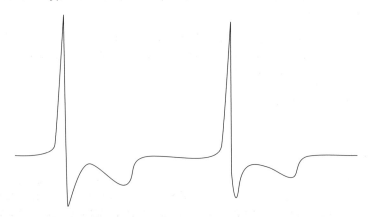

Comment on the biochemistry results provided?

The urea and creatinine are elevated and the serum potassium is raised.

What are the causes of an elevated serum potassium?

The causes may be broadly grouped into:

Inadequate excretion

- Renal failure
- Potassium sparing diuretics: amiloride, triamterene, spironalactone
- ACE inhibitors
- Acidosis.

Increased extraneous potassium

- Transfusion of stored blood

Increased release from cells

- Rhabdomyolysis
- Tumour lysis
- Succinylcholine
- Digoxin poisoning
- Diabetic ketoacidosis.

How would you manage the hyperkalaemia?

Hyperkalaemia in this patient is probably due to a combination of potassium sparing diuretics and renal impairment secondary to a low GFR as a result of cardiac insufficiency. Normalisation of her potassium may be achieved through omission of the potassium sparing diuretics. Her digoxin levels should be checked and her cardiac failure treated.

Hyperkalaemia of greater than 7 mmol/l is a medical emergency needing immediate treatment:

- Myocardial protection: 10 ml of 10% calcium chloride
- Glucose and insulin as an infusion with regular estimations of serum potassium and blood glucose.
- Correction of acidosis
- Nebulised salbutamol.

What causes creatinine to rise?

There will either be an increase in creatinine production or a reduction in renal function and therefore handling of the creatinine load. Serum creatinine will increase in cases of rhabdomyolysis, high muscle mass or even excess red meat ingestion.

Decreased tubular secretion can be caused by drugs, e.g. trimethoprim or cimetidine.

What is the cause and significance of the heart murmur in this case?

The description of the murmur and the enlarged left atrium as well as the presence of atrial fibrillation suggests mixed mitral valve disease.

The presence of a cardiac murmur in the face of symptoms of cardiac failure warrants further investigation of the cause of the murmur. She would also require prophylaxis against infective endocarditis prior to an invasive procedure.

The European Society of Cardiology has set guidelines that define which cardiac conditions antimicrobial prophylaxis is indicated for:

- Complex congenital cyanotic heart disease
- Prosthetic heart valves
- Previous infective endocarditis
- Surgically constructed conduits – systemic or pulmonary
- Acquired valvular heart disease
- Mitral valve prolapse with regurgitation or severe valve thickening
- Non-cyanotic congenital heart disease (except secundum type ASD) including bicuspid aortic valves
- Hypertrophic cardiomyopathy.

Define heart failure?

Heart failure occurs when the heart is unable to maintain a cardiac output sufficient to meet the metabolic demands of the body. The syndrome is characterised by breathlessness, fatigue and oedema. Objective evidence, preferably in the form of echocardiography, of cardiac dysfunction should be present.

What are the principles of managing heart failure?

Establish that the patient has heart failure according to the definition above. Assess the severity of presenting symptoms and determine the cause and any exacerbating factors. Identify other diseases which are relevant to the management of heart failure as well as assessing complicating factors, e.g. renal failure.
Choose appropriate management.

Would you administer a general anaesthetic?

No. Her untreated heart failure and abnormal biochemistry pose an unacceptable risk.

Describe the commonly performed local anaesthetic blocks for ophthalmic surgery?

Modified retro-bulbar block
A 24 mm 25 g needle is inserted inferotemporally lateral to the lateral limbus with the patient looking straight ahead. The needle may be inserted percutaneously through the lower eyelid or through the conjunctival reflection. Once the needle has been inserted 10–15 mm vertically into the eye

parallel to the floor of the orbit (pass the equator of the globe), it is redirected superomedially to enter the muscle cone. 4–5 ml of local anaesthetic is injected.

Peri-bulbar block
The peri-bulbar block differs from the modified retro-bulbar block in that the needle is not directed superomedially once the equator of the globe has been passed. The injection is therefore made extraconally close to the orbital wall beyond the equator of the globe into the peri-bulbar space. The patient looks straight ahead and topical local anaesthetic is applied prior to needle insertion. 5–10 ml of local anaesthetic is injected.

The optic nerve runs in the medial half of the orbit. The retro-bulbar block risks damage to the optic nerve if the needle strays medially. The peri-bulbar approach ensures safety of the optic nerve.

Sub-tenon's block
Topical local anaesthetic is instilled into the eye as well as aqueous iodine. The eyelids are held apart with a speculum and the patient is asked to look upwards and outwards.

This block involves making an incision into the inferomedial aspect of the conjunctiva using a round tip spring scissors (Westcott's). The conjunctiva is elevated prior to the incision being made with a non-toothed forceps (Moorfield's). A sub-tenon's needle is inserted into the incision made and advanced posteriorly along the sclera. 4–6 ml of 2% lidocaine are delivered posterior to the equator of the globe.

Comment on the dose of warfarin in a smallish lady giving an INR of 1.6. What drugs interact with warfarin?

This is a substantial dose, which is not achieving a therapeutic INR.

Warfarin may be potentiated by drugs that inhibit hepatic drug metabolism, e.g. metronidazole, amiodarone and imipramine.

The effectiveness of warfarin may be reduced by drugs that induce cytochrome P450 enzymes, e.g. barbiturates, griseofulvin. Some parenteral feeds and vitamin preparations may contain vitamin K, thereby antagonising the action of warfarin. Drugs like cholystyramine may bind to warfarin in the gut.

Bibliography
Fauci AS, Braunwald E, Isselbacher KJ. et al. (1998). *Harrison's Principles of Internal Medicine*, 14th Edition. Singapore: McGraw-Hill.

Fuster V, Ryden L. (2001). Management of atrial fibrillation. *European Heart Journal*, **22**, 1852–923.

Hamilton R C, (1995). Techniques of orbital regional anaesthesia. *British Journal of Anaesthesia*, **75**, 88–92.

Horstkotte D, Follath F, Gutschik E et al. (2004). Guidelines on the prevention, diagnosis and treatment of infective endocarditis. *European Heart Journal*, **25**, 267–76.

Kumar PJ, Clark ML. (2002). *Clinical Medicine*, 5th edition. London: WB Saunders.

Swedberg K, (Chairperson), Cleland J, Dargie H, et al. (2005). Chronic heart failure. *European Heart Journal*, **26**, 1115–40.

Long Case 17

'The one about the guy with chronic back pain'

A 77-year-old man presents to the chronic pain clinic with severe back pain. He has a background history of prostate cancer. The back pain is of more than 6 months' duration and is associated with stabbing pain which radiates to his left foot.

Medications	Ibuprofen	400 mg t.d.s
	Paracetamol	1 g q.d.s.
	Gabapentin	100 mg t.d.s

O/E	Frail.
	No evidence of recent weight loss.
	No lymphadenopathy or oedema.
	Musculoskeletal examination: no scars or deformities over his back.
	Tender over the supraspinal muscles bilaterally.
	Restricted extension and lateral rotation but normal forward flexion.
	Normal tone and power in the lower limbs with an absent ankle reflex on the left.
	Straight leg raise test positive on the left with intact sensation.

What are the important issues in this case?

Back pain in the elderly may have a sinister cause, particularly with a history of cancer. This pain is chronic and has features of nerve root irritation on history and examination.

What are the three main diagnostic categories which patients with back pain fall into?

■ Serious spinal pathology
■ Chronic lower back pain
■ Nerve root (radicular) pain.

What is meant by red flags in the context of back pain? Can you provide examples?

The presence of red flags suggests **serious spinal pathology**

■ Patient age <20 and >55
■ History of significant trauma
■ Constant progressive pain worse when lying down – particularly in the thoracic spine
■ Structural deformity

- History of cancer
- Drug abuse
- Use of steroids
- Widespread neurological signs, such as recent onset of bladder dysfunction, saddle anaesthesia, progressive sensory loss with or without motor loss in the distribution of nerve roots
- Marked restriction of lumbar flexion (<5 cm)
- Fever
- Unexplained weight loss and systemically unwell.

What are the possible differential diagnoses in a patient presenting with back pain?

The differential diagnosis includes conditions, which may be either **intraspinal** or **extraspinal**. A thorough history and examination will provide clues as to which specific pathology may be present.
Intraspinal causes:

- Infection (abscess, discitis)
- Neoplasm
- Arachnoiditis
- Ruptured inter-vertebral disc.
  Extraspinal causes are varied and pain may result from pathologies relating to the:

Abdomen	Peritoneal cavity neoplasm
Retro-peritoneal space	Aortic aneurysm, neoplasia
Pelvis	Gynaecological disorders
Orthopaedic	Hip arthritis
Vascular	Insufficiency
Aneurysm	
Neurological	Neuropathy

What are yellow flag risk factors in acute back pain and what do they suggest?

Yellow flags are **psychosocial risk factors** which suggest an increased likelihood of developing chronic disability – they include:

- Belief that back pain is harmful or potentially severely disabling.
- Fear avoidance behaviour and reduced activity levels.
- Tendency to low mood and withdrawal from social interaction.
- An expectation of passive treatment(s) rather than a belief that active participation will help.

What investigations would you perform in this patient?

Lumbar spine radiography
Not recommended for low back pain in the absence of red flags even if the pain has persisted for 6 weeks. Lumbar spine radiography has a low yield in

terms of useful findings and suffers from a disparity with regard to interpretation between clinicians. There is a poor correlation between pain and changes found on X-ray. Plain radiographs are good at showing the lytic lesions of multiple myeloma.

Bone scans

Bone scans do not have a place in the diagnostic evaluation of back pain in the absence of red flags. It can be difficult to distinguish degenerative disease from bone metastases.

Magnetic resonance imaging and CT

Radiological evidence of disc and bony abnormalities are found in the normal asymptomatic population and are only weakly associated with back pain.

Radiological evidence of prolapsed intervertebral discs occurs in over 25% of asymptomatic subjects. MRI is considered the gold standard for investigating spinal abnormalities.

CT is superior to MRI in detecting bone tumours in flat bones such as the pelvis, whilst MRI is superior for imaging long bones and the spine. CT is unreliable in the diagnosis of disc lesions, but CT myelography may be used in patients who are unable to have an MRI scan.

What treatment modalities are available for the management of chronic back pain?

- Pharmacology
- Physical therapies
- Surgery
- Injection therapies
- Neuromodulation
- Complementary therapies
- Psychological therapies.

Pharmacology

- Tricyclic antidepressants and anti-convulsants – for neuropathic pain. Tricyclic antidepressants are particularly useful where pain is causing sleep disturbance because of their sedative side effects.
- Paracetamol: no evidence of benefit but low likelihood of harm.
- NSAIDS: moderate evidence for efficacy.
- Opiates should be titrated against the level of chronic lower back pain and should be prescribed as part of a multimodal interdisciplinary treatment plan. Benefits of opioid therapy may include an increased ability to interact with family, function in the household and improved sleep.

Injection techniques

Epidural steroid injections which can be:

■ Interlaminar – moderate evidence for short term relief (NNT of 7,3 for 75% pain relief in the short term 1–60 days) and limited for long-term relief (NNT of 13 for greater than 50% pain relief in the long term 12 weeks to 1 year).
■ Transforaminal – strong evidence for short- and long-term relief.

Chronic mechanical lower back pain.

■ Facet joint injections
■ Radiofrequency lumbar facet denervation
■ Botulinum toxin A injections.

A Cochrane review summarized the evidence for injection therapy by saying that facet joint, epidural and local injection therapy has not yet been shown to be effective nor has it shown to be ineffective. A solid evidence base is lacking; however there is no justification for abandoning injection therapy in patients with chronic lower back pain.

Neuromodulation
Transcutaneous electrical nerve stimulation (TENS) is widely used and is relatively safe. However there is no conclusive evidence for its effectiveness in chronic pain according to a Cochrane review (Carrol, D *et al.* 2002).

Psychological therapies
Cognitive behavioural therapy (CBT) is effective in reducing the pain experience and improving positive behavioural expression, appraisal and coping in patients with chronic pain.

Physical therapies
The avoidance of immobility and the participation in physical exercise is essential in the rehabilitation of the chronic back pain sufferer who exists in a cycle, which consists of avoiding activity through fear of pain. This results in weakness of musculature from disuse leading to disability and depression causing further pain. Improving spinal muscle strength is likely to improve symptoms.

An MRI scan report shows metastatic disease to his lumbar vertebrae. What treatment modalities are used to treat metastatic bone pain?

Initial management will focus on analgesia according to the **WHO analgesic ladder. Non-steroidal anti-inflammatory drugs** are used in metastatic bone pain, based on the role that prostaglandins play in this pathology.

Radiotherapy plays a central role in the management of metastatic bone pain particularly where the pain is localised. A meta-analysis of radiotherapy for metastatic bone pain demonstrated that 27% of patients achieved complete pain relief at 1 month (NNT 3,9) and 29% achieved at least 50% pain relief at 1 month post-radiotherapy (NNT 3,6).

Widespread bone metastases may be treated with **chemotherapy.**

Prostate and other hormone sensitive cancers may be treated with **hormone manipulation.**

Bibliography

Jensen TS, Wilson PR, Rice ASC. (2003). *Clinical Pain Management: Chronic Pain*. London, UK: Arnold.

Moore A, Edwards J, Barden J, McQuay H. (2003). *Bandolier's Little Book of Pain*. Oxford, UK: Oxford University Press.

Stannard C, Booth S. (2004). *Pain*, 2nd edition. London, UK: Elsevier Limited.

Sykes N, Fallon MT, Patt RB. (2003). *Clinical Pain Management: Cancer Pain*. London, UK: Arnold.

Addendum

NICE Clinical Guideline 88. Low back pain: Early management of persistent non-specific low back pain. May 2009.

This guidline has altered the principles of management of low back pain to include the following:

- an exercise programme
- a course of manual therapy
- a course of acupuncture

Long Case 18

'The one about the smoker with bellyache and sepsis'

A 50-year-old man is admitted to hospital with severe abdominal pain and right upper quadrant tenderness. He is in his late 50s, smokes 20 cigarettes per day and has previously been a heavy drinker.

O/E		
	Respiratory rate	23 breaths/min
	Heart rate	110 beats/min
	Blood Pressure	90/60
	Temperature	38.5 °C
Investigations	Hb	11 g/dl
	WCC	20×10^9/l
	Neutrophils	14×10^9/l
	Platelets	98×10^9/l
	Na	140 mmol/l
	K	4.0 mmol/l
	Urea	8.6 mmol/l
	Creatinine	156 μmol/l
	AST	120 IU/l (normal range 10–40)
	ALT	110 IU/l (normal range 5–40)
	Alk Phos	98 IU/l (normal range 25–115)
	Bilirubin	32 mg/dl (normal range <17).

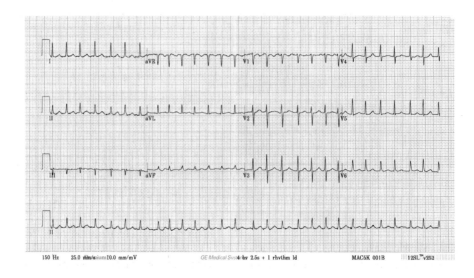

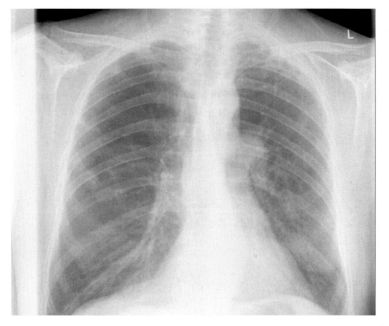

1. Can you summarise the case?

This 50-year-old gentleman, with a history of smoking and alcohol abuse, presents with evidence of severe sepsis. He satisfies all four criteria that comprise the systemic inflammatory response syndrome (SIRS). The significantly raised white cell count and the clinical signs suggest an intra-abdominal infective process. He is hypotensive and has some end-organ dysfunction as evidenced by a raised urea and creatinine. He has abnormal liver function tests, which are likely to be related to the right upper quadrant pain. He is also thrombocytopaenic, mildly anaemic and has atrial fibrillation with a rapid ventricular response.

> **Society of Critical Care Medicine / American College of Chest Physicians Definitions.**
>
> **SIRS** — Diagnosed if two or more of the following are present:
> - Temp >38 °C or <36 °C
> - HR > 90 bpm
> - RR > 20 bpm
> - WCC <4 or > 12 x 10^9/l
>
> **Sepsis**   - SIRS plus signs of infection
> **Severe sepsis**   - Sepsis associated with organ dysfunction
> **Septic shock**   - Severe sepsis with hypotension despite adequate fluid resuscitation.

The ECG shows atrial fibrillation with a ventricular response rate of about 160 beats per minute.

The CXR is an PA film. There are bullae in both upper zones. The lung fields are clear.

2. What are the possible differential diagnoses?
The most likely diagnosis is acute pancreatitis or biliary sepsis, for example:

- Ascending cholangitis
- Acute cholecystitis
- Empyema of the gallbladder

Other differential diagnoses would include:

- Perforated peptic ulcer
- Acute myocardial infarction.

3. What do you think about the white cell count?
He has a raised white cell count with a neutrophilia, indicating an acute infective process.

4. What further investigations would you perform?
- Arterial blood gas analysis
- Serum amylase
- Abdominal ultrasound scan or CT scan
- Troponin T
- Two sets of blood cultures as well as urine and sputum cultures
- PT and APTT.

5. Do you think the patient requires further resuscitation?
A diagnosis of severe sepsis necessitates early, aggressive resuscitation. A key paper by Rivers *et al.* (2001) looked at exactly this type of scenario and showed that those patients who were resuscitated promptly to specific haemodynamic indices had a significantly improved survival at 28 and 60 days. These

parameters have since been included in the surviving sepsis campaign guidelines.

Targets for resuscitation in the Rivers study were:

- MAP > 65 mmHg
- CVP 8–12 mmHg
- Haematocrit >30%
- ScvO$_2$ (central venous oxygen saturation) >70%
  Fluids, vasopressors, inotropes and blood transfusions were used to achieve these targets.
- Broad spectrum antibiotics should be administered in the first hour and these should cover the common Gram-negative pathogens that cause biliary sepsis, e.g. *E coli*, *Klebsiella* and *Pseudomonas*.

Simultaneously with resuscitation, invasive monitoring should be placed, i.e. an arterial line and a multi-lumen central venous catheter. Oxygen therapy must be initiated and consideration should be given to intubation depending in part on the arterial blood gas results.

6. Where would you want this to take place?
The patient should be admitted to an intensive care area. However, resuscitation should not be delayed while this is arranged.

7. On CT scan he has a perforated gallbladder and biliary peritonitis. The surgeon on call wants to take him to theatre immediately – when would you be happy to anaesthetise him?
Anaesthetising an inadequately resuscitated patient risks catastrophic cardiovascular compromise on induction of anaesthesia. The timing of surgery is therefore a balance between achieving adequate organ perfusion and the need to eradicate the source of the sepsis. Restoration of an adequate circulating volume, a MAP > 65 mmHg and cardiovascular stability would be desirable. This operation is life-saving and he should go to theatre as soon as he is resuscitated.

8. How would you proceed?
- Once in the anaesthetic room, having taken a brief anaesthetic history and assessed the airway, I would ensure that invasive monitoring was in situ in addition to the usual minimum monitoring standards.
- Trained assistance, readily available cardiovascular drugs (particularly a vasopressor such as metaraminol) and a fast running drip would be required.
- I would perform a modified rapid sequence induction. After 3 minutes of pre-oxygenation, I would give 100 mcg of fentanyl and a titrated dose of thiopentone followed by suxamethonium, being aware of the likely effect of the drugs on the patient's blood pressure.
- Anaesthesia could be maintained with isoflurane in oxygen and air, with fentanyl for intra-operative analgesia.

- Maintenance of an adequate MAP and CVP using clear fluids, blood and vasopressors according to the Rivers criteria are reasonable goals.
- Multimodal intra-operative analgesia using opioids and paracetamol should be used. NSAIDS should be avoided in this patient because of their effects on renal function. The presence of sepsis militates against performing an epidural in this patient.
- Even though at present the patient is pyrexial, devices such as fluid warmers and a forced-air warming blanket should be in place to prevent hypothermia.
- The blood bank should be informed if the patient had a coagulopathy in case blood products are required.
- Being aware of the lung bullae, the airway pressures should be kept low and a lung-protective ventilation strategy may also help to address any subsequent associated lung injury.
- During the case, the blood gases should be monitored and this may help to determine whether the patient can be extubated at the end of the case.
- The patient should be returned to the intensive care unit.

9. The patient is transferred to ICU where he develops severe sepsis. What therapeutic strategies are employed on critical care units in patients with severe sepsis?

In recent years the European Society of Critical Care Medicine, amongst others, have developed the **surviving sepsis campaign**. This initiative comprises a set of evidence-based recommendations looking at many aspects of the management of patients with severe sepsis. As well as incorporating the Rivers' parameters already mentioned, other aspects addressed are:

- **Ventilation:** Low (6 ml/kg) as opposed to high (12 ml/kg) tidal volumes have been shown to decrease the mortality rate by 9% as well as lowering levels of cytokines and decreasing end-organ dysfunction in patients with acute lung injury. There is no difference in mortality between patients treated with high levels of PEEP and the levels used by the ARDS Clinical Trials Network Group.
- **Activated protein C:** The mechanism of action whereby APC improves outcome is unknown. The modulation of coagulation may not be the primary mechanism underlying the anti-hypotensive effect of APC. APC also has anti-inflammatory and anti-apoptotic effects. Considering the evidence from the trials below, it appears to be effective in patients with a high risk of death and severe sepsis (NNT 7.7).

    PROWESS (Recombinant APC Worldwide Evaluation in Severe Sepsis.)

    ADDRESS (the administration of drotrecogin alfa in early stage severe sepsis) – No benefit in low risk groups. This has led to debate about the efficacy of APC and a further large-scale trial is planned.

    ENHANCE (Extended Evaluation of Recombinant Human Activated Protein C United States).

PROWESS inclusion criteria

Severe sepsis based on a modified version of the ACCP-SCCM 1992 guidelines
Documented or suspected infection
At least three SIRS criteria
Evidence of at least one acute (<24 h) organ dysfunction.
Specifically:
o **Infection**: Known or suspected to have infection with at least one of the following:

- White blood cells present in a sterile site
- Perforated viscus
- Radiographic evidence of pneumonia plus purulent sputum
- High risk for infection (e.g. ascending cholangitis).

o **Modified SIRS criteria**:

- Patient had at least three of the four criteria.

o **Organ or system dysfunction**: At least one of the following five criteria:

- CVS: systolic blood pressure of 90 mm Hg or less, or mean arterial pressure of 70 mm Hg or less for at least 1 hour, despite adequate fluid resuscitation, adequate intravascular volume or use of vasopressors.
- Renal: urine output less than 0.5 ml/kg per hour for 1 hour despite adequate fluid resuscitation.
- Respiratory: ratio of $PaO_2:FIO_2$ of 250 or less if other organ dysfunction, or 200 or less if the lung was the only dysfunctional organ.
- Rheumatologic: platelet count of $80 \times 10^3/mm^3$ or less, or a decrease by 50% in the preceding 3 days.
- Unexplained metabolic acidosis: pH of 7.30 or less, or base deficit of at least 5 mmol/l with lactate more than 1.5 times above the upper limit of normal.

Contraindications to APC (according to PROWESS)

- Trauma or surgery within the last 12 hours
- Active haemorrhage
- Concurrent anticoagulation
- Thrombocytopaenia (platelets <30 000/ cubic mm)
- Recent stroke.

Intensive insulin therapy
Hyperglycaemia has the following deleterious effects in sepsis:

- Procoagulant
- Induces apoptosis
- Increases the risk of infection
- Impairs neutrophil function
- Impairs wound healing

▓ Increased risk of death.

Insulin has anti-inflammatory, anti-apoptotic and anticoagulant effects. Van Den Berghe (2006) randomised intubated surgical patients who were not septic to receive intensive insulin therapy to maintain blood glucose between 4.4–6.1 mmol/l or 10–11.1 mmol/l and demonstrated increased survival for those in the former group especially those with ICU stays of more than 5 days. This effect was not seen in a study of medical patients and demonstrated increased risk of death in patients with ICU stays of less than 3 days. The role of intensive insulin therapy in patients with sepsis needs to be evaluated.

Corticosteroids in patients with sepsis who require critical care
Early 48 hour course of corticosteroids does not improve survival in severe sepsis (level 1 evidence)

Other therapies in patients with sepsis

▓ Enteral nutrition
▓ Stress ulcer prophylaxis
▓ Avoidance of neuromuscular blockers
▓ Sedation breaks
▓ Minimise the use of steroids
▓ DVT prophylaxis where appropriate.

Bibliography
Bernard GR, Vincent JL, Laterre PF et al. (2001). Efficacy and safety of recombinant human activated protein C for severe sepsis. New England Journal of Medicine, **344**, 699–709.

Jackson WL. (2005). Should we use etomidate as an induction agent for endotracheal intubation in patients with septic shock? A critical appraisal. Chest **127**, 1031–8.

Rivers E (2001). Early goal-directed therapy in the treatment of severe sepsis and septic shock. New England Journal of Medicine, **345**, 1368–77.

Russell JA. (2006). Management of sepsis. New England Journal of Medicine, **355**, 1699–713.

Van Den Berghe G, Wilmer A, Hermans G. et al. (2006). Intensive insulin therapy in the medical ICU. New England Journal of Medicine, **354**, 449–61.

www.survivingsepsis.org.

Long Case 19

'The one about atrial fibrillation post AAA repair'

You see a 70-year-old man 4 days after he has undergone abdominal aortic aneurysm repair. His past medical history includes a transient ischaemic attack, non-insulin-dependent diabetes mellitus, hypertension and shortness of breath on exertion.

The CXR shows pulmonary oedema, cardiomegaly and right lower lobe collapse with tracheal deviation.

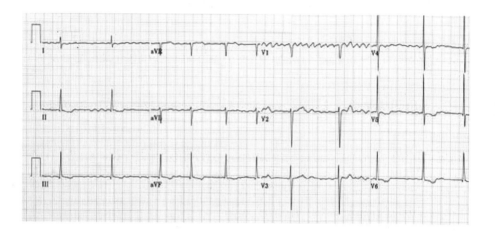

Na	131	mmol/l	(136−148)
K	3.6	mmol/l	(3.8−5.0)
Urea	13.2	mmol/l	(2.5−6.5)
Creatinine	131	μmol/l	(60−120)
Calcium	2.41	mmol/l	(2.12−2.63)
AST	22	IU/l	(7−40)
Total protein	70	g/l	(60−80)
Albumin	41	g/l	(30−52)
Bilirubin	11	μmol/l	(3−17)
Alkaline phos	54	IU/l	(50−130)
RBC	4.29	x10¹²/l	(3.80−5.80)
Hb	13.0	g/dl	(11.5−16.5)
PCV	0.370		(0.37−0.47)
MCV	86.5	fl	(79−97)
MCH	30.4	pg	(27.0−32.0)

MCHC	35.1	g/dl	(32.0–36.0)
RDW	13.7		(11.5–16.0)
PLT	188	x10⁹/l	(150–400)
MPV	10.1	fl	(6.5–9.5)
WCC	12.1	x10⁹/l	(4.0–11.0)
Neutrophils	11.58	x10⁹/l	(2.5–7.5)

1. Tell me about the ECG

The rate is approximately 80 bpm, but the rhythm is irregularly irregular. There are flutter waves seen in the V1 rhythm strip. The axis is normal. There are no Q waves and the QRS width is normal. There is evidence of infero-lateral ischaemia shown by the inverted and biphasic T waves in this territory (II, III, aVF and V3–V6). There is borderline LVH by voltage criteria.

2. What is atrial fibrillation?

- **Supra-ventricular arrhythmia** characterized by the complete absence of co-ordinated atrial contractions.
- No discernable p-waves.
- The ventricular response rate depends on the conduction of the AV node.

3. What is the difference between atrial fibrillation and flutter?

- Flutter is a more organised and regular form of atrial activity.
- Classically with an atrial rate of 300 bpm.
- 'Saw toothed' flutter waves are present on the ECG.
- The ventricular response depends on conduction through the AV node.
- The classic ECG has 2:1 block, hence a ventricular rate of 150 bpm.

4. Discuss the electrolyte results – are these typical of such patients post-op?

The post-operative electrolytes are influenced by many different factors

- Pre-op levels
- Drug therapy
- Renal function
- Iatrogenic fluid management
- Stress response to surgery.
- The sodium is often low due to water retention in excess of sodium causing a dilutional state. There may have been hypotonic fluids administered.
- The potassium may not have been adequately replaced, or the patient may be chronically depleted due to chronic diuretic administration. Insulin and catecholamines cause uptake of potassium into cells and may have been administered.

■ The urea and creatinine are slightly elevated, which probably represents pre-existing reno-vascular disease in this arteriopath. Compromised renal blood flow post-op should be assessed by monitoring the urine output and serial results. A period of renal ischaemia may have occurred intra-operatively due to clamping of the aorta if the disease involved the origins of the renal arteries.

5. What are the possible causes of the AF?

The commonest causes in the peri-operative period relate to changes in fluid and electrolyte balance, the response to surgery and systemic inflammation. Omission of regular cardiac drugs such as β-blockers is also an important causative factor.

Causes of atrial fibrillation
In the peri-operative setting:

■ Hypovolaemia
■ Systemic inflammation/S.I.R.S./ 'hyperadrenergic' state
■ Electrolyte abnormalities especially low potassium or magnesium
■ Withdrawal of β-blockers
■ Following cardiac surgery.

Other more 'medical' causes:

■ Structural heart disease (ASD or mitral valve disease)
■ Ischaemic heart disease
■ Thyrotoxicosis
■ Excess caffeine or alcohol (acute or chronic)
■ Pulmonary embolism
■ Pneumonia
■ Pericarditis.

'Lone AF' is AF in the absence of any demonstrable medical cause, but this is not usually diagnosed in the peri-operative period.
    Loss of the atrial 'kick' as it contracts and empties into the LV can reduce LV filling (and hence CO) by 10%–20% with a normal ventricle. LV filling may be reduced by 40%–50% in those with a 'stiff' ventricle (diastolic dysfunction), e.g. with aortic stenosis.
    The disorganised contractions of the atria cause stasis of blood and the risk of thromboembolism. There is a 3%–7% annual risk of thromboembolic CVA.

---

6. How would you identify the causes in this situation?

Knowledge of the patient's history and an assessment of volume status and electrolytes would help to identify the cause. An ECG should be performed to help exclude acute ischaemia.

In the context of major vascular surgery, systemic inflammation and a heightened adrenergic state are likely to play a major role. This may explain why β-blockers are efficacious in this setting.

7. What other ways do you know to identify AF?
- The pulse will be irregularly irregular.
- An absence of p waves on the ECG monitor.
- No 'a wave' in the jugular venous pulsation as this is caused by sinus atrial contraction.
- Chaotic atrial activity can be seen on echocardiography.

8. Discuss AF management in the intensive care unit

> Assess for **cardiovascular compromise,** and resuscitate simultaneously if needed. **Oxygen** should be administered, continual **ECG monitoring** instituted and **IV access** secured.

- Signs of cardiovascular compromise requiring urgent intervention are
  - Systolic BP < 90 mmHg
  - Signs of heart failure
  - Chest pain
  - HR > 150 bpm.
- If these signs are present, then urgent **synchronised DC cardioversion** is required. An attempt to correct electrolyte and volume abnormalities should be made concurrently.
- In the stable patient, restoration of sinus rhythm is the aim. This can be done electrically or pharmacologically.

9. What drugs would you administer?
If the onset is within 7 days and the patient does not have any underlying ischaemic heart disease or ventricular dysfunction, then Vaughan–Williams Class Ic drugs are appropriate, such as **propafenone** or **flecanide**. Otherwise, a class III drug such as **amiodarone** is recommended.

10. The medics get involved and suggest DC cardioversion (DCC). Assuming that this patient is cardiovascularly stable, is it safe to proceed with DCC now?
There are a number of points to consider:

- General anaesthetic assessment and fasting times.
- When did the AF start (history of palpitations or recording on monitor) and is it acute or chronic?
- What is the likelihood of an **atrial thrombus** which could be embolised by reverting the atria to sinus rhythm?
- What is the ventricular rate now? – may need pacing after cardioversion if the rate is below 60 bpm.

■ Has there been an ischaemic episode?

> **Cardioversion and Anticoagulation**
> Cardioversion should only be attempted without anticoagulation if the duration of the AF is less than 48 hours. If the duration is unknown or longer than this, then 3–4 weeks of anticoagulation (INR 2–3) is required to reduce the incidence of clot embolisation. If there is a contra-indication to anticoagulation, or if the cardioversion is deemed necessary more urgently, then an echocardiogram is needed to exclude thrombus in the atrium and atrial appendage.

11. How would you anaesthetise him for cardioversion?

This should be done in a critical care or theatre area with the usual preparation, equipment and assistance needed for any routine anaesthetic. Someone independent should be present to perform the defibrillation, preferably with a hands-free device.

Elective cardioversion has been done under conscious sedation without any adverse effects, but the usual technique is to use a sleep dose of propofol following pre-oxygenation. One could maintain the airway with a facemask or an LMA.

12. Would you use any invasive monitoring?

This would be influenced by the patient's cardiovascular response to the general anaesthetic 4 days previously and by the current cardiovascular stability. If there is any serious doubt about cardiovascular performance or reserve, an arterial line should be given consideration, but this is a short procedure and the cardiac output should improve with the restoration of sinus rhythm.

13. If the patient had a pacemaker in situ or an implantable cardiac defibrillator, is it safe to administer a shock?

Yes. You should place the paddles as far away as possible from the device and preferably in the anterior–posterior position.

14. If the patient did not cardiovert, what would you do?

You can try an AP shock. If this fails, try a period of 4–6 weeks of medical therapy and anticoagulation. If the patient is still in AF, then a further trial of DCC is reasonable.

If a second DCC is unsuccessful, then rate control is the next step to improve symptoms and reduce ventricular failure.

15. What drugs would you use here then?

Drugs that block AV conduction such as β-blockers, the non-dihydropyridine calcium channel blockers (verapamil or diltiazem) or digoxin.

16. Are there any times when you wouldn't use these drugs for a patient presenting with a supra-ventricular tachycardia?

Patients who have pre-excitation syndromes with an accessory conduction pathway between the atria and ventricles (such as in the **Wolff–Parkinson–White syndrome**) should **not be given AV node blocking drugs** if they develop an SVT. This will promote the atrial impulses to travel directly to the ventricle at up to 300 bpm via the accessory pathway. The drugs of choice are amiodarone, flecainide or procainamide.

Bibliography

Bajpai A, Rowland E. (2006). Atrial fibrillation. *Continuing Education in Anaesthesia, Critical Care and Pain.* **6**(6), 219–24.

Fuster V, Ryden L, Goldman L. *et al.* (2001). ACC/AHA/ESC guidelines for the management of patients with atrial fibrillation: Executive summary. *Circulation*, **104**, 2118–50.

Nolan J. (2005). Peri-arrest arrythmias. *Resus Council (UK) Guidelines*. www.resus.org.uk/pages.

Long Case 20

'The one about pre-op assessment of IHD'

A 67-year-old man is scheduled for an elective abdominal aortic aneurysm repair. He has had hypertension for about 8 years and occasional exertional angina for about 3 years.

Medication	Trandolapril	4 mg once daily
	Atenolol	50 mg once daily
	ISMN	5 mg once daily

Clinical examination	Heart rate 70 bpm
	BP 160/90 mmHg
	JVP not elevated.
	Scattered crackles at both lung bases

Investigations	Normal FBC and U & E

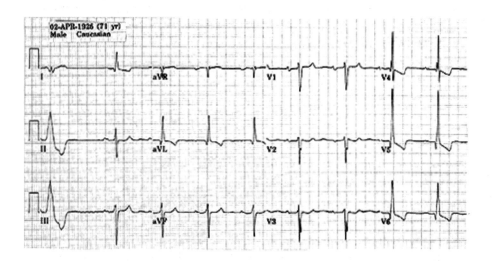

02-APR-1926 (71 yr)
Male Caucasian

1. Can you summarise this case?

This is a 67-year-old arteriopath with significant history of ischaemic heart disease and poorly controlled hypertension. He is scheduled to undergo major vascular surgery. Regarding his medication, if there are no contraindications, he should probably be on a statin and aspirin. From his chest examination, there is a small possibility that he has pulmonary oedema. His other investigations are unremarkable, other than an ischaemic ECG with strain pattern. He is at high risk of major peri-operative cardiac events.

2. Talk me through his ECG

The rate is 60 bpm and the rhythm is sinus as evidenced by the p waves before each QRS complex. There is one ventricular ectopic. There is left axis deviation. The PR interval is normal and there are no pathological Q waves. The R wave in V5 is >35 mm and there is down-sloping ST depression in the lateral chest leads and leads I and aVL. These findings would be consistent with left ventricular hypertrophy with a strain pattern. This would be compatible with a history of ischaemic heart disease and hypertension.

3. What do you think of the clinical findings?

Clinical examination reveals chest signs, which could possibly indicate LVF or a chest infection. Scattered bibasal crackles are, however, not uncommon and his JVP is not elevated and there is no mention of other clinical signs of cardiac failure such as tachypnoea, pitting oedema, a gallop rhythm or ascites. His WCC is not elevated and there are no reported symptoms to support a diagnosis of a lower respiratory tract infection. A chest X-ray would assess his cardiac size and help to distinguish between a cardiac and a respiratory cause.

4. Do you think his blood pressure is adequately controlled?

No. The British Hypertension Society recommends, for patients with diabetes, renal impairment or established cardiovascular disease (the case here) a target of ≤130/80 mm Hg. A knowledge of previous blood pressure readings would help ascertain if this is a 'one-off' high, or if the BP has been elevated for some time. He is already established on an ACE inhibitor, a β-blocker and a nitrate. Non-compliance with his medication should also be considered as a cause of the poor control of his blood pressure.

He has other risk factors for cardiovascular disease and a history of angina that makes chronic blood pressure control even more important. If time permits, adding a thiazide diuretic or a calcium channel antagonist to his regime may help long-term control.

If the surgery is urgent, then there are increased risks of cardiovascular events including MI, LVF, intracerebral haemorrhage and renal failure. Perfusion pressures will have to be maintained at higher levels than normal.

See British Hypertension Society / NICE guidelines (*Clinical guideline 34,* June 2006) and see short question on uncontrolled hypertension.

5. What do you think about the risk of him having a peri-operative cardiac event?

The risk is high. Evaluation of cardiovascular risk for elective surgery involves:

■ Identification of risk factors and potentially correctable co-morbidity
■ Appropriate intervention to reduce risk and improve outcome.

Goldman et al. (1978) were the first to use **scoring systems** to stratify the risk of peri-operative cardiac events by assigning points based on clinical risk factors and combining these with surgical factors. This type of system has been used since 1978 and works well to identify high-risk patients, but is less useful for intermediate or low risk patients and doesn't give guidance for peri-operative assessment.

The **Revised Cardiac Risk Index** performs best in studies that have compared risk indices head-to-head. This system is widely used. This patient would score points for a high-risk surgical procedure (AAA), a history of ischaemic heart disease and a history of congestive cardiac failure (crackles in both lungs). This would make him Class IV with a risk of 11% of a major cardiac event.

Revised Cardiac Risk Index (*Circulation* 1999, **100**, 1043–49)
Each risk factor is assigned one point.
High-risk surgical procedures

■ Intraperitoneal
■ Intrathoracic
■ Supra-inguinal vascular.

History of ischaemic heart disease

■ History of myocardial infarction
■ History of positive exercise test
■ Current complain of chest pain considered secondary to myocardial ischaemia
■ Use of nitrate therapy
■ ECG with pathological Q waves.

History of congestive heart failure

■ Pulmonary oedema
■ Paroxysmal nocturnal dyspnoea
■ Bilateral rales or S3 gallop
■ Chest radiograph showing pulmonary vascular redistribution.

History of cerebrovascular disease

■ History of transient ischaemic attack or stroke

Pre-operative treatment with insulin
Pre-operative serum creatinine > 2.0 mg/dl (= 177 μmol/l)

RISK OF MAJOR CARDIAC EVENT

Points	Class	Risk
0	I	0.4%
1	II	0.9%
2	III	6.6%
3 or more	IV	11%

ACC/AHA 2007 *Guidelines on Peri-operative Cardiovascular Evaluation and Care for Non-cardiac Surgery*
'Intervention is rarely necessary to simply lower the risk of surgery unless such intervention is indicated irrespective of the pre-operative context.'
Major clinical risk factors: – considered to represent major clinical risk

- Unstable coronary syndromes
  - Unstable / severe angina
  - Recent MI (<1 month)
- Decompensated heart failure
- Significant arrhythmias (e.g. VT , uncontrolled AF, third-degree block)
- Severe valvular heart disease.

Clinical risk factors: (derived from the Revised Cardiac Risk Index, except type of surgery)

- Mild, stable angina
- Previous MI by history or pathologic Q waves (>1 month)
- Compensated or prior heart failure
- Diabetes mellitus (particularly insulin-dependent)
- Renal insufficiency.

Minor predictors (e.g. age, abnormal ECG, uncontrolled hypertension) – not incorporated into recommendations.

For several years now, the **American College of Cardiology and the American Heart Association (ACC/AHA)** have produced guidelines that provide a framework for considering cardiac risk in non-cardiac surgery (most recently updated in 2007). It is not a scoring system, but looks critically at the evidence and risks/benefits of different pre-operative investigations and treatments for patients with various risk factors.

6. How do you assess functional capacity?
This can be assessed by history of exercise tolerance, or more formally with exercise testing in a monitored environment. Functional capacity can be assessed using the Duke Activity Status Index. Patients who can't sustain 4 METs of activity have poor outcomes following major surgery.

Classification of functional capacity

1—4 METs Poor   Eating, dressing, walking around the house.
4—7 METs Moderate Climbing one flight of stairs, walking on the
                                flat at 4 mph
7—10 METs Good   Carrying shopping upstairs, cycling, jogging
>10 METs Excellent

Functional capacity assessment

- **Cardiopulmonary exercise (CPX) testing**
- **Exercise ECG testing**
  - Detects myocardial ischaemia with ST changes or hypotension
  - No good if can't exercise, e.g. arthritis, or interpret ECG, e.g. LBBB, digoxin.
- **Pharmacological stress testing**
  - Thallium – taken up by perfused heart muscle
  - Dipyridamole acts as coronary vasodilator
  - Permanent cold spots demonstrate un-perfused myocardium
  - Reversible cold spots demonstrate impaired coronary flow.
- **Dobutamine stress echocardiography**
- Looks for new or worsening wall motion abnormalities implying ischaemia.
- Time consuming.

Functional capacity and METs

METs are metabolic equivalents and are multiples of the basal metabolic rate (assumed to be 3.5 ml/kg per min).

Stair climbing is not standardised, but climbing two flights of stairs is considered to demand at least 4 METs.

VO_{2max} is the point when oxygen uptake plateaus during exercise, despite increasing work. The *anaerobic threshold* is the point where extra oxygen-independent metabolism is required to sustain performance. This can be determined by lactate or CO_2 measurement. The point where lactate or CO_2 (ventilation) start to rise exponentially is the lactate or ventilation threshold and, although these points are not exactly the same, the ventilatory threshold is easily reproducible, and is accepted to be the anaerobic threshold in pre-op testing.

CPX testing is cardiopulmonary exercise testing, usually done on a bicycle, with ECG and expired gas monitoring. It is expensive and time consuming, but research has shown it to be a valuable predictor of cardiovascular functional reserve for major surgery. More units are getting access to these testing facilities in the UK.

7. What further assessments would you like in this case?

There are various algorithms for determining the course of action based on the pre-op assessment and the urgency for surgery. I would take the stepwise approach to peri-operative cardiac assessment recommended by the ACC/AHA taskforce. Namely:

1. **Determine the urgency of the surgery**. In this case how big is the aneurysm and what is the likelihood of rupture?
2. **Does the patient have one of the major cardiac risk factors?** It doesn't sound like he has decompensated heart failure but the bibasal crackles are cause for concern. He has a history of angina and the stability of his symptoms would need to be ascertained.
3. **Is the patient undergoing low-risk surgery?** – No.
4. **Does the patient have good functional capacity without symptoms?**
5. If the patient has **poor functional capacity**, is **symptomatic**, or has **unknown functional capacity**, then the presence of active clinical risk factors will determine the need for further evaluation.

Cardiac risk stratification for non-cardiac surgical procedures

Risk stratification	Procedure examples
Vascular (reported cardiac risk often more than 5%)	Aortic and other major vascular surgery Peripheral vascular surgery
Intermediate (reported cardiac risk generally 1% to 5%)	Intraperitoneal and intrathoracic surgery Carotid endarterectomy Head and neck surgery Orthopaedic surgery Prostate surgery
Low (reported cardiac risk generally less than 1%)	Endoscopic procedures Superficial procedure Cataract surgery Breast surgery Ambulatory surgery

---

- He should have functional capacity testing (exercise ECG, CPX testing), unless his physical performance is excellent as assessed by history (e.g. Duke Activity Status Index.)
- Depending on the result of this, he may require coronary angiography.
- Any intervention indicated by the testing should be done prior to surgery (e.g. PTCA or CABG).
- Indications are the same as for those patients not undergoing surgery.
- Elective surgery should be delayed for 3 months following CABG.

> It is worth noting that functional investigations reveal critical coronary stenoses and not all peri-operative MIs are associated with such lesions.

8. Would you continue his atenolol?

Yes. β-blockers should be continued in patients undergoing surgery who are receiving β-blockers to treat angina, symptomatic arrhythmias, hypertension, or other ACC/AHA Class I guideline indications. Recent studies have shown that preventing peri-operative myocardial ischaemia with pharmacological interventions reduces the risk of myocardial infarction. Treatment with β-blockers is of benefit in those with proven coronary artery disease who are undergoing major surgery. The other combinations of cardiac risk and surgical stratification are less clear and judgements should be made on an individual basis. Most patients do tolerate acute β-blockade well, although gradual treatment introduced over a few weeks is preferable. Some patients will experience bradycardias and some, including those with new LV wall motion abnormalities, will develop LV failure.

> See short question on ischaemic heart disease

9. What about his other medications?

■ ACE inhibitors improve survival in those who have impaired LV function, diabetes and ischaemic heart disease. Data regarding their use peri-operatively is inconclusive but the current recommendation is to stop them the day before surgery to avoid adverse haemodynamic changes intra-operatively. They should then be re-introduced gradually post-op.

■ The nitrate should be continued.

10. What about this man's pre-operative investigations? What do you want to do? Would you delay surgery to get them done?

He is having high risk surgery (>5% mortality) and has active clinical risk factors for cardiovascular disease (stable angina.) He should have his functional capacity assessed, ideally by CPX testing, thallium or exercise ECG, especially if his history of exercise tolerance is poor. If these tests indicated coronary ischaemia, he should have an angiogram. Surgery should be delayed to facilitate these investigations and would afford the opportunity to control his hypertension.

11. Let's assume he has excellent exercise tolerance and he comes back with controlled blood pressure after the addition of a calcium channel blocker. How would you anaesthetise him?

This operation requires general anaesthesia and has the potential for major blood loss and fluid shifts.

- A sedative pre-medication such as temazepam would be useful in controlling any anxiety pre-operatively.
- Ensure his usual cardiac drugs given on the morning of surgery (except ACE inhibitor).
- Standard basic monitoring should be supplemented with an arterial line and two large bore cannulate sited prior to induction.
- Site a thoracic epidural prior to induction for post-operative analgesia (see box).
- Induction with fentanyl 2 mcg/kg, slow bolus of propofol to 3 mg/kg, and then muscle relaxant such as Atracurium 0.5 mg/kg assuming he is fasted, with no reflux, and a normal airway assessment.
- I would maintain him with a volatile anaesthetic in oxygen and air
- A central line is useful as an indication of filling and to allow the use of vasopressors.
- Additional haemodynamic (flow) monitoring would be useful, e.g. oesophageal doppler or pulse-contour analysis.

12. Are you concerned about anything you may have to give with regards to his epidural?

Heparin is given during these cases and there is potential for an epidural bleed. The risk of this must be balanced with the risk of post-operative pain, which will be significant in a population who are arteriopaths. The risk is very low especially given the time period that is likely to elapse between siting the epidural and administering the heparin. It should be remembered that heparin is not a fibrinolytic agent.

Bibliography
Biccard BM. (2005). Relationship between the inability to climb two flights of stairs and outcome after major surgery: implications for the pre-operative assessment of functional capacity. *Anaesthesia*, **60**, 588–93.

Fleisher LA, ACC/AHA (2007). Guidelines on Perioperative Cardiovascular Evaluation and Care for Noncardiac Surgery. http://www.acc.org/clinical/guidelines/perio/dirIndex.htm.

Fleisher L, Beckman JA, Brown KA. *et al*. ACC/AHA (2006). Guideline Update on Perioperative Cardiovascular Evaluation for Noncardiac Surgery: Focused Update on Perioperative Beta-Blocker Therapy. A Report of the American College of Cardiology/American Heart Association Task Force on Practice Guidelines. www.acc.org/clinical/guidelines/perio_betablocker.pdf.

Goldman L, Caldera DL, Nussbaum SR. *et al*. (1978). Cardiac risk factors and complications in non-cardiac surgery. *Medicine*, **57**, 357–70.

Mangano DT, Layug EL, Wallace A, Tateo I. (1996). Effect of atenolol on mortality and cardiovascular morbidity after noncardiac surgery. *New England Journal of Medicine*, **335**, 1713–20.

Older P, Hall A. (2004). Clinical review: how to identify high-risk surgical patients. *Critical Care*, **8**(5), 369–72.

Older P, Hall A, Hader R. (1999). Cardiopulmonary exercise testing as a screening test for perioperative management of major surgery in the elderly. *Chest*, **116**(2), 355–62. http://www.bhsoc.org/NICE_BHS_Guidelines.stm.

Long Case 21

'The one about the manic depressive for a dental clearance'

A 45-yr-old male with a 29-year history of manic depression presents for a full dental clearance. He has had anaesthetics for multiple electroconvulsive therapy treatments in the past. He is a heavy smoker and a recently diagnosed hypertensive.

Medication Imipramine 150 mg daily (like amitriptyline TCA)
Lithium carbonate 400 mg daily
Flupentixol decanoate 100 mg every 4 weeks IM
Chlorpromazine Hydrochloride 150 mg daily
Amlodipine 10 mg daily

On examination Unkempt
Height 170 cm, Weight 110 kg (BMI 38)
Dry mouth and fine resting tremor
Loose teeth
BP 150/90, HR — 80 bpm
CVS — Normal
RS — widespread wheeze

Na	133	mmol/l	(136–148)
K	4.2	mmol/l	(3.8–5.0)
Urea	14.0	mmol/l	(2.5–6.5)
Creatinine	160	μmol/l	(60–120)
Hb	12.0	g/dl	(11.5–16.5)
MCV	88.9	fl	(79–97)
MCH	32.4	pg	(27.0–32.0)
MCHC	33.1	g/dl	(32.0–36.0)
PLT	221	×10⁹/l	(150–400)
WCC	11.0	×10⁹/l	(4.0–11.0)
Lithium level	1.0	mmol/l	(reference 0.4–1.0 mmol/l)

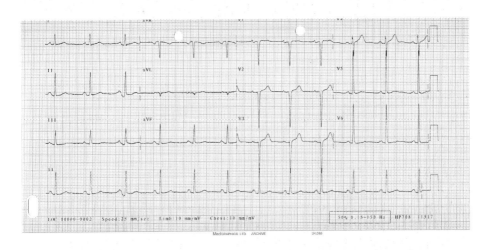

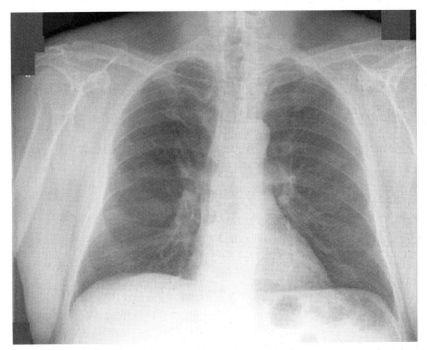

1. What are the problems with this patient?

There are several issues. This man takes multiple medications for the treatment of manic depression, he is obese with hypertension, renal impairment and possibly respiratory disease. In addition, he may have a difficult airway. This would need formal assessment with a combination of bedside tests. His obesity along with any airways disease will reduce his respiratory reserve and FRC. This, in turn, will reduce the amount of time available under anaesthesia to deal with a potentially difficult airway due to rapid desaturation. As a middle-aged heavy smoker, he is at risk of ischaemic heart disease and his ECG indicates left ventricular hypertrophy. He may have poorly controlled hypertension and his compliance with medication may not be reliable. The renal impairment may reflect end-organ damage from hypertension, intrinsic reno-vascular disease or may be associated with the lithium therapy.

2. What are the problems due to smoking?

Smoking is a risk factor for arterial disease including ischaemic heart disease. The respiratory effects include destruction of the alveoli and cilia, which can lead to COPD, emphysema and poor clearance of the copious amounts of mucus produced. The airways will be more irritable during manipulation, resulting in an increased risk of bronchospasm and laryngospasm during anaesthesia. Smokers are more prone to atelectasis and post-operative respiratory infections. COHb levels will be increased, often to 10%–15%, which impairs the oxygen carrying capacity of the blood. Finally, cigarette smoke contains nicotine, which stimulates the sympathetic nervous system, and carcinogens that increase the risk of lung and laryngeal neoplasia, in particular.

3. How do you classify obesity?

See short question on obesity.

4. What are the anaesthetic implications of obesity?

See short question on obesity.

5. Tell me about his anti-psychotic drugs and how they work.

He is on a combination of anti-psychotic drugs including a depot preparation, which may be to help with compliance.

Lithium is used in the treatment and maintenance of mania and bipolar disorder and acts as a 'mood stabiliser'. Lithium alters neuronal sodium transport and probably affects serotonin, noradrenaline and glutamate transmission. It has a narrow therapeutic range and levels must be carefully monitored. It becomes more active if the serum sodium concentration drops, so care must be taken when giving diuretics concurrently.

Flupentixol (previously spelt flupenthixol) specifically antagonises D1 and D2 dopamine and serotonin receptors. It is an older 'typical' anti-psychotic, but is useful as it can be given by depot injection.

Chlorpromazine is another older 'typical' anti-psychotic and has sedative, anticholinergic and antidopaminergic effects. It also causes hypotension and has anti-emetic properties.

Imipramine is a tricyclic anti-depressant. This group of drugs has an unknown mechanism of action. They probably work by inhibiting the re-uptake of noradrenaline, dopamine, or serotonin by nerve cells.

6. What are the other drugs used to treat this condition?

Newer 'atypical' anti-psychotics such as clozapine or olanzipine have similar actions, but a reduced incidence of extra-pyramidal side effects, especially tardive dyskinesia. Benzodiazepines can be used for anxiety and anti-depressants or anti-convulsants for features resistant to other treatments.

7. Run through the investigations for me

▪ There is mild hyponatraemia and significant renal impairment. The FBC is normal, but the lithium level is at the upper limit of normal which may be explained by the renal impairment. Lithium's action is increased by hyponatraemia.

▪ The ECG shows sinus rhythm with left axis deviation. There is marked LVH with a strain pattern.

▪ The CXR is a PA film and is adequately penetrated. The lung fields are clear and the heart outline is normal.

8. What are the likely causes of his renal impairment?

The usual causes of **pre-renal** problems are hypovolaemia or renal artery stenosis. Intrinsic **renal causes** such as glomerulonephritis, drug nephropathies, interstitial nephritis or small vessel arterial disease are possible aetiologies and **post-renal** obstruction could be caused by stones, clots or tumour. Ultrasound imaging of the renal tract, urine analysis and serial results may help to identify the cause. The most likely cause from the history given – is lithium.

9. Is he fit for his anaesthetic today?

No. There are a number of outstanding issues. Firstly, his exercise tolerance needs to be assessed by history initially and then dynamic testing if necessary. He may have significant COPD. Pulmonary function tests would help to diagnose this and also allow the opportunity to assess the degree of reversibility of any bronchospasm. He may benefit from inhaled bronchodilators to improve his respiratory function. Serial measurements of blood pressure should be made by his primary care physician and further treatment instituted if necessary. He should also be encouraged to lose weight and stop smoking. Finally, a psychiatrist should review his anti-psychotic medication.

10. Let us say he sees a physician and comes back on inhalers that improve his exercise tolerance. His airway looks normal and blood pressure is controlled. How are you going to anaesthetise him? Talk me through induction and maintenance.

This man needs to be intubated due to his obesity and this may need to be via the nasal route depending on the requirements of the dental surgeon. A vasoconstrictor might need to be applied to the nose first. After establishing routine monitoring and intravenous access, he should be pre-oxygenated sat up at about 20° for a full 5 minutes. He could be induced with fentanyl 1mcg/kg and propofol to effect, followed by a muscle relaxant such as rocurinium 0.5 mg/kg, once facemask ventilation is established. Maintenance with Sevoflurane in a 70/30 mixture of oxygen and nitrous oxide will minimise airway irritation and allow rapid wake-up at the end of surgery.

11. Would you let him breathe spontaneously?

No. His obesity is likely to result in atelectasis and desaturation. He may also have **central hypopnoea**, which will be exacerbated by the opioid leading to an inadequate minute volume if left to breathe spontaneously. IPPV with PEEP and a reduced I:E ratio would be the best ventilatory strategy to avoid this. The lighter plane of anaesthesia required for spontaneous ventilation may cause problems with laryngospasm and bronchospasm.

12. What are the other options to anaesthetise for this surgery?

Depending on the extent of the surgery, the surgeon and the patient, it is possible to perform the operation on a nasal mask, an LMA or an oral endotracheal tube. The masks do not protect the airway fully from soiling, and in this obese patient, an endotracheal tube is the safest way to proceed.

13. In recovery post-operatively, the patient is confused. How would you approach this problem?

This should be approached in a systematic manner, ensuring firstly that the airway is patent and that the respiratory effort is adequate enough to avoid hypoxia or hypercarbia.

See short question on post-operative confusion.

14. What would you do for post-operative analgesia?

- Pain following dental extractions is usually managed by simple multi-modal analgesia with paracetamol and NSAIDs if they are not contra-indicated.
- The dental surgeons usually use local anaesthetic with a vasoconstrictor to control bleeding, but this helps with post-op analgesia.
- Dexamethasone is sometimes used to control oedema, particularly if the extractions are traumatic, and this can help to control inflammation.
- Opioid analgesia can be used in recovery if pain control is not adequate.

15. How would you monitor his renal function in the post-operative period?

The most useful guide is urine output and this can be measured hourly if there is a concern.

Serial creatinine, urea and electrolytes will give an indication of the kidney's ability to excrete and maintain homeostasis.

The actual values may not be as useful as the trends due to his size.

A measure of glomerular filtration rate (GFR) is the best way of assessing performance and this can be estimated from a formula or calculated by collecting the urine over a 24-hour period.

The Cockcroft–Gault formula

$$Creatinine\ clearance = \frac{(140 - age) \times weight\,(kg) \times 1.23 \times (0.85\ if\ female)}{Creat\,[\mu mol/l]}$$

Bibliography

Allman K, Wilson I. (2002). *Oxford Handbook of Anaesthesia* (Oxford Handbooks) 2nd edition. Oxford University Press. ISBN: 0192632736.

British National Formulary No. 53 (March 2007) Section 4.2.1. Antipsychotic drugs.

Cockcroft D, Gault M. (1976). Prediction of creatinine clearance from serum creatinine. *Nephron*, **16**(1), 31–41.

Lane S, Saunder D, Schofield A, Padmanabhan R, Hildreth A, Laws D. (2005). A prospective randomised controlled trial comparing efficacy of pre-oxygenation in the 20 degree head-up vs supine position. *Anaesthesia*, **60**, 1064–7.

Long Case 22

'The one about the unconscious O/D in A&E'

You are called to the accident and emergency department to see a 20-year-old with suspected suicidal overdose. No history is available from the patient. Relatives give a history of suicidal overdose of unknown tablets 6 hours ago.

Examination	GCS	5/15
	HR	120 bpm
	BP	96/41 mmHg

Investigations	Sodium	141	mmol/l
	Potassium	3.9	mmol/l
	Urea	4.1	mmol/l
	Creatinine	62	μmol/l
	Hb	13.8	g/dl
	WCC	4.7	$\times 10^9$/l
	Plts	310	$\times 10^9$/l
	pH	7.28	
	PO_2	12.2	kPa
	PCO_2	3.8	kPa
	BE	-6	
	Paracetamol	170	mg/l
	Salicylates	Not detected	

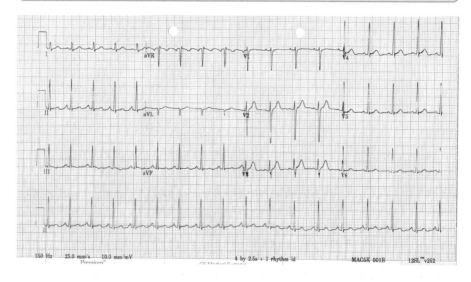

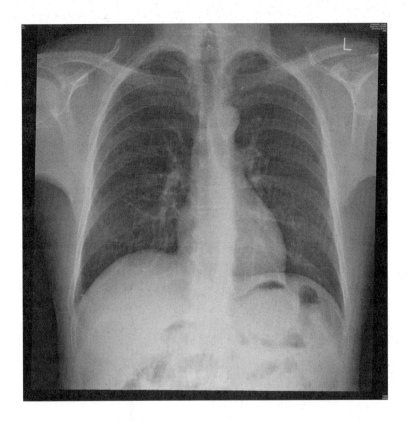

Can you summarise this case and your key concerns?

This 20-year-old patient has taken an overdose of unknown medications. She has a depressed GCS, sinus tachycardia, metabolic acidosis, and elevated plasma paracetamol levels.

The GCS is less than 8/15 therefore airway protection by endotracheal intubation is indicated. While the paracetamol levels are raised, and will require treatment, this does not explain the depressed conscious level. Ingestion of other medications should be considered and the presence of metabolic acidosis and tachycardia may suggest tricyclic antidepressants.

Outline your initial assessment and management of the patient?

I would adopt an ABC approach to initial assessment and management. Airway:

■ GCS <8/15 requiring airway protection. Endotracheal intubation with rapid sequence induction and cricoid pressure. Full monitoring and trained assistance should be in place and pre-oxygenation performed. Induction with thiopentone and suxamethonium is appropriate with sedation maintained with propofol or midazolam if required. A nasogastric tube should be sited and gastric contents aspirated to reduce aspiration risk and removed unabsorbed medication.

Breathing:

■ Ventilation with 100% oxygen. Care to prevent hypoventilation as hypercapnia will worsen acidosis. Consider hyperventilation if tricyclic overdose.

Circulation:

■ Sinus tachycardia and mild hypotension may be due to drugs taken, A fluid bolus may be considered to restore circulating volume if vasodilation is suspected.

Specific management of the overdose will depend on the agents taken. Activated charcoal may be given to awake patients or via the NG tube if overdose occurred within 1 hour. The paracetamol levels are elevated and will require specific treatment. If a tricyclic overdose is suspected, then additional management should also be considered.

Tell me how GCS is broken down?

The Glasgow Coma Score		
Eye opening	Spontaneous	4
	To speech	3
	To pain	2
	Nil	1
Verbal response	Orientated	5
	Confused	4
	Inappropriate words	3
	Sounds	2
	Nil	1
Motor response	Obeys commands	6
	Localises to pain	5
	Withdrawal	4
	Abnormal flexion	3
	Extension	2
	Nil	1

Tell me about paracetamol overdose?

The toxic effects of paracetamol overdose are caused by the minor metabolite **N-acetyl-*p*-benzo-quinone imine (NAPQI)** formed by the action of cytochrome P450. Normally, this is conjugated with **glutathione** (a tripeptide and an anti-oxidant) in the liver to a non-toxic metabolite and excreted by the kidneys. In overdose glutathione may be exhausted, resulting in hepatic and renal damage.

In the acute overdose the patient may be asymptomatic or complain of nausea and vomiting. Liver necrosis may develop with right subcostal pain and tenderness and acute hepatic failure characterised by encephalopathy and coagulopathy. Renal failure may develop.

Management is guided by paracetamol plasma levels and is dependent on time of overdose. Nomograms of plasma paracetamol levels are available in the BNF. Patients above the treatment line should be treated with acetyl cystiene. Patients at high risk due to enzyme induction or reduced glutathione reserves are treated above a lower treatment line.

	High risk groups	
P450 induction	Carbamazepine	
	Phenytoin	
	Rifampicin	
	Alcohol	
	Barbiturates	
Reduced glutathione	Malnourished patients;	Anorexia
		Alcoholism
		HIV

Acetyl cysteine is given intravenously diluted in 5% glucose. The infusion runs for 20 hours and 15 min. The dose is as follows:

- 150 mg/kg in 200 ml over 15 min
- 50 mg/kg in 500 ml over 4 hours
- 100 mg/kg in 1000 ml over 16 hours.

Evidence of hepatic failure may lead to the infusion being continued over this period after discussion with a local liver centre. Liver transplantation may be required.

What are the indications for liver transplantation?

The King's College Hospital prognostic criteria can be used to identify patients with a poor outcome following paracetamol-induced fulminant hepatic failure (0.98 positive predictive value). Those criteria are:
Either arterial pH <7.3 (or <7.25 if N-acetyl cysteine)
or all three of:

- PT >100 s (INR >6.5)
- Creatinine >300
- Grade III encephalopathy.

Grades of encephalopathy	
Grade I	Euphoria/depression, mild confusion
Grade II	Lethargy, moderate confusion, asterixis
Grade III	Somnolence, marked confusion, asterixis
Grade IV	Coma

What are the features of tricyclic antidepressant overdose?

Symptoms:

- Dry mouth
- Blurred vision
- Confusions or depressed conscious level

Signs:

- Anticholinergic features;
  - Dilated pupils
  - Dry mouth
  - Flushing
  - Tachycardia
- Coma
- Respiratory depression
- Hypotension
- Hyperreflexia
- Seizures
- Cardiac conduction abnormalities (prolonged QRS duration)
- Arrhythmias
- Metabolic acidosis
- Urinary retention

How would you manage this?

- **Activated charcoal** orally should be given if the patient is conscious.
- If, however, the GCS is depressed **airway control** and protection with endotracheal intubation is necessary
- Any **seizures** should be managed with intravenous **benzodiazepines**.
- QRS prolongation (>1.0 ms) is a particular worry in tricyclic overdose and is associated with the onset of arrhythmias. Increasing the arterial pH >7.45 reduces the free portion of the drug and cardiac binding. This may be achieved by **hyperventilation** or by **bicarbonate administration** (8.4% 25–50 ml aliquots).
- **Cardiac monitoring** should be continued for at least 12 hours. Anti-arrhythmic drugs are best avoided.
- Patients with significant overdose are best nursed in a **critical care** setting.

Bibliography

Bovill JG, Howie MB. (1999). *Clinical Pharmacology for Anaesthetists*. Harcourt Publishers.
Lai WK, Murphy N. (2004). Management of acute liver failure. *BJA CEPD*, **4**(2), 40–3.
Marrero J, Matinez F, Hyzy R. (2005). Advances in critical care hepatology. *American Journal of Respiratory and Critical Care Medicine* **168**(12), 1421–5.
Oh TE. (1977). *Intensive Care Manual* 1997. Oxford, UK: Butterworth-Heinemann.

Long Case 23

'The one about a craniotomy in a patient with neurofibromatosis'

You are asked to anaesthetise a 32-year-old man for a craniotomy to remove an occipital space-occupying lesion. He was admitted 5 days ago with fits and visual disturbance. He has been fit free since admission.

PMSH	Neurofibromatosis		
	Lung resection for bilateral bullae 4 years ago		
Social History	20 per day smoker		
	10 units of alcohol per week		
Drugs	Phenytoin 100 mg TDS		
Examination	Heart rate 100 bpm		
	BP 140/66		
	Chest clear		
	Right inferior homonymous hemianopia		
Investigations	Sodium	131	mmol/l
	Potassium	4.1	mmol/l
	Urea	4.3	mmol/l
	Creatinine	84	μmol/l
	CRP	85	
	Billirubin	12	μmol/l
	Alk Phos	173	IU/l
	AST	32	IU/l
	GGT	52	
	Hb	14.2	g/dl
	WCC	7.3	x10^9/l
	Plts	178	x10^9/l
	ESR	50	

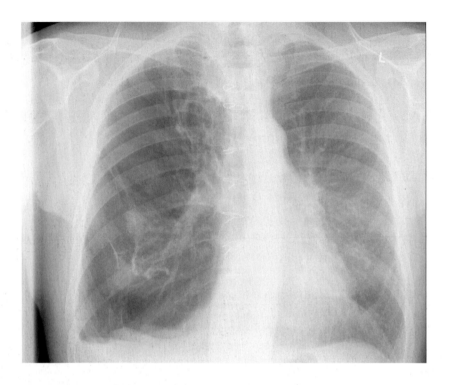

The chest X-ray
In the exam, the chest X-ray for this question was reported to show features of neurofibromatosis in addition to multiple bullae and signs of previous bilateral lung resections. The chest X-ray here shows sternal wires indicating a previous sternotomy and surgical clips and a pleural reaction in the right lower zone from a prior lung resection.

Chest X-ray signs of neurofibromatosis

- Often there are none
- Fibrosis
- Chest wall and pulmonary neurofibromas
- Paraspinal masses (intrathoracic meningocoele)
- Rib notching (neurofibromas on intercostal nerves)
- 'Ribbon ribs' – the ribs look twisted
- Kyphoscoliosis.

1. Can you summarise this case?

This is a 32-year-old man with neurofibromatosis and bullous lung disease presenting for urgent resection of a cerebral space-occupying lesion that is causing neurological symptoms. His fits have been controlled pre-operatively; however, there are concerns regarding his ECG, raised inflammatory markers and bullous lung disease.

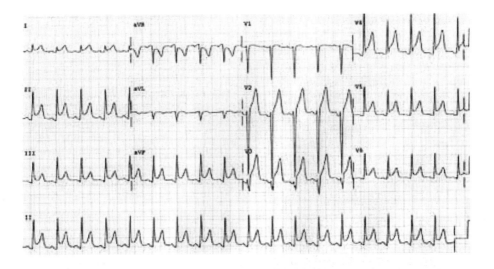

Neurofibromatosis	Autosomal dominant 1:3000 Type 1 (peripheral) Chromosome 17 Type 2 (central) Chromosome 22
Signs	Skin tumours Café-au-lait patches (>5) Neural tumours (central and peripheral neurofibromas, meningiomas, gliomas, neuromas) Multiple associated abnormalities (scoliosis, phaemochromocytoma, pulmonary fibrosis, cardiomyopathy, renal artery stenosis)

2. Is this case urgent?

Yes, as the patient has developed neurological features and the resection
should be done urgently. It is not, however, an emergency and the operation
can be delayed while further investigation and management of his medical
problems is performed as an inpatient.

3. Can you summarise his investigations?

The blood tests show a mild hyponatraemia and raised inflammatory markers
(ESR 50, CRP 85).
The ECG shows:

- Rate 120–130
- Rhythm sinus
- Axis ~ +60–70°
- The P waves and the QRS complexes are normal. There is widespread ST
  elevation.

In summary, the ECG shows evidence of pericarditis. The differential diagnosis would be massive AMI. ST elevation can also occur in left ventricular aneurysm.

The chest X-ray shows multiple bullae in both lung fields. The CTR is normal. The mediastinum is normal. There are no bony or soft tissue abnormalities.

> This chest X-ray report refers to the X-ray remembered from the exam.

4. What are your concerns?

My two main concerns are the ECG evidence of pericarditis and the bullous lung disease.

- Regarding the ECG, I would perform a detailed cardiovascular examination and arrange an urgent cardiology review. An echocardiogram should be performed to assess cardiac function and presence of pericardial fluid. If a significant effusion is present, pericardiocentesis should be considered pre-operatively. Raised cardiac enzymes may indicate myocarditis or infarction.
- Regarding the CXR, the presence of multiple bullae pose a risk of pneumothorax during positive pressure ventilation. As this will be a neurosurgical procedure in the prone position, this will be unavoidable; however, avoidance of high inspiratory pressures and volumes should be considered.

Causes of pericarditis

- Viral (Coxackie)
- Post infarction
- Uraemia
- Connective tissue disease
- Malignancy
- Rheumatic fever
- TB
- Bacterial (Staphylococcus, Haemophilus influenzae)

5. Would you proceed with the case immediately?

No. I would arrange urgent cardiology review and investigation. There is time to optimise the patient before surgery.

Key principles of neuroanaesthesia:

- Maintenance of cerebral perfusion pressure. $CPP = MAP - (ICP + CVP)$
- Prevention of BP surges (intubation, pins, emergence) to limit bleeding and ICP
- Still patient

- Rapid wake-up with little residual sedation to allow assessment post-op
- Anti-emesis
- Risk of air embolism
- Limitation of ICP (slack brain):
  - Low normal $PaCO_2$
  - Normal oxygenation
  - Head up position
  - Prevention of coughing or straining
  - Mannitol
  - Avoidance of agents which increase ICP (Ketamine, N_2O, and to some degree volatiles)
  - Reduced cerebral metabolic rate (anaesthetic agents)
  - Management of fits (increases $CMRO_2$ and ICP)
  - Prevent hyperthermia.

6. The patient has been seen and optimised by the cardiologists; how would you proceed with the anaesthetic?

Pre-operatively:

- Assessment and optimisation has been done.
- Standard fasting.
- Explanation of anaesthetic plan to patient.
- Discussion with surgeon regarding positioning of patient and degree of intracranial mass effect expected. May require pre-operative steroids to reduce oedema.

Induction:

- Full anaesthetic monitoring and trained assistance.
- Arterial line and wide bore access should be sited before induction to limit haemodynamic instability. Emergency drugs including pressors should be prepared.
- Pre-oxygenation. May take longer than normal due to lung disease.
- Induction with remifentanil, propofol, and atracurium would be appropriate. Remifentanil infusion may be established with a 1 mcg/kg bolus over 1 minute; however, this may cause bradycardia and hypotension. Some anaesthetists start at higher than normal infusion rate (~0.5 mcg/kg per min) until intubation which is then reduced. Anaesthesia should be maintained with either TIVA or a volatile + remifentanil technique.
- If concern regarding fitting, thiopentone may be more appropriate.
- Head up position may help with ventilation, oxygenation, and ICP. Hypotension may complicate.
- Endotracheal intubation with a reinforced tube after time for full muscle relaxation to prevent coughing. Tube should be well secured as patient will

be prone and mouth packs may be considered. Tapes should not impede venous return. Auscultation to exclude endobronchial intubation.

▧ Limitation of pressor response by remifentanil is often adequate, but beta-blockade (esmolol) and intravenous lignocaine have been used.

▧ Central temperature monitoring.

▧ Positive pressure ventilation aiming for a low normal $PaCO_2$ to maintain ICP. Increased respiratory rate with low tidal volumes should be considered to limit the pneumothorax risk in this patient.

▧ A central line should be sited to assist with haemodynamic monitoring and support.

Positioning:

▧ Prone
  ● Eye protection and padding.
  ● Secure reinforced endotracheal tube.
  ● 6-person team (head, feet, two on each side).
  ● Patient rolled, with arms by side, onto arms of people by side.
  ● Care to avoid rotation of head.
  ● Chest and pelvis supported with abdomen free.
  ● Face down or to side with care to avoid pressure to eyes and facial nerve.
  ● Arms to side or brought up together towards head with care to avoid brachial plexus injury.
  ● Care regarding padding of pressure areas.
▧ Head up
  ● Hypotension due to pooling of blood in dependent areas.
  ● Increased risk of air embolism.
▧ Pins
  ● Will require increased depth of anaesthesia and analgesia as very stimulating.

Adverse effects of prone position

▧ Reduced access to airway.
▧ Increased airway pressures if abdomen splinted.
▧ Reduced venous return if increased abdominal pressure.
▧ Displacement of tubes and lines during proning.
▧ Injuries during turning (neck).
▧ Brachial plexus injuries if arms abducted.
▧ Compression injuries:
  ● Eye (retinal artery causing blindness)
  ● Facial nerve
  ● Ulnar nerve at elbow
  ● Lateral cutaneous nerve of the thigh.

Maintenance:

▧ TIVA

- Propofol TCI with remifentanil
- Reduce $CMRO_2$ and maintain auto-regulation reducing ICP
- Easily titrated during different phases of surgery
- Possible free radical scavenging by propofol
- Rapid smooth emergence
- Reduced PONV
- Risk of awareness if i.v. dislodged.

- Volatile + remifentanil
  - Sevoflurane or isoflurane in oxygen air (N_2O should be avoided as it increases ICP and would increase the risk and size of pneumothorax in this patient).
  - Do not significantly effect autoregulation in the normal clinical range.
  - Halothane best avoided as most increase in ICP.
  - Some concern regarding desflurane also (may also increase coughing).
  - Animal models suggest that pre-conditioning and reduced apoptosis may occur in hypoxic injury. Thought to via calcium release from intracellular stores.
  - Comparable wake-up times with sevoflurane and TIVA.

- Neuromuscular blockade to prevent coughing and straining. Remifentanil also helps to prevent this.
- Normal saline maintenance. Hypertonic saline may help to reduce oedema. Avoid dextrose containing solutions.
- Maintain normothermia.
- Mannitol 0.5–1.0 mg/kg of 10% or 20% if cerebral oedema.

Emergence:

- If significant oedema, then the patient may be best left asleep and allowed to recover in intensive care.
- Maintain anaesthesia until supine and out of pins.
- 100% oxygen
- Anti-emesis (ondansetron, dexamethasone).
- Reverse neuromuscular blockade with monitoring.
- Stop anaesthesia.
- Extubation may be undertaken deep to limit coughing, but awake intubation ensures airway protection and allows assessment of neurological status.
- Pressor responses should be managed with intravenous beta-blockade (e.g. esmolol).

Analgesia:

- Local to scalp.
- i.v. paracetamol
- Codeine i.m. (thought to produce less sedation than morphine).
- Morphine i.v. (may causes sedation and pain post-craniotomy often minor).

Post-operative care:

- Best performed in a high dependency setting.

▨ May require intensive care with sedation and ventilation if oedema or reduced conscious level post-operatively.

Bibliography

Bicker PE, Fahlman CS. (2006). The inhaled anaesthetic, isoflurane, enhances Ca dependent survival signalling in cortical neurons and modulates MAP kinases, apoptosis proteins and transcription factor during hypoxia. *Anaesthesia and Analgesia*, **103**(2), 419–29.

Deakin CD. (1998). *Clinical Notes for the FRCA*. Edinburgh: Churchill Livingstone.

Kumar P, Clark M. (1994). *Clinical Medicine*. Baillière-Tindall.

Nasu I, Yokoo N, Takaoda S *et al*. (2006). The dose-dependent effects of isoflurane on outcome from severe forebrain ischemia in the rat. *Anaesthesia and Analgesia*, **103**(2), 413–17.

Long Case 24

'The one about the head-injured patient'

> This long question has some overlap with the short questions on 'intracranial pressure' and 'raised intracranial pressure therapy'. It is included for completeness.

You are called to Accident and Emergency to see a 20-year-old male. He has been brought in by ambulance after falling from a second-floor window. He is on a spinal board with neck immobilisation in place. He is making incomprehensible moaning noises and will not open his eyes even to pain. He responds to sternal rub with abnormal flexion only.

Observations	HR	125 bpm
	BP	87/45 mmHg
	Sats	94% on 15 l/min O_2 via a mask with reservoir bag
CXR		Demonstrates bilateral pneumothoraces

1. Would you like to summarise this case?

This is a young man who has sustained a significant fall, resulting in a severe head injury with a depressed conscious level. He is tachycardic and hypotensive suggesting the possibility of other injuries. He is only saturating at 94% on 15 litres of oxygen and his chest X-ray shows bilateral pneumothoraces.

Head injury grading	GCS	Grade
	13–15	Mild
	9–12	Moderate
	<8	Severe

2. How would you manage this patient acutely?

I would adopt an ABC approach to this patient.
Airway:

- In the event of the airway being obstructed, jaw thrust **not chin lift** should be used as there is the strong possibility of a C-spine injury.
- Nasal airways are best avoided as there is a risk of a base of skull fracture.

- GCS is <8 (E1 S2 M3 = 6), therefore intubation will be required to protect the airway. This should be performed with a rapid sequence induction, cricoid pressure and manual in line stabilisation of the C-spine.
- The cervical spine should be protected with collar, blocks, and tapes.

Breathing:

- Continue 100% oxygen.
- Bilateral intercostal chest drain insertion to drain pneumothoraces.
- Maintenance of low normal carbon dioxide (4 – 4.5 kPa) when ventilated (head injury).

Circulation:

- Patient is tachycardic and hypotensive suggesting blood loss from other injuries.
- Two large bore (14 or 16 gauge) cannulae should be sited.
- Blood should be sent for FBC, U+Es, glucose, and urgent cross match (6 units).
- Fluid resuscitation should be commenced with warmed Hartmann's solution.
- A urinary catheter should be sited unless there is evidence of significant pelvic injury.

Disability:

- GCS is low and urgent CT head should be arranged (to be performed after anaesthesia and intubation)
- Significant delay should be avoided.

Exposure:

- Head-to-toe evaluation.
- Log roll.
- Trauma series X-rays (C-spine, chest, pelvis).
- Assessment for sites of blood loss;
  - Long bone injuries,
  - Pelvic trauma,
  - Intra-abdominal bleeding (FAST scan),
  - Thoracic injury (NB tension pneumothorax).

3. What is cerebral perfusion pressure and how may it be calculated?

Cerebral perfusion pressure is calculated by subtracting the intracranial pressure from the mean arterial pressure **(CPP = MAP – ICP). The normal CPP is 80–100 mmHg**.

Evidence suggests that outcome can be improved by maintaining CPP > 70 mmHg in head-injured patients. In practice, this means maintaining MAP in the range 90–100 mmHg until ICP monitoring is instituted.

Intracranial pressure (ICP)

Normal	ICP < 10−15 mmHg
Intracranial hypertension	ICP > 15−20 mmHg
Treatment threshold	ICP > 20−25 mmHg

4. What is the Monro Kellie doctrine?

The Monro (1783) Kellie (1824) doctrine states that the cranium is a 'rigid box' containing 'nearly incompressible brain', CSF and blood. Any increase in the volume of any of these components will therefore increase intracranial pressure. Furthermore, any increase in the volume of one element must occur at the expense of another.

Intracranial volume in adults   ~ 1500 ml
- Blood 10% (~150 ml)
- CSF 5%−10% (~75 ml)
- Brain 80−85%

5. What happens to intracranial pressure as volume increases?

As intracranial volume increases, CSF is shunted into the spinal canal and the dural sinuses are compressed. More long-term compensation occurs due to reduced CSF production. When these compensatory mechanisms are overwhelmed, a sudden dramatic rise in ICP results.

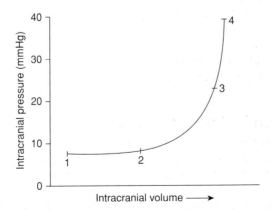

Figure taken from Pinnock, Lin & Smith, (2003). *Fundamentals of Anaesthesia*, 2nd edition, © 2003 Greenwich Medical Media Ltd. Reproduced with permission.

> To be able to quickly draw some of these graphs may be very useful in the exam.

6. What is cerebral auto-regulation and how is it thought to occur?

Normal cerebral blood flow is ~50 ml/100 g per min (15%–20% of cardiac output). Cerebral auto-regulation describes how cerebral blood flow is kept constant over a wide range of mean arterial pressures (typically MAPs ~ 50–150 mmHg).

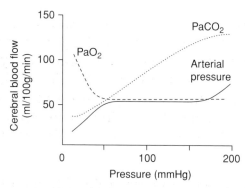

Figure taken from Pinnock, Lin & Smith, (2003). *Fundamentals of Anaesthesia*, 2nd edition, © 2003 Greenwich Medical Media Ltd. Reproduced with permission.

There are several theories of how auto-regulation occurs:

■ **Myogenic**; direct response by smooth muscle to changes in perfusion pressure.
■ **Metabolic**; response to the change in CO_2, O_2, pH, and K^+ levels alter blood flow.
■ **Tissue**; increased blood flow increases interstitial fluid which compresses blood vessels.

7. What factors can be controlled to improve outcome following head injury?

The key principle in the management of the head injured patient is the prevention of **secondary brain injury**. There are several simple key principles involved to try and keep local physiology as normal as possible. These are:

■ **Normotension**   Maintain MAP > 90 mmHg (CPP > 70 mmHg)
■ **Normoxia** SpO_2 < 90% associated with worse outcome.
■ **Normocapnia** $PaCO_2$ 4–4.5 kPa. Cerebral blood flow is linearly related to $PaCO_2$ in the range 3 kPa–10 kPa, therefore hypercapnia should be avoided. Hyperventilation may reduce already compromised cerebral blood flow and should also be avoided.

■ **Normothermia**   Increases in temperature will increase cerebral metabolic rate and, as such, increase cerebral blood flow and oxygen demand. Resetting of the hypothalamic temperature limits may make this problematic and may require surface cooling and paralysis. The role of mild hypothermia in sub-groups of head-injured patients has shown some promising results, but there is no global consensus on its use.

■ **Normoglycaemia**   Hyperglycaemia may increase cerebral metabolic rate.

■ **Seizure control**   Seizures are associated with greatly increased cerebral metabolic rate, oxygen demand and ICP.

8. After intubation, a further two litres of normal saline and insertion of the intercostal drains, the patient's heart rate is now 90 bpm, blood pressure 130/70 and his oxygen saturation is 97%. Ultrasound of his abdomen is negative, and there are no other major injuries detected on examination or trauma series. What is your priority now?

Now the patient is stable, an urgent CT scan should be performed of the patient's head.

9. The scan shows an acute extra-dural haematoma. What would you do next?

The priority now is to arrange for emergency neurosurgical evacuation of the haematoma. If neurosurgery is not available in my centre, then an emergency transfer should be arranged. Delays for central line insertion and other non-essential procedures should be avoided. The transfer should be completed in under 4 hours.

10. After emergency craniotomy and evacuation, the patient is transferred to intensive care with an ICP monitor in situ. The ICP is reading 30 mmHg. What are the therapeutic options for reducing ICP?

The options available are either medical or surgical and their use will depend on the developing clinical situation.

Medical:

■ 30–45 degree head up.
■ Deepen sedation (propofol or midazolam).
■ Thiopentone infusion (to bring about burst suppression).
■ Neuromuscular blockade.
■ Mannitol – 0.25–1 g/kg of 20%. Monitor osmolarity (target 300–310 mosm/l). May precipitate hyperosmolar renal failure if too high.
■ Maintain CO_2 4–4.5 kPa.
■ Maintain temp < 37 °C.
■ Control seizure activity.

Surgical:

- CSF drainage.
- Decompressive bifrontal craniectomy.
- Removal of contusions.
- Lobectomy.

Bibliography

Deakin CD. (1998). *Clinical Notes for the FRCA*. Edinburgh, UK: Churchill Livingstone.

Girling K. (2004). Management of head injury in the intensive-care unit. *BJA CEPD*, **4**(2), 52–6.

Mishra LD, Rajkumar N, Hancock SM. (2006). Current controversies in neuroanaesthesia, head injury management and neuro critical care. *BJA CEPD* **6**(2), 79–82.

Long Case 25

'The one about the trauma patient in accident and emergency'

You are called to accident and emergency to help with a 53-year-old female after a road traffic accident. The patient had been involved in a head-on collision with a lorry and had a prolonged extraction at the scene due to entrapment. Oxygen is being administered via a mask with a reservoir bag. Two 16G lines have been inserted and 500 ml of saline is being infused. A right-sided chest drain has been inserted by Accident and Emergency staff. A CT scan of her neck and brain are normal. The secondary survey has revealed a fractured left femur, fractured pelvis and a positive diagnostic peritoneal lavage (DPL).

Observations	HR	105 bpm
	BP	100/45 mmHg
	RR	40 bpm
	Sats	98%
	GCS	15/15
	Chest	Paradoxical chest movements on right side with reduced air entry

Investigations	Hb	11.0 g/dl
	WCC	8.6×10^9/l
	Plts	189×10^9/l
	Na	142 mmol/l
	K	4.3 mmol/l
	U	12.2 mmol/l
	Creat	97 μmol/l
	Glu	11 mmol/l
	pH	7.31
	PCO_2	4.9 kPa
	PO_2	18.3 kPa
	BE	−7

1. Would you like to summarise this case?

This is a 53-year-old female with multiple injuries following a road traffic accident. She has a normal GCS and has had her neck radiologically cleared. There is evidence of chest trauma with a clinical flail segment on the right and a treated traumatic pneumothorax. Her respiratory rate is elevated, suggesting an element of respiratory distress. Haemodynamically, she has a mild tachycardia and a metabolic acidosis suggesting hypovolaemia. There are major orthopaedic injuries that will require stabilisation and evidence of abdominal bleeding on DPL.

2. Why do you think the blood glucose is raised?

The glucose will be raised secondary to the stress response, which is the name given to the metabolic and hormonal changes which follow injury or trauma. It is a systemic response encompassing neuro-endocrine, immunological and haematological effects.

> **Endocrine stress response**
> Increased:
>
> ■ Growth hormone
> ■ ACTH
> ■ Prolactin
> ■ Vasopressin
> ■ Catecholamines
> ■ Cortisol
> ■ Aldosterone
> ■ Glucagon
> ■ Renin.
>
> Decreased:
>
> ■ Insulin
> ■ Testosterone
> ■ Oestrogen
> ■ T3.

3. Why do you think the urea is raised?

There are several possibilities:

■ Pre-existing
■ Bleeding into the gut lumen
■ Though early, it could represent pre-renal failure due to hypovolaemia.
■ It may be due to renal impairment from rhabdomyolysis as a result of the prolonged entrapment although again, this would be early.

4. Are you concerned about the haemoglobin level?

The haemoglobin level is adequate, but there is evidence of hypovolaemia suggesting significant blood loss and further haemodilution will occur both spontaneously and due to fluid resuscitation. Therefore, while the laboratory haemoglobin concentration is normal, the actual level of total haemoglobin available for oxygen delivery will be low.

The injuries documented are associated with significant blood loss and transfusion is likely to be needed after initial volume resuscitation.

> **Blood loss from orthopaedic injuries**
> ▨ Fractured humerus   Up to 750 ml
> ▨ Fractured tibia   Up to 750 ml
> ▨ Fractured femur   Up to 1500 ml
> ▨ Fractured pelvis   Several litres

5. Why is the patient acidotic?

The acidosis is likely to be a lactic acidosis secondary to tissue hypoperfusion.

6. Why do you think the $PaCO_2$ is normal despite the rapid respiratory rate?

While the rate is elevated, effective ventilation will be compromised by:

▨ Rapid shallow breathing due to pain from rib fractures
▨ Diaphragmatic splinting from abdominal injury
▨ Paradoxical chest movements from flail segment
▨ V/Q mismatch from pulmonary contusions and collapsed lung
▨ Increased alveolar dead space due to hypovolaemia.

7. What is the significance of the chest injuries?

The chest injuries are multiple rib fractures with a right-sided flail segment, a traumatic pneumothorax, and probable pulmonary contusions. The patient has signs of respiratory distress with a very high respiratory rate and a PaO_2 of only 18.3 kPa on 15 litres per minute from a mask with reservoir bag (FiO_2 0.8–0.85). In addition, pulmonary contusions may worsen over the first 12–24 hours. The patient will require early intubation and ventilation. Efforts should be made to correct haemodynamic instability prior to induction.

> **ATLS Guidelines for pulmonary contusions**
> 'Patients with significant hypoxia (i.e. $PaO_2 \leq 8.6$ kPa or sats $\leq 90\%$ on room air) should be intubated and ventilated within the first hour after injury.'

8. How would you assess the adequacy of the intercostal chest drain?

▨ Clinical improvement in respiratory symptoms, oxygenation, and air entry
▨ CXR showing re-expansion and adequate position
▨ Drain bubbling on insertion and swinging with respiration

9. How would you assess the degree of blood loss?

Blood loss may be estimated by the observations on initial presentation by the ATLS classification.

	Class 1	Class 2	Class 3	Class 4
Blood loss	≤750 ml or ≤15%	750–1500 ml or 15%–30%	1500–2000 ml or 30%–40%	>2000 ml or >40%
Pulse rate	<100	>100	>120	>140
Blood pressure	Normal	Normal	Decreased	Decreased
Pulse pressure	Normal or increased	Decreased	Decreased	Decreased
Respiratory rate	14–20	20–30	30–40	>35
Urine output ml/hr	>30	20–30	5–15	Negligible
Mental status	Slightly anxious	Mildly anxious	Anxious, confused	Confused, lethargic

10. What fluid would you give to resuscitate the patient?

This patient has Class 2–3 haemorrhage and may be experiencing ongoing blood loss. The options for fluid are:

- Crystalloid; Hartmann's in 3:1 ratio to blood loss – adequate for Class 1 and 2 haemorrhage and initial resuscitation of higher classes.
- Colloid; 1:1 ratio with blood loss – no proven benefit over crystalloid
- Blood; Appropriate for class 3 and 4 haemorrhage – will be required with this patient.

11. What are the surgical priorities with this lady?

- **Control of intra-abdominal bleeding.** If the patient is stable further imaging may be performed first (CT scan). DPL is 98% sensitive but non-specific. If the patient is unstable, exploratory laparotomy should be performed.
- **Stabilisation of fractured pelvis.** May be performed initially with a sheet wrapped around the pelvis, a vacuum device or pneumatic anti-shock garments. Formal stabilisation with external fixation should be performed early, when other more immediately life-threatening injuries have been treated.
- **Stabilisation of fractured femur.** Can be achieved with a traction splint such as the Thomas splint and later with traction on a calcaneal pin.

12. How would you anaesthetise this patient?

- An anaesthetic history should be sought from the patient.
- A period of pre-optimisation would be ideal to ensure adequate fluid resuscitation, although on-going bleeding may mandate induction while still haemodynamically unstable.
- Trained assistance.
- Adequate preparation would include a machine check, availability of suction, a range of airway adjuncts, vasopressors and inotropes, a rapid delivery fluid warmer (such as the 'Level 1' infusor) as well as warming blankets. Liaison with blood bank would be sensible.

- Full anaesthetic monitoring, including capnography, are mandatory and an arterial line should be sited prior to induction.
- Other essential monitoring would include a urinary catheter after induction (caution regarding pelvic fractures) and temperature probe
- Central venous access may be gained immediately after induction to help guide fluid administration.
- The patient should be pre-oxygenated for 3 minutes and then anaesthetised with a rapid sequence induction. Suxamethonium should be used. There are a number of choices for induction agent, each with potential advantages and disadvantages.
  - **Thiopentone** may unmask hypovolaemia, has negative inotropic effects and causes vasodilatation.
  - **Etomidate** may give better haemodynamic stability, but inhibits cortical synthesis via 11β-hydroxylase and is associated with decreased survival when used as induction agent in patients with sepsis (CORTICUS).
  - **Ketamine** is associated with greater stability, but it has a longer induction time.
  - **Propofol** causes significant hypotension and is inappropriate in this situation.
- Maintenance of anaesthesia would be with a volatile agent in oxygen – oxygen and air when stable.
- Analgesia can be provided by fentanyl, which may offer greater haemodynamic stability than morphine.
- Post-operatively, the patient will require ventilation on **intensive care.**

References

ATLS Manual 7th edition 2004.

Burton D, Nicholson G, Hall GM. (2004). Endocrine and metabolic response to surgery. *Continuing Education in Anaesthesia, Critical Care and Pain* **4**(5), 144–7.

Saayman A, Findlay GP. (2003). The management of blunt thoracic trauma. *Continuing Education in Anaesthesia, Critical Care and Pain* **3**(6), 171–4.

A system for interpreting and presenting chest X-rays

When faced with a chest X-ray in the heat of the examination, it is vital to have a system of interpretation and presentation, particularly if the diagnosis does not jump out at you.

It is always difficult to know whether to present an X-ray starting with the diagnosis and following up with the supporting findings, or whether to use your system to present the findings and *then* reach a diagnosis.

For example: 'This chest X-ray shows the features of mitral stenosis which are . . .' *or* 'There is a double heart border and calcification . . . These features suggest a diagnosis of mitral stenosis.'

In the Long Case you will have had a chance to view the chest X-ray and can therefore be more confident mentioning a diagnosis first. If the abnormality or diagnosis is 'barn-door' (e.g. large, cavitating lesion), then the examiners may not be impressed if you take 5 minutes to mention it! In the Short Cases you may be given chest X-rays that are more of a 'spot diagnosis' (such as pneumothorax) and you should try to mention the gross abnormality first. You should then use your system to make sure you do not miss other abnormalities (such as a bilateral pneumothorax!). Other chest X-rays may be more subtle (such as features of cardiac failure) and these may be better dealt with by using the systematic approach.

A suggested framework

Names/sex	Look for breast shadows.
Date	
PA/AP, lateral film	Clues: written on the film, 'mobile', scapulae, intubated, monitoring.
Orientation, i.e. left/right	
Rotation	Look at the heads of the clavicles.
Penetration	Can you see the thoracic spine through the heart?
ET tube/tracheostomy	Comment on presence and position.
Lines, etc.	Comment on presence and position.
	CVP – tip should be above the level of the carina. This ensures that it is outside the pericardium.
	PA catheter – the tip should be in the mid-zone.
	N/G, chest drains, ECG leads

The Clinical Anaesthesia Viva Book, Second edition, ed. Julian M. Barker, Simon L. Maguire and Simon J. Mills. © J. M. Barker, S. L. Maguire, S. J. Mills 2009.

Heart and mediastinum	Position, C/T ratio (not with AP), borders
Lungs	Expansion, hila-right higher than left normally.
Bones and soft tissues	Fractures, metastases, surgical emphysema, etc.
'Areas easily missed'	Apices, behind the heart, below the diaphragm, the hila

An answer may begin:

'This is a chest X-ray of a female patient taken on **/**/**. It is an AP film as the patient is intubated. The film is not rotated and the penetration is adequate. The tip of the endotracheal tube is correctly placed. There is a central venous line in the right internal jugular vein and the tip lies in an appropriate position above the level of the carina. I cannot comment accurately on the heart size because of the projection of the film. There is no mediastinal shift. However, there is a small apical pneumothorax on the right, possibly as a consequence of insertion of the CVP line. The lung fields are otherwise clear.'

This approach is clearly not appropriate if you are presented with an obvious tension pneumothorax. In that situation it may be better to say:

'This is a left tension pneumothorax. There is a large left-sided pneumothorax with gross mediastinal shift...'

In summary, it may be best to tailor the technique of presentation to the type of abnormality seen and how confident you are about it.

Appendix 2

Interpretation of commonly occurring PFTs

Obstructive picture $\downarrow$ FEV$_1$
$\downarrow$ FVC
$\downarrow$ FEV$_1$/FVC ratio (normally around 75%)
$\downarrow$ FEF$_{25-75}$ (forced expiratory flow)
$\downarrow$ / $\rightarrow$ DL$_{CO}$
(FEF$_{25-75}$ is representative of small airways

Restrictive picture $\downarrow$ FEV$_1$
$\downarrow$ FVC
$\uparrow$ FEV$_1$/FVC ratio
$\downarrow$ / $\rightarrow$ DL$_{CO}$

Interpretation of DL$_{CO}$ and K$_{CO}$

- Carbon monoxide transfer factor (DL$_{CO}$) is reduced in conditions that damage the alveolar capillary membrane, e.g. pulmonary fibrosis and in conditions where lung surface area is reduced, e.g. emphysema and pneumonectomy. It is also reduced in anaemia and ventilation/perfusion mismatch.
- K$_{CO}$ (= DL$_{CO}$ corrected for lung volume) remains low in pulmonary fibrosis but is higher in emphysema and pneumonectomy, where it is the total lung surface area that is reduced.

Flow–volume loops in large airway obstruction

Variable extra-thoracic obstruction, e.g. goitre
- Inspiratory limb flattened (normally semicircular) as trachea collapses on inspiration.
- Expiration OK as trachea 'pushed' open.

Variable intra-thoracic obstruction
- Expiratory limb flattened as trachea 'pushed' closed.
- Inspiratory limb OK as trachea 'pulled' open.

Fixed large airway obstruction
- Both inspiratory and expiratory limbs are flattened.

The Clinical Anaesthesia Viva Book, Second edition, ed. Julian M. Barker, Simon L. Maguire and Simon J. Mills. © J. M. Barker, S. L. Maguire, S. J. Mills 2009.

Index

WITHDRAWN
BRITISH MEDICAL ASSOCIATION LIBRARY
BMA Library